HEALTH PROMOTION

Achieving High-Level Wellness in the Later Years

Third Edition

HEALTH PROMOTION

Achieving High-Level Wellness
in the Later Years

Third Edition

Michael L. Teague
University of Iowa

Valerie L. McGhee
Wichita State University

David M. Rosenthal
University of Iowa

David Kearns
University of Iowa

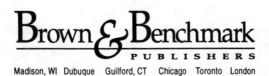

Brown & Benchmark
PUBLISHERS

Madison, WI Dubuque Guilford, CT Chicago Toronto London
Mexico City Caracas Buenos Aires Madrid Bogotá Sydney

ISBN 0-697-26268-5

Printed in the United States of America

10 9 8 7 6 5 4 3 2 1

TABLE OF CONTENTS

ACKNOWLEDGMENTS

To Valerie McGhee's family, Mike, Caitlin, and Devin. To Valerie's parents, Paul and Ginger, for their wisdom, compassion, and optimism. To Michael Teague's mother, Mildred, and late father, Donald, for encouraging their children to live above mediocrity. To Dave Rosenthal's family, Jane, Daniel and Rebecca for always being supportive of his work. To his mother Gertrude (Trude, Gert) Asch Rosenthal and father Samuel Rosenthal, who despite all the odds always believed in what their son did. To Joyce Murphy and Joy Fry for taking the time to type this manuscript and always being patient. Finally, to Harry Nathan Asch, Dave's grandfather and Anna Kaplowitz, his grandmother-in-law, who shared his room and house before they died. To David Kearns' parents, Charles and Darlene, for all that they have done and all that they continue to do. To his friends, Michael Berger, James Kochalka, and Sean O'Sullivan, for their persistent encouragement over the years. And to Anna Dahlke, his grandmother, for her wonderful spirit, her cherry pies, and all that she has taught him about "successful aging." His love, always.

PREFACE

Health promotion initiatives for older adults in the 1980s were mixed more with words of "hope" than action. There is hope, however, that the disinterest and misguided presumptions behind health promotion efforts for older adults will erode in the 1990s. Much of this hope is based on the Healthy People 2000: National Health Promotion and Disease Prevention Objectives (U.S. Department of Health and Human Services, 1990) report. This report contains a number of challenging health objectives that may entice the active involvement of allied health profession efforts to initiate health promotion programs for older adults. The theme of the Healthy People 2000 report for older adults is independence and vitality in later life. Underlying this theme is the concept that health promotion goes beyond disease prevention by regarding health as more than simply the absence of disease.

Health promotion draws from the concepts of holistic health, wellness, self-care, and health prevention. Essentially, health promotion may be defined as the science and art of helping people alter their lifestyles to move toward optimal health. This continuum definition of health promotion is illustrated in Figure 1.

The left end of Figure 1's continuum represents premature death or a state of extreme illness. The right end represents optimal health or well-being. The midpoint is a neutral point or a state of no discernible illness or well-being. Medicine has traditionally focused on the left side of the continuum by working with patients who have symptoms of disease or disabilities. Once an individual reaches the midpoint or neutral point of wellness, traditional medicine has few tools to assist this individual in reaching optimal well-being.

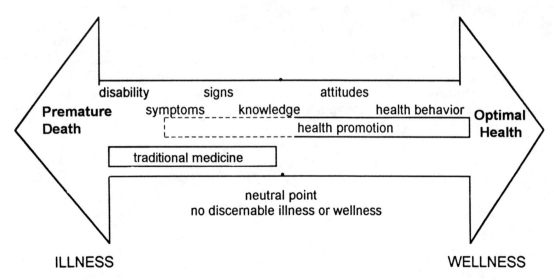

Figure 1. Health continuum.

Health promotion has traditionally focused on the right side of the Figure 1 continuum by working with people who may be described as overtly healthy. The tools of health promotion are the changing of knowledge, beliefs, attitudes, and lifestyle practices and behaviors that reduce health risks and promote optimal health, that is, physical, emo-tional, spiritual, intellectual, and social health.

Recently, health promotion efforts have been directed toward the left side of the continuum as well, by focusing on the rehabilitation of sick patients. For example, exercise programs have been used with cardiac, stroke, or musculoskeleton problems; and nutrition programs have focused on diabetes, osteoporosis, obesity and biochem-ical dysfunction. However, the point is that regardless of a client's or patient's health condition, the goal of health promotion is to help people move toward a state of optimal health. This book examines this dual role of health promotion (i.e., working on the right and left side of Figure 1) as it applies to the elderly.

Yet, Figure 1 would suggest that health promotion generally is an integrated, techno-logical field. To the contrary, health promotion is in its infancy. The practitioners of health promotion include physicians, nurses, recreation therapists, exercise scientists, nutritionists, social workers, physical therapists, and health educators. Each of these professions has experienced some success in health promotion by applying the know-ledge of their exclusive disciplines. Unfortunately, most professionals who practice some dimension of health promotion do not understand the interdisciplinary nature of the field.

If we permit this exclusiveness to continue, the issues of professional turf and how to separate wellness from medicine will impede the future development of health promo-tion programs for the elderly. For example, certification in exercise science leads to more fragmentation in the field and more battles over turf. Payment for services on a fee-for-services basis will encourage further licensing and fuel inflation. The point is that a full range of service providers, both licensed and unlicensed, need to participate in the structuring of health promotion programs for the elderly. Thus the health promotion skills and knowledge evident in this book should be taught and incorporated into existing professional categories in a broadened aging network.

CHAPTER 1

HEALTH PROMOTION FOR THE ELDERLY:
NEED FOR A NEW PERSPECTIVE

Health promotion programs for the elderly cannot be separated from the larger issues of health care, of America's policy choices in regard to aging, or the social, economic, and political environments that govern policy choices. The dominant view among yesterday's and today's policy makers is that health services, especially high-cost, medically based technology, can solve the "aging" problem. Although the attention devoted to the biological and biomedical aspects of aging is important, this exclusive emphasis has diverted attention from the significant influence of multiple social, behavioral, and environmental factors on aging.

Health promotion signifies a shift from a biomedical definition and model of health and disease toward a view that encompasses the social and physical environment, as well as individual lifestyle and behavior. The authors address this paradigm shift from a medical model to a broader health model and its impact on health promotion programs for the elderly. Specifically, we will focus on: (1) older adults and the health care crises, (2) cost-extrapolation projections for future Medicare and nursing home health care, (3) movement toward a new health paradigm, (4) the new rhetoric that surrounds health promotion programs for older adults, and (5) the theory underlying health promotion programs for containing health care costs.

THE HEALTH CARE CRISIS

Estes, Gerard, Zones and Swan (1984) describe the 1980s as an "era of crisis"; e.g., fiscal crisis, energy crisis, productivity crisis, education crisis, health care crisis. Crises provide an important impetus for future policy action and, often, broad discretion by government. Actions by government that may be ordinarily opposed are often readily accepted by the public in response to a crisis. Berger and Luckmann (1966) have called such crises "the social construction of reality." In reference to the health care crisis, Estes et al. (1984) add

> A reality once perceived, comes to exist because others believe and act as if it is real. Policy actions and social consequences flow from such definitions and perceptions, although they may represent only partial realities. Thus we have crises of health care and crises of aging. (p. 94)

The health care crisis, and the role of the elderly in this crisis, has been a source of stormy debate in the 1980s. Paradoxically, the aspect of America's special circumstances that seems to require explanation is less the fact of the cost explosion associated with an aging society than the indignant reaction to this crisis.

Health Costs

In 1965, Americans spent approximately $39 billion for medical needs of all kinds. This expenditure amounted to 5.9% of the gross national product (GNP). By 1979 total health care expenditure increased to $212 billion which was slightly less than 9% of the GNP. Health costs in 1984 reached $387 billion (10.8% of GNP) and rose to $425 billion in 1986. Today, health care expenditures are topping the $500 billion mark (11% of GNP). Under our present trend, the annual health care bill will hit a trillion dollars in the early 1990s (15% of GNP) and continue to double every six to seven years thereafter.

A key impact of rising health care costs has been the dramatic increase in health benefit premiums. Health insurance premiums soared in 1989 (22% increase) and are projected to soar even more in 1990. Some firms expect premium increases of 40 to 50%. Factoring in dental plans and Health Maintenance Organizations (HMOs), total health benefit costs increased nearly 17% from $2,354 in 1988 to $2,748 in 1989. Health analysts project that health benefits will surpass $3,200 per employee in 1990--a 23% increase (Thompson, 1989). Califano (1986) described how this soaring cost in health care bills and insurance premiums impacts our economy:

> We pay more for health care than for chrome or upholstered bucket seats when we buy a car. In 1984 the auto industry had to sell at least 500,000 cars and trucks just to pay its health care bills. For each $500 day a patient spends in the hospital, some $30 of the bill goes to pay health benefits for hospital employees. Three cents of the cost of each fast-food hamburger we buy goes to the health industry. A new automobile tire costing $57 includes $2 for health care; a $200 airline ticket, $4. Health benefits for active and retired employees account for $60 of the cost of every metric ton of aluminum ALCOA produces.
>
> Health costs are a large part of the reason why America still can't compete with foreign steel. The United States spent $1,580 per person on health care in 1984—far more than the next highest outlay, West Germany's $900 per person, three times more than Japan's $500, and four times Great Britain's $400. Yet, in each of those nations, health care is sophisticated and modern. Life expectancy is just as high as in the United States and infant mortality is lower. (p. 59)

Medicare and Medicaid

In the 1960s, Congress recognized that America's elderly faced a significant gap between the medical care they needed and what they could afford. Medicare and Medicaid were enacted to close the gap. The rationale behind the Medicare and

Medicaid program was for the government to protect the economic standing of the elderly during their declining years. But like the elderly they protect, Medicare and Medicaid have become less "healthy" with age.

Both Medicare and Medicaid paved the way to a healthier nation and an increased quality of life for older adults. But in 1988 Medicare spending increased 7.7% ($179.9 billion). Hospital spending rose 1.9% and physician spending increased by 18.9%. Medicare was responsible for 27% of hospital bills and 22% of physician bills. Growth in the elderly population and the continued expansion of health services will almost triple the number of hospital days for patients over 65 by the year 2000. The share of hospital beds for the elderly will increase from 30% to 58%. It should not be surprising that the Medicare trustees estimate that the program's health insurance will be bankrupt in the 1990s unless significant changes are forthcoming.

The Medicaid system is also falling on hard times. Medicaid was primarily designed for poor people who qualify under the Aid to Families with Dependent Children (AFDC) and Supplementary Security Income (SSI). AFDC children and parents represent 70% of Medicaid recipients, but they receive less than 30% of the program's funds. The aged, blind, and disabled make up the remaining 30% of recipients and consume over 70% of all Medicaid spending. Medicaid's share of our overall health care expense ranged between 10 and 11% in the 1980s. Americans spend in excess of $42 billion annually in nursing home care, with the government assuming approximately 48% of this tab (mostly through Medicaid).

COST-EXTRAPOLATION AND FUTURE HEALTH CARE COSTS

Escalating health care costs are of immense concern to local, state and national governments. Inflation of hospital and health care provider costs, the emergence of new diseases such as AIDS, and the development of new therapeutic modalities and medical technology are principal factors behind escalating health care costs. In this chapter, however, our focus is on another factor that has and will continue to have a dramatic impact on health care costs in the coming decades: aging of the aged. The "aging of the aged" refers to those individuals aged 85 years and above. This "old-old" segment of society is the fastest-growing age group in the United States.

Chronic Conditions in Old Age

Older adults are afflicted less by acute conditions than young adults. But they are afflicted much more often by chronic conditions, such as heart disease and arthritis. More than 80% of the elderly suffer from at least one chronic condition, and almost 50% report two or more such conditions. Approximately 24% of older people living in the community have severe chronic conditions that prevent them from carrying on one or more major daily life activities (Public Health Service, 1989). The prevalence of chronic conditions and subsequent daily activity limitations increase with age (Table 1-1). People age 85 and older represent only 7% of people age 65 and older but "constitute

19 to 37% of people dependent in home management activities, 18 to 26% of people dependent in personal care activities, 27% percent of people dependent in mobility activities, and 16% of people who were incontinent daily" (Public Health Service, 1989, p. 7-7). These dreary statistics portray a very clear picture of the impact of poor health in the later years.

Projecting Future Health Costs for Medicare and Nursing Homes

Schneider and Guralnik (1990) used the current U.S. Census Bureau projections for the growth of the "old-old" age group to project future costs for Medicare and nursing homes. These projections were based on low-mortality, middle-mortality, and high-mortality assumptions that affect the growth of older age groups (Figure 1-1).

Figure 1-2 provides an overview of the impact of an aging America on Medicare costs. We caution that interpretations from Figure 1-2 should be guarded. Projecting future health care costs from Census Bureau data has many limitations (projected number of individuals age 65 and older, estimates of morbidity at specific ages, estimated health care costs at different ages for specific conditions). Nevertheless, policy makers use projections from Census Bureau data to formulate plans and justify programs. Average annual Medicare costs in 1987 were $2,017 for individuals aged 65 to 74 and $3,215 for those aged 85 years and above. These costs, using the middle-mortality assumption, will nearly double (using 1987 dollars) by the year 2020. By the year 2040, the level of Medicare spending for the age 65 and older population may range from $147 billion (low-mortality assumption) to $212 billion (high-mortality assumption). This three-fold increase in Medicare costs is based on 1987 dollars.[1]

Schneider and Guralnik's (1990) projection for nursing home care costs is even more alarming (Figure 1-3). In 1985 dollars, the cost of nursing home care could rise to between $84 billion (low-mortality assumption) and $139 billion (high-mortality assumption) by the year 2040. The reader should note that approximately 40 percent of current nursing home costs are reimbursed by the federal government through Medicaid. It is quite conceivable that government expenditure for nursing home cost may reach $56 billion (40% of 139 billion).

---

[1]In 2031 the first baby boomer will turn 85 years old. By 2040, the average age of the baby boomer will be 85 years old.

Table 1-1. Functional limitations of the elderly residing in communities (not in nursing homes or institutions), United States, 1984 (in thousands, except percent). Covers persons 65 years old and over who were living in communities outside of nursing homes or other institutions (civilian noninstitutional population).

Functional Limitation	Persons 65 years and over	65-74 years old			75-84 years old			85 years and over	Living	
	Total	Male	Female	Total	Male	Female	Total		Alone	others
Total, 65 years and over	26,433	16,288	7,075	9,213	8,429	3,128	5,121	1,897	8,397	18,036
Percent with difficulty in										
Walking	18.7	14.2	12.9	15.1	22.9	18.3	25.7	39.9	20.4	17.9
Getting outside	9.6	5.6	4.5	6.5	12.3	7.5	15.3	31.3	9.7	9.5
Bathing or showering	9.8	6.4	5.7	6.9	12.3	9.2	14.2	27.9	9.9	9.7
Transferring	8.0	6.1	4.8	7.0	9.2	6.0	11.2	19.3	8.8	7.6
Dressing	6.2	4.3	4.4	4.2	7.6	7.3	7.7	16.6	5.0	6.8
Using toilet	4.3	2.6	2.4	2.7	5.4	3.6	6.5	14.1	3.4	4.7
Eating	1.8	1.2	1.5	.9	2.5	2.5	2.4	4.4	1.2	2.1
Preparing meals	7.1	4.0	3.0	4.8	8.8	6.0	10.5	26.1	6.0	7.6
Shopping for personal items	11.3	6.4	4.6	7.8	15.0	9.6	18.4	37.0	11.9	11.0
Managing money	5.1	2.2	2.8	1.8	6.3	5.4	6.8	24.0	4.0	5.5
Using the telephone	4.8	2.7	3.5	2.0	6.0	7.9	4.8	17.5	2.6	5.8
Doing heavy housework	23.8	18.6	11.2	24.3	28.7	15.9	36.4	47.8	28.0	21.9
Doing light housework	7.1	4.3	3.5	5.0	8.9	6.2	10.5	23.6	6.6	7.4
Percent not performing activity										
Preparing meals	5.2	4.6	9.8	.5	5.5	12.0	1.6	8.9	1.1	7.1
Shopping for personal items	2.0	1.1	1.9	.5	2.5	2.9	2.3	7.5	2.2	1.9
Managing money	1.9	1.3	1.6	1.1	2.2	2.1	2.2	5.9	.8	2.4
Using the telephone	.8	.5	.8	.3	.9	1.4	.6	2.1	.8	.7
Doing heavy housework	9.7	8.1	12.7	4.6	11.5	16.3	8.6	15.9	7.1	11.0
Doing light housework	3.5	2.8	6.1	.3	4.0	7.8	1.7	7.1	.7	4.8

Source: Judah Matras, *Dependency, Obligations, and Entitlements: A New Sociology of Aging, the Life Course, and the Elderly*, 1990, p. 291. Reprinted by permission of Prentice-Hall, Englewood Cliffs, NJ.

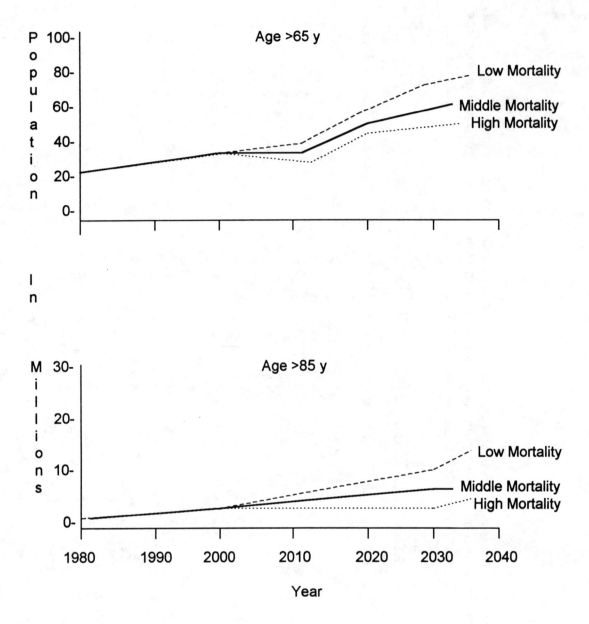

Figure 1-1. Projected growth of the population aged 85 years and above. Projections are based on low- (Series 9), middle- (Series 14), and high- (Series 19) mortality assumptions from the U.S. Bureau of Census.

From *Dependency, Obligations, Entitlements* by Matras, Judah, c 1990. Reprinted by permission of Prentice-Hall, Inc., Upper Saddle River, NJ.

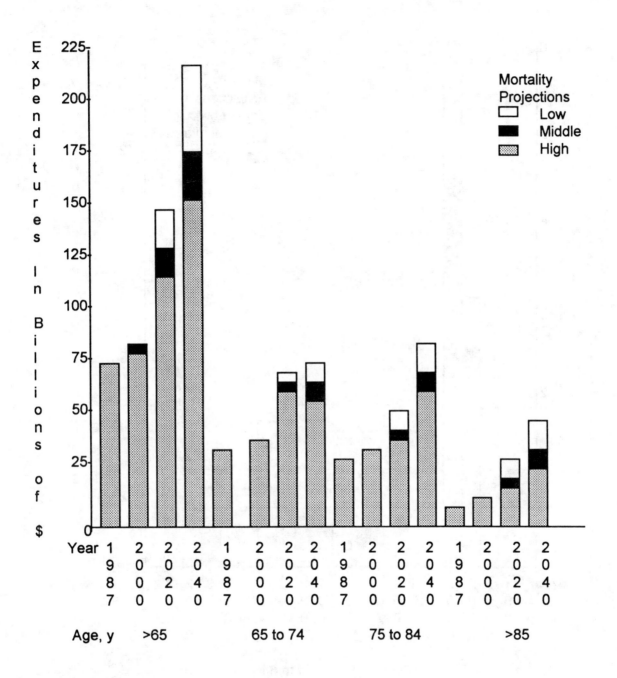

Figure 1-2. Actual (1987) and projected Medicare expenses in 1987 dollars by age group. Average Medicare expenses per person were obtained from data from the Health Care Financing Administration. Cost projections are based on low- (Series 9), middle- (Series 14), and high- (Series 19) mortality assumptions from the U.S. Bureau of Census. Source: E. L. Schneider and J. M. Guralnik. The Aging of America: Impact on Health Care Costs, *JAMA*, (263), May 2, 1990, p. 2337. Copyright 1990, American Medical Association.

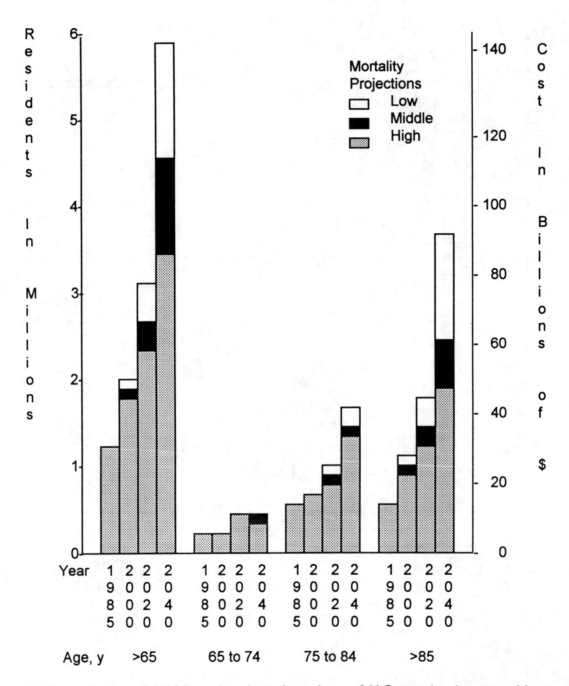

Figure 1-3. Actual (1985) and projected numbers of U.S. nursing home residents and costs in 1985 dollars by age group. The numbers of nursing home residents in 1985 are from the National Nursing Home Survey, and the costs per resident are from the Health Care Financing Administration. Projected numbers of residents and costs are based on low- (Series 9), middle- (Series 14), and high- (Series 19) mortality assumptions from the U.S. Bureau of the Census and 1985 costs.

Source: Data from E. L. Schneider and J. M. Guralnik, "The Aging of America: Impact on Health Care Costs" in *JAMA* (263), May 2, 1990.

Rising Prevalence of Disability and Future Health Costs

The Schneider and Guralnik (1990) projections for Medicare and nursing home care costs assume that the level of disability and utilization of nursing home beds will remain stable over the coming decades. However, two specific age-dependent disorders that contribute significantly to disability and long-term care needs seriously question this assumption. Thus, Schneider and Guralnik (1990) also provide a projection impact on Medicare and nursing home costs based on the rising prevalence of moderate to severe dementias and hip fractures. Figures 1-4 and 1-5 provide an overview of these projections.

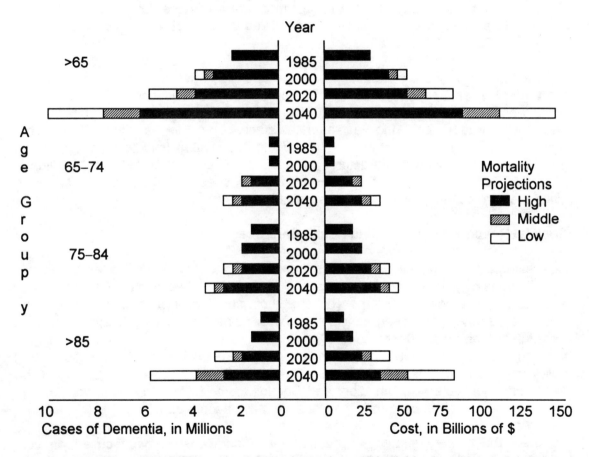

Figure 1-4. Actual (1987) and projected number of individuals with moderate and severe dementia and costs in 1985 dollars for care by age group. These numbers are calculated by applying estimated age-specific prevalence rates of dementia in the community and in nursing homes. Costs for dementia are calculated for cases both in the community and in nursing homes. Projected numbers of affected individuals and costs are based on low- (Series 9), middle- (Series 14), and high- (Series 19) mortality assumptions from the U.S. Bureau of the Census and 1985 costs. Source: E.L. Schneider and J.M. Guralnik. The Aging of America: Impact on Health Care Costs, *JAMA*,(263), May 2, 1990, p. 2339. Copyright 1990, American Medical Association.

Dementias increase rapidly with age, from 3% at ages 65 to 74 to 9% at ages 75 to 84 and 28% at ages 85 and older. Moreover, the prevalence of dementia in nursing homes is much higher (range 47% to 56%) than in community dwellings. Hu and Cartright (1986) estimate that the cost of care for a dementia person treated at home is $11,735 per year and $22,548 per year in nursing homes. The cost of care for moderate to severe dementias in 1985 was $35.8 billion. This cost, in 1985 dollars, will range from 92 billion (low-mortality assumption) to $149 billion in 2040 (Figure 1-4). Schneider and Guralnik (1990) write,

> These numbers approach the magnitude of current federal deficits. If the expenditures for all levels of dementia were used for these calculations instead of those for just moderate to severe dementia, the future costs for this condition would exceed the largest federal deficits. (p. 2039)

Hip fractures increase exponentially with age and also have a devastating impact on the lives of older Americans. By age 85 and above, the incidence of hip fracture for white women is 2%. Approximately 20% of older adults experiencing a hip fracture succumb to death within one year after the fracture, and an additional 20% do not regain mobility without assistance. The modest assumption (middle mortality) shows that health care costs for hip fractures will rise from $1.6 billion in 1987 to $6 billion in 2040 (1987 dollars) (Figure 1-5). Moreover, these cost estimates are very conservative since they are based only on acute hospitalization costs.

Societal Response to Escalating Health Care Costs

Cost-extrapolation projections, such as those envisioned by Schneider and Guralnik, have increasingly led to vocal suggestions for rationing health care costs for older Americans. Ex-Colorado Governor Richard Lamm and Daniel Callahan (Director of the Hastings Institute) have been principal spokespersons for rationing health care costs for adults in their late 70s, or early 80s. For example, Lamm and Callahan suggest that medical care be limited only to relieve suffering. Despite their contention, most policy makers recognize the pitfalls in rationing health care costs by age. But if the health costs projected by Schneider and Guralnik come to fruition, the unpopular age rationing stance posed by Lamm and Callahan may become popular.

To date, the primary strategy to control health care costs have focused on cost containment such as Health Maintenance Organizations, Diagnostic Related Group reimbursement, and increased obligation by the individual to contribute to cost-share health insurance plans. Early returns suggest that these measures have not been successful in the late 1980s.

Schneider and Guralnik (1990) note that one positive approach to reducing health care costs in the future is to mobilize research resources to concentrate on common diseases that lead to long-term disability in the old-old population. For example, only 0.1 to 0.2 cents are spent on basic research for Alzheimer's disease for every dollar

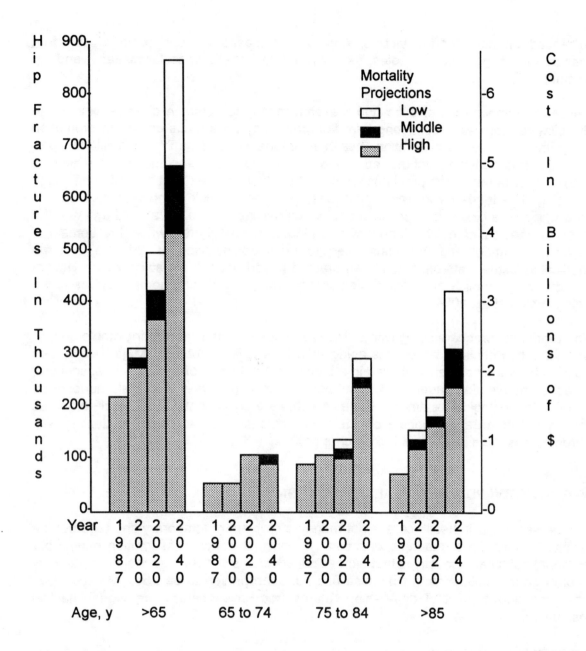

Figure 1-5. Actual 1987 and projected hip fractures and costs in 1987 dollars by age group. Age-specific prevalence rates for hip fractures are from the national Hospital Discharge Survey; and the costs were calculated from Medicare payment schedules for this diagnosis. The costs include only acute hospitalization and surgeons' fees. Projected numbers of hip fractures and costs are based on low- (Series 9), middle- (Series 14), and high- (Series 19) mortality assumptions from the U.S. Bureau of the Census and 1985 costs. Source: E. L. Schneider and J. M. Guralnik. The Aging of America: Impact on Health Care Costs, *JAMA* (263), May 2, 1990, p. 2339. Copyright 1990, American Medical Association.

expensed on care for the victims. Additional diseases in need of more sufficient research funding include diabetes, osteoarthritis, peripheral vascular disease, and hip fractures.

Despite the importance of allocating research money to common diseases leading to disability, a more successful long-term approach may be a focus on health promotion programs; i.e., health prevention, health maintenance and health rehabilitation programs. An underlying point missed in health rationing and cost-containment strategies is that many of the health problems faced by the elderly are a result of a societal image of aging. The tendency in American society has been to link aging with diseases, to view aging as a biological process of decay and decline, and to equate old age with the need for medical care. This tendency has placed aging squarely within the domain of medical treatment and has contributed to the medicalization of old age. A large medical-industrial enterprise has been created based upon this medicalization view of aging through publicly subsidized, high-cost hospital and nursing home services to the aging (Estes et al., 1984).

The tendency to equate aging with a disease arises from this view of inevitable decline and thus, by definition, associates aging as a bio-medical problem. Major health care policies for the elderly are reflected in a biomedical definition of health; i.e., absence of disease. Intervention under a biological perspective is generally wholesale adoption of medical technological treatment. But as health care costs continue to escalate and as the impact of an aging population fuels this increase, our approach to dealing with chronic illness and disability will likely change.

MOVING TOWARD A NEW HEALTH PARADIGM

The present crisis in health care is not merely a problem of temporary shortage but the result of moving in a dead-end direction. A principal working assumption behind our present health care industry is that biomedical advances correlate strongly with the lofty goal of good health. Yet, this premise has not been proven to be true. Moreover, we have reached a point of diminishing returns from investment in traditional medical institutions.

Tragedy of the Commons

Garrett Hardin's (1968) term, "The Tragedy of the Commons," is very descriptive of today's health care crisis. To Hardin, the Tragedy of the Commons stems from the incompatibility of individual choice and group survival. In colonial days, each farmer traditionally acquired wealth by increased use of the commons—that is, the New England village green–which served as a common grazing area. The system worked as long as the number of cattle being grazed was not too large, but if each individual exercised his right to over-graze his livestock, there would be no more room and no more grass. Continued escalation in use eventually led to depletion, and the result was impoverishment. Without a new morality, the commons would be ruined.

The relationship of the health consumer and morality is comparable to that of the farmer and the commons. Without a new morality, the finite limits of the medical care system will be surpassed and collapse will result. For example, the escalation in the two major government health care programs, Medicare and Medicaid, has already resulted in a bulging of the seams of the federal budget and a threat to the commons—the American public.

Construction of health policy for the elderly has led to an acute, curative, hospital-based system which favors older people, resulting in the medicalization of aging. The medicalization of aging has both denied the significant role that social and economic factors play in determining the health status of the elderly and underplayed the role that health promotion can play in health status. Aging brings with it more susceptibility to illness. This heightened susceptibility implies more medical care for both chronic and terminal conditions which, in turn, require more hospital care, more health care professionals and administrators, and escalating health costs and insurance reimbursement. The end result is a health care crisis and an aging crisis.

Our life saving technology of the past four decades has outstripped our health-preserving technology, and the net effect has been to worsen the people's health. Chronic disease has become an inescapable part of our lives and will continue to increase as the American population ages. Moreover, if current trends continue, by the year 2000 an estimated 50% of our federal health care expenditures will be devoted to the care and treatment of the older population (American Hospital Association, 1985). To avoid this crisis in health care and aging, health care organizations must be willing to change traditional modes of care to deal effectively with chronic diseases and conditions of aging. There are strong signs that such a shift is emerging among health care providers and consumers.

History of the Paradigm Shift

John McKnight, Director of the Center for Urban Affairs at Northwestern University, provides an understandable perspective of health paradigms by dividing health history into three areas: (1) Engineering Era, (2) Medical Era, and (3) Post-Medical Era. Health promotion is assumed to be part of the Post-Medical Era (McKnight, 1982).

Engineering Era. The Engineering Era prevailed in the 18th and 19th centuries. Human relations created massive new health threats as the rural populace moved to urban centers. Three principal strategies were employed by public health advocates to manage or cure acute diseases: (1) production systems, delivery and distribution of adequate food supplies to starved populations, (2) pasteurization of food and (3) sewer and water systems for sanitation practices. By the close of the Engineering Era, the public health profession was burgeoning.

Medical Era. The Medical Era dominated the 1920s to the 1960s. Allopathic medicine emerged as the dominant system and added three major contributions to public health: (1) development of vaccines, (2) creation of large-scale medical enterprises for drug administration and disease treatment, and (3) advances from medical technology. The Medical Era interested itself in acute or infectious diseases.

Three major problems in the health field that emerged in the 1970s and 1980s have now merged into a larger and more complex series of problems for health policy. They are (1) increasingly chronic character of illnesses suffered by the total population, (2) increasing emphasis, both within and outside the medical profession, on problems of quality of life, and (3) the increasing attention being given to the organization of health care, focusing on improving the quality of care and reducing costs. In particular, current models of health care organization, procedures for assessing quality of care, and assumptions of quality of life are being reevaluated in light of the substantial differences between acute and chronic diseases. This reevaluation has moved American society into a Post-Medical Era or Health Field Era.

Post-Medical Era. The Post-Medical Era is generally recognized to have begun after 1960 and may be appropriately described as the Health Field Era. The practice of medicine in the latter stages of the Medical Era and the beginning stages of the Health Field Era have largely relied on the advancements of high technology medicine. The problem in acute disease is proper diagnosis and the delivery of more-or-less well understood treatment technology. The patient is expected to be back on his or her feet within days or weeks, needing little in the way of ancillary services.

Managing Chronic Illness

Payment in the acute care system is based on the model of exchange in the marketplace and exceptionally expensive treatment is expected to be handled by some form of health insurance. Under this highly specialized and technically oriented health system, the world is divided into the world of the sick, and the world of the well. Although the rising costs of the acute health care system are debated, a closer look at this debate reveals that participants do not grapple directly with the real issue—the increasingly chronic and unresolvable character of illness.

Chronic illness cannot be "cured" but must be "managed." This differentiation between curing and managing makes chronic diseases different in many respects from acute diseases, the model upon which our present health care system is traditionally based. The health field today, however, generally agrees that the four major determinants of physical well-being are: (1) individual lifestyle (smoking, exercise); (2) social organization (stress); (3) physical environment (pollution, workplace); and (4) economic status (poverty, overconsumption). The Health Field Era, therefore, has called for a paradigm represented by different tools, actors, interests, and a different understanding of life.

It is not that allopathic medicine has failed, but that health determinants must be addressed by the individual and the society in which the individual lives. Although the elderly have a viable need for acute medical care, their major requirement is a continuum of services for managing or preventing the disabling conditions of chronic diseases. Providing this continuum of services has led to a renewed interest in health promotion programs.

HEALTH PROMOTION AND THE ELDERLY: THE NEW RHETORIC

Until recently, the elderly were not included in the new wave of health promotion programs. Minkler and Fullerton (1980) identified four principal reasons behind this exclusion. First, the focus on life extension and the elderly is generally perceived as not having a future. Second, health promotion programs focus on reducing risk factors associated with premature mortality and morbidity, whereas the elderly have already lived beyond the premature demarcation point. Third, the image of health promotion is viewed as advancing "youthfulness," and thus older adults do not fit this image. Fourth, the focus on controlling chronic disease is an irrelevant goal for the elderly since many of them already have one or more chronic conditions that limits their level of functioning. Somers, Kleinman, and Clark (1982) would add the shared public and professional belief that it is already too late for the elderly and they should be content with enjoying what they have without any lifestyle intervention.

1981 White House Conference on Aging

There were signs in the 1980s that health promotion activities for the elderly were receiving interest. The 1981 White House Conference on Aging (U.S. Department of Health and Human Services, 1982) devoted one of its 14 task force committees solely to promotion and maintenance of wellness. Specifically, the Committee on Promotion and Maintenance of Wellness made six recommendations. First, accrediting bodies for educational training programs for certain professions (e.g., physicians, nurses, therapists) should require courses on geriatrics and health promotion. Second, federal, state, and local governments should develop and disseminate educational materials on health promotion for the elderly. Third, the nation's health policy should include improving the health of all Americans, especially the elderly, containing health care costs, and focusing direct attention on health promotion and disease prevention. Fourth, additional emphasis must be placed on behavioral and lifestyle modifications within the control of the individual. Fifth, the health care system needs to be restructured to take advantage of wellness and prevention services. And sixth, a comprehensive review is needed of prevention-oriented health screening procedures for the elderly to determine medical efficacy. The intent of the review was to provide effective and cost-efficient health procedures (Weiler, 1986).

Health Objectives for the Nation

Based upon the 1979 publication of Healthy People: The Surgeon General's Report on Health Promotion and Disease Prevention (U.S. Department of Health and Human Services), a companion report was produced to provide a strategic focus for pursuit of national health objectives, the 1980 publication The 1990 Health Objectives for the Nation. This Public Health Service (PHS) used this report to set out 226 national objectives that addressed improvements in health status, risk reduction, public and professional awareness, health services and protective measures, and surveillance and evaluation efforts to measure attainment of specified objectives. The 226 health objectives were categorized in 15 priority areas under the headings of preventive services, health protection, and health promotion. Drawing on the 1981 White House Conference on Aging, the explicit goal for the elderly under the 1990 report was to reduce the average annual number of days of restricted activity by 20%, a reduction from 39 days to less than 30 days.

1995 White House Conference on Aging

May 2–5, 1995, the White House Conference on Aging (WHCoA) was held in Washington, D.C., with 2,217 delegates who represented all 50 states, the territories and the District of Columbia. The delegates were selected by members of Congress, Governors, and the national aging organizations and were predominately Democrats.

Over 50 resolutions were adopted which will help shape the nation's age policy for the next decade. The 1995 White House Conference on Aging was the fourth in United States history, the first since 1981 and the last of the 20th century. The WHCoA was authorized by the 1992 Amendments to the Older Americans Act and was signed by President Clinton on February 17, 1994. Forty of the adopted resolutions were synthesized from recommendations received from the more than 800 pre-Conference events. The remaining 10 resolutions were introduced by delegates at the Conference. On May 5 the delegates voted to make the following resolutions their top 10 priorities:

1. Keeping the Social Security Sound for Now and for the Future.
2. Preserving the Integrity of the Older Americans Act.
3. Preserving the Nature of Medicaid.
4. Reauthorization of the Older Americans Act.
5. Ensuring the Future of the Medicare Program.
6. Increase Funding for Alzheimer Research.
7. Preserving Advocacy Functions under the Older Americans Act.
8. Ensuring the Availability of a Broad Spectrum of Services.
9. Financing and Providing Long-term Care and Services.
10. Acknowledging the Contribution of Older Volunteers.

Appendix A contains the recommendations related to health promotion as they applied to the aforementioned 10 priorities.

It has been suggested to many that the 1995 WHCoA of delegates overwhelmingly voted to maintain the status quo without any apparent concern about the rising costs of the nation's budget deficit and its long-term effects on future generations. It appeared as if these delegates wanted to maintain and even expand benefits and services provided by such programs as Medicare/Medicaid, Social Security, and the Older Americans Act, even though the child poverty level has reached its highest level in over 30 years. One in five of all voters in the 1992 elections were older adults. This large representation in older delegates raised concerns among other adults that the older delegate constituency was motivated for self-interest rather than societal needs.

The 1990 Health Objectives were used in the 1980s to spotlight problems, set priorities, and allocate resources at the local, state, and national levels. Although progress was made toward these objectives, this progress was of minimal concern to the elderly. The 1990 Health Objectives, to the exclusion of older adults, focused primarily on premature mortality and morbidity. But as we enter the 1990s there is a renewed opportunity to focus more directly on older adults. The Healthy People 2000: National Health Promotion and Disease Prevention Objectives moves in that direction (U.S. Department of Health and Human Services, 1990).

Year 2000 Health Objectives

The Healthy People 2000 objectives parallel the 1990 health objectives in the comprehensiveness of health issues it addresses. However, the draft review for this report, released in September 1989 for public review, is much broader in terms of scope of participation. Moreover, the Year 2000 priority includes vitality and independence of older people as a priority concern. This concern is based on a better understanding of the aging process. Research makes evident that a great deal of the physical decline prevalent among the elderly is due less to aging per se than to an absence of comprehensive disease prevention strategies. The most prevalent chronic diseases and conditions in later life derive from faulty lifestyle and environmental factors, factors for which effective health promotion interventions often exist.

Earlier in this chapter, we emphasized that the leading chronic conditions for older people were arthritis, hypertensive disease, heart conditions, hearing impairments, and dementia. The rates for these diseases, in most cases, are much higher for the elderly than for people ages 45 through 64. Due to these conditions, older adults experience more hospitalizations, visit physicians more frequently, and consume more prescription and over-the-counter drugs than the general population. Although health behaviors practiced earlier in life can certainly influence the status of health later in life, growing evidence shows that health promotion interventions even later in life can produce health benefits and a higher quality of life. More research, however, is needed to determine when interventions are effective for "preventing the onset or ameliorating the course of disease and what outcomes have the most impact on functional independence and quality of life" (Public Health Service, 1989, p. 7-2). The Public Health Service adds that the lack of a conceptual framework for health promotion and disease prevention for older adults has hindered past research efforts.

The taxonomy of prevention in common usage which looks at interventions as primary, secondary, and tertiary--aims at reductions in morbidity and premature mortality--is inadequate in addressing the complex interactions of disease and disability in older people. If the goal is to extend active life expectancy, as most experts agree, the challenge is not solely on how to prolong life but how to maintain the health and quality of life of older people. For many in the aging population, a pressing need is protection of functional capacity, either from progression of disease-associated morbidity or from unrelated co-morbidity or disability. To be able to maximize independence and quality of life, a comprehensive approach is needed (Public Health Service, 1989, p. 7-2).

In Chapter 2, we present a conceptual foundation for health promotion programs that respond to the functional needs of older adults. The objectives for older adults contained in the Healthy People 2000 report (Appendix A) will fit under this conceptual framework.

There was little question that efforts by the 1981 White House Conference on Aging and the 1990 Health Objectives for the Nation laid the ideological groundwork for health promotion programs directed toward the elderly. But the lack of secure policies and funding for such programs in the 1980s made the development of health promotion programs for the elderly more rhetoric than substance. The Healthy People 2000 report and its obvious cross-cutting areas for the "independence" and "vitality" objectives specified for the elderly provide a more promising outlook. Moreover, the Center for Disease Control's (CDC) Planned Approach to Community Health (PATCH) program will be used to define and refine local community action and public health activities for attaining the Year 2000 health objectives. The CDC's publication Healthy Communities 2000: Model Standards may serve as a guiding framework for local entities.

THEORY UNDERLYING HEALTH PROMOTION AND HEALTH CARE COST CONTAINMENT

The current theory underlying the health promotion movement in this country is as follows: As a nation, we are dying from very different diseases than we were at the turn of the century. In the early 1900s infectious diseases were the major causes of morbidity and mortality. These infectious diseases were principally related to such health issues as polluted water and lack of sewage disposal. Today, the consequences of such conditions (e.g., pneumonia, tuberculosis) have been virtually eliminated and the primary causes of mortality and morbidity are what may be called "diseases of choice"–chronic diseases such as heart disease, cancer, and diabetes. Factors contributing to chronic diseases are lifestyle habits. Yet, the health community has responded to the dramatic shift by continuing to treat the new chronic diseases with traditional methods–that is, to identify symptoms and causes once the illness has occurred and then seek its cure. This approach has proven to be less effective with chronic diseases than it was with infectious diseases.

Active Life Expectancy

In 1986, the remaining life expectancy for men was approximately 14.8 years and 18.98 years for women at age 65. The overall average life expectancy at age 65 for the total population was 16.8 years, up from 15.2 years reported in 1970. But the simple prolongation of life does not make a valuable contribution to the health of elderly people unless the gain in quantity years is represented by quality years of life. The term "active life expectancy" is now used as a measure for quality, years characterized by good health, illness, impairment, and disability.

Figure 1-6 illustrates a model of age-related changes of survival curves and active life-expectancy. The area between the three curves displays the amount of time expected to be lived in a given health status. The "A" area of the curve, under the morbidity curve, is considered years free from disability. Morbidity (B), years without significant disability, consists of the area between the B and C curves. The area above the C curve is considered to be years of significant disability. The horizontal lines l_1 and l_2 represent two hypothetical individuals. l_1 is a person who lives 45 years of healthy life (A_1), 3 years of morbidity (B_1), and 7 years of disability (C_1) before succumbing to death at age 55. l_2 lives 60 years of healthy life, 5 years of morbidity, and 12 years of disability before incurring death at age 77.

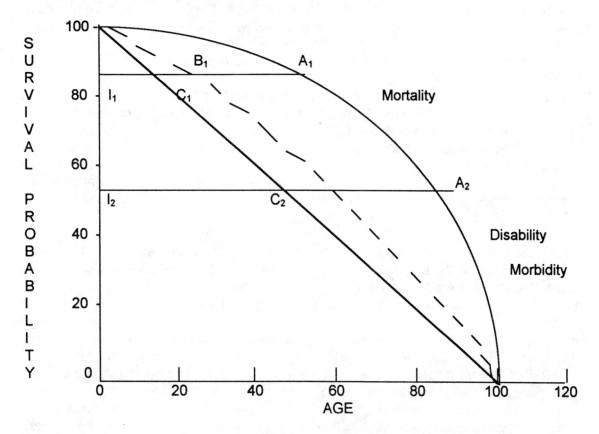

Figure 1-6. A model of age-related change in health, function, and survival: For the population and for two hypothetical individuals, l_1 and l_2. Legend: Outermost Curve = Total Life Expectancy; Intermediate Curve = Healthy Life Expectancy; Innermost Curve = Active Life Expectancy.

Source: Data based on "The Uses of Epidemiology in the Study of the Elderly" in *Technical Report Series 806*, figure 3, page 261. World Health Organization, Geneva.

Calculating QALY

The active life years (curve A) is a summary measure of health that combines mortality (quantity of life) and morbidity (quality of life) into a single measure. Although several approaches have been used for combining mortality and morbidity, the quality-adjusted life years (QALY) has emerged as the popular calculation measure. The QALY uses a life-expectancy model consisting of two sets of data. First, a life table of the population is used as an indicator of the proportion of people living and dying in each age interval and the average number of years remaining at each age interval. Second, point-in-time estimates of well-being of a population are used to represent individual functioning (psychomotor, cognitive, affective). As examples, affective functioning may refer to limitations in performing social roles; psychomotor functioning may be a measure of bed confinement or mobility limitation. Point-in-time measures are multiplied times the number of years of life remaining at each age interval in the life table as an estimate of QALY. For example, life expectancy at birth in 1987 was 74.9 years. If the overall point-in-time estimate for well-being is 80% (0.8), the .8 x 74.9 will equal 60 years of healthy life. This means the remaining 15 years are spent in morbidity and disability.

The Public Health Service is presently pursuing a point-in-time estimate of well-being that can be used as a nationally representative index for QALY calculation. In the meantime, the Public Health Service (1989) report used an 0.8 estimate for QALY. This index yielded a baseline estimate of life expectancy at birth of 60 years of healthy life and approximately 15 years of ill health or life dysfunction. The goal is to increase active life expectancy at birth to at least 65 years. This goal may be attained by increasing life expectancy from 74.9 years to 81.2 or by raising the QALY index to 0.87. Attainment of this objective will likely require both actions.

Older adults were also recognized in the Healthy People 2000 report under a QALY objective. Specifically, the objective is to increase active life expectancy (QALY) at age 65 to at least 14 years for men and 16 years for women. In 1986, "approximately 82% (12.0 of 14.8 years) of expected additional years for men age 65 and older, and approximately 73% (13.7 or 18.98 years) of expected additional years for women age 65 and older, were expected to be active" (Public Health Service, 1989, p. 7-6). For the age 85 and older group, 2.7 of 5.8 (46%) total years of life expectancy for men and 2.4 of 7.2 (33%) years for women were expected to be active. The decrease in active life expectancy years for the 85 and older group is partly due to the expected years to be lived in an institution, that is, 1.05 years for men and 2.20 years for women. Additionally, the small percentage of QALY years for females is partially due to their extended years of life expectancy.

Boon or Drain

The consequences of aging are diverse. But one consequence that tends to permeate most discussions is rising health care costs and the impact of an aging America on these costs. Given that older adults require more services from our health care system, will battle lines form between generations for health care resources? Will health rationing become a reality? What ethical, political, and economical principles will be used to distribute health care resources? Will the American public be willing to devote an additional 5 to 10% of the GNP to health care? The answers to these questions will not come easily.

One course of action that would be the simplest to implement stands out: continuation of present policy that is based on the medical model. The medical model relies on curative medicine, institution-based long-term care, and fee-for-service reimbursement that is underwritten through government expenditures. The demographic projections, advancing medical technology, and increasing service demand leading to even higher health care costs threaten the continuance of our present "medical model" system. New or complementary models, such as health promotion, are likely to be introduced. The Public Health Service Objective for an increase in quality adjusted life years is a good indicator of more innovative health care approaches.

Future of Health Care Services for Older Adults

There is no doubt that Medicare, Medicaid, and the Older Americans Act programs have significantly helped to improve the health and economic security for older adults. However, our society is faced with a major challenge of "can we afford the cost" of providing health care at the same level we have in the past? Because the life expectancy of the elderly in the United States has increased and because our technology has continued to make significant strides, we are faced with an increasing gross national product of expenditure for health care. In 1995 alone, Medicare represented about 11.5% of the federal outlays and Medicaid approximately 5.7%. There is a general concern about the federal and state budgets for these programs and for the insolvency facing the Medicare Hospital Insurance Trust Fund. In 1995, total spending by Medicare on persons age 65 and older was about $155 billion and in excess of $46 billion for Medicaid. Medicare and Medicaid constitute about 17.4% of the federal budget and 3.8% of the GDP in the United States. Moreover, both of these programs will conceivably grow by about 10% in the near future. Medicare and Medicaid cover approximately 63% of the majority of health care expenses for our older Americans. But, older adults are still effected by major gaps in Medicare and Medicaid for covering costs of prescription drugs, hearing aids, eyeglasses, most disease prevention programs, health promotion services and long-term care. Often, the cost of supplementary health insurance is prohibitive for many older adults. Although the cost for supplemental health insurance is high, about three-quarters of older adults have some form of private supplemental coverage, even if they limit spending in other areas.

Our health care system is fragmented and difficult to maneuver at best. In-patient hospitalizations are fewer than any time in history and the length of stays are shorter. Older adults find themselves less able to take care of themselves at home, but may not have the means to access the long-term care system. The annual cost of long-term care exceeds $30,000 and is prohibitive for most people. For this reason, we are seeing a surge in private insurance for long-term care; about 2 million policies are sold each year. But, the financial burden for long-term care insurance is feasible for a very small minority of seniors. Since the cost of policies rises with advanced age, the future of health care services for the elderly is facing increased political pressure to reduce spending. Physicians and hospitals are feeling the pinch of lower payment levels for both Medicare and Medicaid patients as compared to the private sector. Payment levels under Medicaid, for example, are already so low that if further cuts were incurred, the entire program would be compromised. Public policy makers anticipate that the beneficiaries of Medicare will experience higher cost-sharing measures such as increased co-payment premiums.

Older adults can anticipate that the expansion of managed care will have a vital impact on their health care services. Medical care expenditures have skyrocketed due to such factors as consumer expectations, technology, our focus on diagnosis and cure, and a third party payment structure which makes our medical care appear free. As a society, we have realized that it has become critical to differentiate between health care and medical care. The individual's health, lifestyle, and ability to understand their health problems become critical to the financial success of managed care systems. For example, capitated managed care offers economic incentives to focus on health by stressing self-care practices. In essence, the American health care system is in the process of building a system that incorporates information management systems, negotiates risk-sharing arrangements, and controls cost through disease management from a diagnosis specific treatment process to total patient well-being.

Managed Care refers to "health care" and involves health care through a continuum of services. A patient has a primary physician who serves as the "gatekeeper" by referring the patient to specialists only when it is deemed necessary. The ultimate goal is to keep people healthy by using preventive medicine to alleviate the need for more intensive medical care later. The positive aspect of managed care is that there is more effective coordination and support for those with high cost illnesses which benefits both patients and taxpayers. However, to date, managed care plans have had little to no experience in dealing with the specialized older adult population's medical needs; managed care plans have also failed to help ease the financial burdens of the Medicare system. The requirements for reporting both quality and quantity of care are not yet well defined. Even if Medicare and Medicaid continued their fee-for-service system, the private marketplace changes of managed care will influence the availability of services for older adults.

CHAPTER SUMMARY

In sociological terms, a model is defined as a complex integrated system of meaning used to view, interpret, and understand a part of reality. The medical model has served this function well for the type of deviance we call illness or disease. Health, according to the medical model, is the absence of disease. In American society, the medical model is assigned the kind of deviance (disease or illness) for which the physician and allied health professional have assumed the positions of appropriate remediating agents.

The trouble with models, particularly successful models like the medical model, is that it is easy to get trapped inside one. Once inside the model, it is hard to get out or see beyond it. Thus a model tends to be self-reaffirming and self-justifying. As the tenure of the model grows, there is a tendency of the model to explain more and more. For example, since deviance is a social judgment, the medical model has been used to explain such things as retardation, drug addiction, criminal behavior, suicide, alcoholism, and even homosexuality.

When accepted by popular opinion and economic or political imperatives, a model can approach sanctification. The attainment of sanctification makes it difficult to openly question or doubt the truth or wisdom of the model (McClary et al., 1985). Many writers today (Carlyon, 1984; Dychtwald, 1984; Fries & Crapo, 1981) believe that the medical model has been sanctified and has trapped health care providers and consumers inside. The inability to see outside the medical model has set American society up for some serious blunders such as using an acute, curative care hospital system to manage and treat chronic diseases. Yet there are strong signs that a paradigm shift is emerging toward a health field or health promotion model.

The purpose of the emerging health field or health promotion paradigm is to dramatically reduce morbidity and mortality from the major chronic diseases. Although chronic diseases are most often found among the elderly population, it is precisely the elderly who have been most neglected in policies and programs aimed at attaining health promotion and disease prevention. To adequately address the needs of the elderly, the concept of health must be altered. This concept of health must move beyond the idea of total freedom from disease to the ability of the individual to live and function effectively in society and to exercise self-reliance and autonomy to the maximum extent possible (Filner & Williams, 1979). Critical to this expanded definition of health is the broader responsibility of the elderly and the response-ability of society for broader social and economic considerations for health promotion activities.

Whether the trend toward an aging America will be a boon or a drain on the nation is a question that the proliferating field of health promotion is well equipped to address. As the understanding of the aging process has developed, it has become evident that a great deal of the physical decline prevalent among the elderly is due less to aging per se than to an absence of comprehensive disease prevention strategies. The salient point is that an aging body requires more health maintenance than it did in earlier years. Although little effort was devoted toward health promotion initiatives for the elderly in the 1980s, the Healthy People 2000 objectives provide a strong impetus for future program development.

CHAPTER 2

HEALTH PROMOTION: CONCEPTS AND DIMENSIONS

Seldom in our history has so much time and energy gone into a fervent debate calling for reform in our nation's health care system. The message conveyed through books, articles, lectures, and television shows, is that we are undergoing a crisis in our health care system. Issues within this crisis have become familiar: escalating and unmanageable costs, waste and inefficiency, overemphasis on technology, and dehumanizing practices. Other aspects are also well publicized. Advancement and sophistication of modern medicine is helping us to know more and to do more about sickness than ever before. Also, equity of access and financing for health is spreading widely among the American population, new forms of health care organizations are being formed, and a consumer-involving rationalization of health systems planning is underway on the local level.

Within this debate about the present and future prospects for health care, one area that has been, in the past, neglected but is now receiving more and more attention is health promotion. The health promotion movement presents itself as a possible focus for agreement between the critics and defenders of health care in this country. Impressive evidence shows that the prevention of disease and injury, and the promotion of positive health efforts, can do much to correct some of the imbalances in the present system.

"Prevention" and "promotion" capture the optimistic interest of professional and layman alike and provide a rallying point for new efforts in health care. Yet the terms and modes of practice in health promotion are incorrectly intermingled, creating much confusion among consumers and health care practitioners. This chapter examines the terminology of health promotion as it applies to the concepts and practices of healthy and chronically ill older adults.

TERMINOLOGY, CONCEPTS, AND MODES OF PRACTICE

The 1979 Healthy People: The Surgeon General's Report on Health Promotion and Disease Prevention (U.S. Department of Health and Human Services, 1979) foreword opens with an explicit distinction between medicine, disease prevention, and health promotion. Health promotion, according to this report, focuses not upon the "ill" or "at risk" but upon the healthy and "tries to help them develop lifestyles that can maintain and enhance that state of well-being." The Surgeon General report then goes on to extol health promotion program activities that are essentially disease prevention by the report's own definition. The confusion between disease prevention and health promotion as depicted in the 1979 Surgeon General report is not unusual. A number of new terms, such as high-level wellness, self-care, holistic health, and disease prevention, have been used in conjunction with the concept of health promotion. These terms have been erroneously interchanged with health promotion, creating confusion for the consumer and the practicing health professional.

High-Level Wellness

Most of us think of ourselves as healthy if we're not in pain, suffering from the flu, or otherwise impaired in any way from normal functioning. A lack of illness symptoms is viewed as a measure of "healthiness." Wellness, however, means much, much more. Wellness is not a static state. There are many levels of wellness, just as there are degrees of illness. For example, we may lack physical symptoms of illness but be bored, depressed, lonely, tense, anxious, or generally unhappy. These emotional states may often set the stage for physical disease by lowering the body's resistance. In other words, diseases and symptoms are not really the problem. They represent the body-mind's attempt to solve a problem—messages from the subconscious to the conscious.

Ryan and Travis (1981, p. 3) use an iceberg analogy to illustrate how we may view health. The tip of the iceberg above the surface level of the water is our actual state of health. Traditional medicine has principally directed its practices toward these visible signs of health. But beneath the surface are different layers—lifestyle behaviors, psychological properties, and philosophical transpersonal areas—requiring different health strategies.

Lifestyle factors include nutrition, fitness, substance dependency, and stress management. Psychological factors refer to questions of what motivates us. For example, why do we persist in lifestyle practices that we know are injurious to our health? How can we foster behavioral change? Finally, the bottom level—spiritual concerns—also determines the health profile at the tip of the iceberg.

The traditional medical model of health care chips away at the surface needs by eliminating disease through treatment. However, wellness means looking below the surface level of health through awareness, education, and growth. Awareness is seeing how you are personally conducting your life. Education means exploring options by looking within ourselves and receiving help from others. Growth means trying out new options. By focusing on self-responsibility, wellness is an expression of, not a substitute for, the best in traditional medical practice.

Self-Care

Implicit in wellness and holistic health is the concept of self-care. As Orem (1980) notes,

> In modern society, adults are expected to be self-reliant and responsi-
> ble for themselves. Most social groups further accent that persons who
> are helpless, sick, aged, handicapped, or otherwise deprived should be

helped in their immediate distress and helped to attain or regain responsibility within their existing capacities. (p. 6)

The concept of self-care assumes that the individual has the knowledge, resources, and motivation to make and apply informed choices about health and lifestyle. Moreover, the self-care concept also assumes that health care resources are distributed equally across socio-cultural-economic lines and that health practices, values, and norms of an individual are similar to those of the health care practitioner.

Since the Medical Era (1920 to 1960), the public has been led to believe that the medical care system is the ultimate and final authority on health. We have come to expect the "quick-fix" or "magic bullet" for all that ails us. Health care providers have been educated to cure illness and often are frustrated when curing is not possible. To date, many health care providers and consumers do not understand the relationship between lifestyle and health. In fact, if the individual assumes self-responsibility, a loss of clinician power and authority threatens health care providers relying on an exclusive curing philosophy (Green, 1985).

Holistic Health

The phrase "holistic health" is often interchanged with wellness, although they do have different meanings. Holism, from the Greek word halos, means whole (person). In reference to health, holistic health may be expanded to mean physical, spiritual, emotional, and mental health. Health in each area results in health of the whole person, whereas illness in any one area creates stress in the other areas.

The geometric triangle provides an excellent analogy of what is meant by holistic health. A triangle is defined as having three sides or corners. If any of these three sides is missing or not connected, the triangle does not exist. Let's assume that the three triangles represent body, mind, and spirit. If we leave out any of the three sides of the triangle, then we no longer have a whole person. Moreover, no matter how much we study one side or one angle of the triangle, we will never know what the properties of the entire triangle are unless we gain knowledge of the other two sides or angles.

One advantage of a triangle analogy to health is that we can clearly see the disadvantage of our tendency to think of the body first. Too many times, we consider only the "body" side of the triangle; once the body seems to be in reasonably good operating condition, we assume that all is well. Yet if the emotional side is disturbed, before long the body will be affected. To carry this thought further, a person may be relatively stable both mentally and physically but without spiritual awareness may have no direction or feeling of purpose in life. Eventually, this spiritual deficit also manifests itself in the other two spheres. Thus, holistic health accounts for the impact and importance of all three sides of the triangle–physical, mental, and spiritual.

Disease Prevention

Because illness frequently serves as a barrier to optimum growth and the realization of personal potential, maintaining an illness-free state through preventive efforts is highly desirable. Prevention can be described as consisting of primary, secondary, and tertiary levels. Each level of prevention requires specific interventions at a distinct point in time relative to the occurrence and processes of disease. Traditionally, the three levels of prevention have been defined as follows:

- Primary prevention refers to preventing the occurrence of disease or injury, for example, influenza immunization.
- Secondary prevention refers to early detection and intervention to curb or retard progression of an illness condition, in order to shorten the duration and severity of a pathogenic condition.
- Tertiary prevention refers to medical surveillance, maintenance and rehabilitation designed to minimize the effect of existing disease, prevent complications and premature deterioration, and return the individual to optimum health, for example, medication for hypertension (Marge, 1988).

The taxonomy of prevention is difficult to apply to chronic diseases of the elderly. A condition may be simultaneously a preventable disease and a precursor (risk factor) for another condition. For example, osteoporosis is a preventable disease but also is a precursor to fractures from accidents (e.g., falling). The key is to recognize that health promotion attempts to maintain current health status or to move to a more desirable level of health. Prevention, probably better described as health-protecting behavior, is a defensive posture or set of actions taken to ward off specific illnesses or their sequence that may threaten the quality of life or longevity (Pender, 1982).

Health Promotion: The Guiding Framework

Defining the term health promotion is imprecise, at best, because of individual ideas of what health actually means. Generally, wellness has been defined as the process of adopting patterns of behavior that can lead to improved health and heightened life satisfaction. Disease prevention may be viewed as health-protecting behaviors directed toward decreasing the probability of encountering illness by active protection of the body against unnecessary stressors or by detection of illness at an early step. In contrast, health-promoting behaviors are directed toward sustaining or increasing the level of well-being, self-actualization, and fulfillment. Health promotion focuses on movement of the individual toward a positively balanced state of increased well-being. Thus the term health promotion implies the application of wellness principles to organizations and institutions.

In an attempt to unify the terms of disease prevention, wellness, and health promotion, the National Council on Aging (NCOA) and the American Hospital Association (AHA) provide a more sophisticated definition of health promotion. The NCOA definition of health promotion is "any combination of health education and related organizational, political, and economic interventions, designed to facilitate behavioral and environmental changes which prevent, delay the occurrence, or minimize the impact of disease or disability while promoting the independence and well-being of older adults" (American Hospital Association, 1985, p. 185). The AHA defines health promotion by including health education and health information: "The process of fostering awareness, influencing attitudes and identifying alternatives so that individuals can make internal choices and change their behavior in order to achieve an optimal level of physical and mental health and improve their physical and social environment" (American Hospital Association, 1985, p. 185).

The core concept of disease prevention is based on health risk factor reduction and prevention. It provides the logic for the variety of prevention activities that have now become a part of health-protection objectives. Yet the core concept of wellness, according to the rhetoric discussed in this section, is self-actualization and personal fulfillment. This core concept enables people to attain a condition of wholeness, happiness, and vitality.

If wellness is the goal of health promotion, we need to use the logic of self-actualization and personal fulfillment as the principal guide to our action. That logic tells us that the barriers to fulfillment of individual potential, such as elevated cholesterol or high blood pressure, are not the only real problems of health. Central to the concerns of health promotion are the ideas of self-care responsibility, wellness, and holistic health. Figure 2-1 describes this relationship.

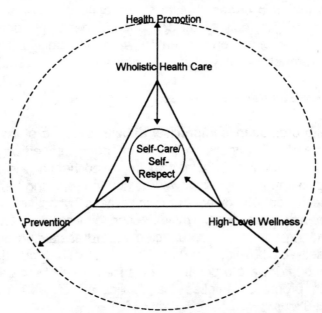

Figure 2-1. The practice model for a healthy life. Developed by K. Green, Health promotion: Its terminology, concepts, and modes of practice. *In* Health Values: Achieving High-Level Wellness, *Vol. 9, No. 3*, May-June, 1985. Reprinted by permission of Slack Incorporated.

Self-care includes all those activities undertaken by the individual to learn how to better take care of oneself, for example, becoming informed about healthy lifestyles. Holistic health requires that the consumer and practicing health professional understand the relationship between the physical, emotional, and spiritual sides of health. Disease prevention requires the practicing of health behaviors that reduce the at-risk factors to ill health. High-level wellness is the internalization of a total lifestyle for the focusing on optimal health rather than on illness. And health promotion provides the guiding framework for putting the concepts and ideas of self-care, holistic health, disease prevention, and wellness into operation (Green, 1985).

Community Health Promotion

The term community health promotion also applies to our discussion. Community health promotion refers to activities directed toward bettering the health of the public, and activities employing resources commonly available to members of the community. It expands beyond the traditional relationship developed between an individual and a health professional to involve a host of agencies, organizations, and institutions in work to enhance people's health. The word community carries with it some implications of scale. Rigid boundaries are very hard to set, but as someone a long time ago put it, "if it feels like a community, it probably is one."

The term health promotion, in our context, simply means to contribute to the advancement of or to further the cause of health. The very open-endedness of the subsequent phrase community health promotion, however it might confuse or worry some, actually provides opportunities for the exercise of creative and imaginative energies. Health promotion programs can be implemented in communities through a wide range of settings (home, school, worksite, health care facilities) by a wide range of techniques (health education, environmental controls, health programs), and under the auspices of a wide array of sponsors (business, labor unions, voluntary agencies, hospitals, public schools, self-care groups).

HEALTH PROMOTION: A CONCEPTUAL MODEL

Health promotion has been popularly defined as "the science and art of helping people alter their lifestyles to move toward optimal health." But this popular definition may be too simple and vague. Goodstadt, Simpson, and Loranger (1987) argue that health promotion should be defined under conceptual and relationship boundaries that establish what should be included and excluded. Additionally, the definition should clearly delineate "contextual uses of works from their broader, common meanings" (p. 61). The broader view of health described in the health continuum presented in the book preface (Figure 1) provides a framework for applying health promotion to both well and non-well older populations. Drawing from this framework, Goodstadt et al. (1987) define health promotion as follows: "Health promotion is the maintenance and enhancement of existing levels of health, through the implementation of effective programs, services and policies" (p. 61).

The Goodstadt et al. (1987) definition provides a conceptual separation between wellness and illness dimensions. This forced divisiveness creates two complementary health maintenance networks: Health Promotion and Health Recovery (Figure 2-2). Primary and secondary prevention objectives fall under the health promotion network. Secondary and tertiary prevention objectives are included in the health recovery network.

Health Maintenance Network

The health promotion network is directed toward well (non-ill) older adults through policies and program services that increase existing health levels. Risk avoidance and risk reduction strategies are employed for this purpose. Risk avoidance strategies (primary prevention) primarily focus on low-risk populations and maintain existing levels of health by inhibiting transition to higher health risks (e.g., drug management programs that prevent substance abuse). Risk reduction programs are targeted toward older adults who are already at risk. The program objective is to help the older adult move into a lower risk category. For example, healthy nutrition practices leading to more accepted blood cholesterol levels are conceptually referred to as secondary prevention–early detection and intervention to curb progression of an illness condition.

The health recovery network targets intervention programs toward the ill older adult. Rehabilitation objectives include "the treatment of the ill, to stabilize their condition, and the introduction of rehabilitation programs to effect a transition to some minimally acceptable level of health" (Goodstadt et al., 1987, p. 61). Thus the health recovery network employs both secondary prevention (early identification and intervention) and tertiary prevention (treatment and rehabilitation) objectives. Edelman and Milio (1986) note that tertiary prevention commences "when a defect or disability is permanent or irreversible" (p. 11). Moreover, the authors also emphasize that the intent is to "minimize the effects of disease and disability by surveillance and maintenance aimed at preventing complications and deteriorations" (p. 11). The goal of tertiary prevention is to return the client to a useful place in society by maximizing remaining functional capacities (Teague, Cipriano, & McGhee, 1990).

Health Maintenance		
Health Promotion Network		Health Recovery Network
Risk avoidance	Risk reduction	
Primary prevention	Secondary prevention	Tertiary Prevention

Figure 2-2. Health maintenance: Health promotion and health recovery networks. Based on the work of M. S. Goodstadt, R. I. Simpson, and P. O. Loranger, "Health promotion: A conceptual integration," *American Journal of Health Promotion*, Winter, 1987, p. 60. Used by permission of the *American Journal of Health Promotion*.

Health Enhancement Network

The health enhancement component comprised in the Goodstadt et al. (1987) definition explains how health promotion extends beyond the traditional prevention and treatment strategies of health maintenance. Two complementary strategies are employed in the health enhancement network:

> Optimization: refers to the narrowing gap between actual and potential levels of wellness in one domain or more. This ideal state, which may never be realized, is defined by the individual's personal goals, potentials, and limitations in the different domains of health. (p. 61)

> Integration: refers to the establishment of a balance of equilibrium among the various domains of health, resulting in an overall or holistic level of wellness in one's life. (p. 61)

Physical health, psychological health, social health, and spiritual health are the four domains addressed under health enhancement. Goodstadt et al. (1987) argue, however, that most health promotion programs have tended to focus on the physical (e.g., fitness) and psychological (e.g., stress management) dimensions to the exclusion of social and spiritual health concerns (i.e., quality of life). This point is of critical importance when designing health promotion programs to meet the diverse needs of older adults.

EXTENDING THE HEALTH PROMOTION MODEL TO REHABILITATION AND AGING

The decline of health and mobility with advancing age demands a search for new alternatives to meet the health needs of older adults. This search for new alternatives has led to increased attention on the role of disease prevention and health promotion for increasing vitality and independence of older people. Research has documented that the so-called signs of "old age" are actually a combination of the effects from disease, the signs of faulty lifestyle practices, and environmental factors. The interplay between these three factors may largely account for the variation between chronological and physiological age in the later years. Part of the difficulty in assessing the relative merits of preventive strategies and health promotion strategies, however, is the lack of agreement on a conceptual foundation for the role that these strategies play in rehabilitation.

The taxonomy of prevention–primary, secondary, and tertiary–aimed at premature mortality and morbidity is inadequate for addressing the complex interactions of disease and disability in older people (Public Health Service, 1989). Extension of life expectancy includes not only the prolonging of life but the extension of quality years in older life, the quality-adjusted life years (QALY). The pressing need for many older adults is protection of functional capacity from progression of disease-associated morbidity or from unrelated co-morbidity or disability.The maximization of independence and quality of life in the later years require a more comprehensive view on how health promotion programs fit into the rehabilitation process. The usefulness components of health promotion in the disability process for older adults is discussed in this section.

Health Maintenance and Disability

The aim of rehabilitation "to restore an individual to his or her former functional and environmental status, or alternatively, to maintain or maximize remaining function" (Williams, 1984, p. xiii) serves as the foundation for care provided to people with disabilities. Some health providers would argue that the rehabilitation aim for older adults is solely focused on maintaining rather than maximizing function. The salient point for our discussion, however, is that the health maintenance component of health promotion has not been fully applied to meet the disability needs of the older population. Failure to distinguish between primary and secondary disabilities has led to this incomplete application.

Although the health recovery network (secondary prevention and tertiary prevention) has been generally applied under the rehabilitation process, the health promotion network has received sparse attention. Marge (1988) argues that this exclusion is due to a general belief by health providers that a client's disability is a static entity. "They [health providers] behave as if the person acquires only one disability and it is their quota for a lifetime." Yet Marge continues, health is a dynamic process whereby disability "should be perceived as a condition undergoing change at all times, from the moment of its acquisition" (p. 30). The dynamic nature of disability establishes the importance of differentiating between primary and secondary disabilities.

Primary disabilities are the first acquired condition. Secondary disabilities directly or indirectly result from a primary disability or occur independently from the primary disability. Marge (1988) further emphasizes that the actual "magnitude and severity of debilitation of the acquired disability is not a factor in the determination of primary and secondary" disability (p. 31). For example, an older adult suffering from rheumatoid arthritis (primary disability) may learn to function effectively but may become severely compromised by a stroke (secondary disability) leaving that person hemophasic and aphasic. The secondary disability, in this example, is more devastating for the older adult than the primary disability. For this reason, it is very important to assess the extent to which a primary disability may place the older client at a greater risk for secondary disabilities.

Despite sparse empirical evidence on secondary disabilities, the prevalence of chronic conditions in later life clearly establishes that older adults are at great risk for secondary disabilities. The leading chronic conditions for older adults are arthritis, hypertensive disease, heart conditions, hearing impairments, and dementia (U.S. Department of Health and Human Services, 1989). Approximately 23% of older adults living in the community have some degree of limitation. Examples of common types of secondary disabilities in later years are identified in Table 2-1.

Table 2-1. Causes and potential for prevention of common secondary disabilities.

Secondary Disabilities	Causes	Outcome
Decubitus ulcers	Inaccessibility to adequate health care, improper seating for those with the disuse syndrome, and lack of continuous personal hygiene.	Preventable.
Genitourinary tract	Inaccessibility to adequate health care, genetic disorders, alcohol and drug abuse, nutritional disorders, lack of personal hygiene, acute and chronic illness.	With the exception of genetic disorders, all other causes are preventable.
Cardiovascular disorders	Alcohol and drug abuse, tobacco use, nutritional disorders, stress, inaccessibility to adequate health care, acute and chronic illness, lack of physical fitness.	Preventable.
Stroke	Lack of physical fitness, nutritional disorders, tobacco use, stress, alcohol and drug abuse, inaccessability to adequate health care (hypertension control).	Preventable.
Musculoskeletal problems	Lack of physical fitness, injuries, stress, genetic disorders, perinatal complications, acute and chronic illness, inaccessibility to adequate health care.	With exception of genetic disorders, all others are preventable.
Arthritis	Speculated lack of physical fitness, nutritional disorders, stress, and possibly genetic disorder.	Unpreventable but certain interventions will delay progress of the disease.
Closed and open head injuries	Injuries, violence, and stress.	Almost all injuries are preventable; some violence is preventable but requires a long period for effective intervention; stress is preventable through treatment of significant maladjustment and modification of a stressful environment.

Spinal cord injury and other physical injuries	Injuries, violence, and stress.	Almost all injuries are preventable; some violence is preventable but requires a long period for effective intervention; stress control is preventable through treatment of significant maladjustment and modification of a stressful environment.
Respiratory problems	Lack of physical fitness, acute and chronic illness, environmental quality problems, alcohol and drug problems, tobacco use, unsanitary living conditions, genetic disorders.	Most of the causes are preventable.
Hearing loss	Genetic disorders, acute and chronic illness, injuries, violence, environmental quality problems (noise pollution).	With the exception of genetic disorders and violence, all all other causes are readily preventable.
Speech and language	Genetic disorders, acute and chronic illness, injuries, environmental quality problems, neurological deficits (such as strokes), cancer, and respiratory problems.	With the exception of genetic disorders and speech and language problems of unknown origin (such as stuttering), the risk for almost all problems can be significantly reduced.
Vision problems	Genetic disorders, acute and chronic illness, injuries, violence, nutritional disorders, environmental quality problems.	With the exception of genetic disorders and violence, all other causes are preventable.
Emotional problems	Genetic disorders, stress, alcohol and drug abuse, deleterious child rearing practices, and deleterious familial-cultural beliefs.	With the exception of genetic disorders, all other causes are preventable.
Skin disorders	Genetic disorders, acute and chronic illness, injuries (fires and burns), nutritional disorders, unsanitary living conditions, and stress.	With the exception of genetic disorders, all other causes are preventable.

From M. Marge, "Health Promotion for Persons with Disabilities: Moving Beyond Rehabilitation" in *American Journal of Health Promotion,* 2(4), 1988. Michael P. O' Donnell Publishers, Rochester Hills, MI. Reprinted by permission.

A close perusal of this table indicates that most of these secondary disabilities are preventable. Disabilities are considered preventable if the probability of acquisition is substantially reduced (Teague et al., 1990). The Committee on Trauma Research elaborates as follows:

> The failure to anticipate and prevent a variety of metabolic, circulatory, respiratory, genitourinary, and musculoskeletal consequences of inactivity and immobility prolongs expensive care, delays active rehabilitation, and leads to failure to regain a state of health and preservation of residual functional capacity for purposeful activity. (Marge 1988, p. 31)

The goals of health maintenance applied to disability in later life include the health objectives under both the health recovery network and the health promotion network. The health promotion network involves the active employment of risk avoidance (primary prevention) and risk reduction (secondary prevention) strategies for preventing secondary disabilities. A working example of this responsibility is the importance of smoking cessation even late in life. Smoking cessation (risk reduction) is very important because this deleterious lifestyle practice complicates existing illnesses prevalent in the older years. For example, smoking decreases the ability of gastric ulcers to heal, has negative effects on bone demineralization, affects mean dosage levels of medications, and reduces the senses of smell and taste that may threaten proper nutritional intake. Moreover, passive smoke can aggravate preexisting chronic heart and obstructive lung diseases.

Risk avoidance strategies may be illustrated by physical activity. An individual suffering from osteoarthritis (potential primary disability) may be tempted to adopt a sedentary lifestyle. Yet sedentary activity may lead to coronary disease, hypertensive disease, diabetes, osteoporosis, or obstructive lung disease, thus resulting in secondary disabilities that are much more serious than the primary disease. Therefore, the encouragement of physical activity throughout life (risk avoidance strategy) is a key dimension in the health promotion network applicable to disability in later life.

Health Enhancement and Disability

The health promotion framework illustrated in Figure 2-3 presents health as a relative concept. Optimal wellness is viewed as an ideal state whereby some rehabilitation is always possible. In reality, however, Goodstadt et al. (1987) state,

> The implementation of rehabilitation may be reasonably limited to only part of the wellness continuum--ceasing somewhere between the region of secondary prevention, after which the strategies of health enhancement become the more important means by which optimal wellness is approached. (p. 62)

Every older adult has unique or different health needs. Yet the health enhancement component has not been an integral part of rehabilitation programs. Despite disability conditions, Brandon (1985) emphasizes that individuals can still potentially excel in a variety of areas:

> Health is a dynamic, ever-changing condition that should be measured in terms of how well individuals live with full use of their available skills or abilities at any point in time. Indeed, the greatest need of all individuals is to function to their fullest in their own unique environment regardless of physical, emotional, or cognitive disabilities. (p. 54)

The inclusion of health enhancement under health recovery may be disturbing to some health providers. Some providers may argue that the principal focus of rehabilitation is to stabilize an unwanted health condition and then restore health to a minimally acceptable level. Attention to the optimization and integration dimensions of health enhancement are not central to stabilization and restoration objectives. Despite this contention, a strong case can be made that actual treatment goals entail long-term movement toward optimal health (i.e., wellness) rather than short-term movement to a symptom-free state. Goodstadt et al. (1987) are quick to acknowledge that movement toward optimal health as a long-term goal is a radical departure from the tertiary philosophy that dominates rehabilitation services today. The implication of health enhancement as a principal rehabilitation goal establishes a link to the health promotion network whereby efforts are made to enhance health in social and spiritual domains as well as psychological and physical domains.

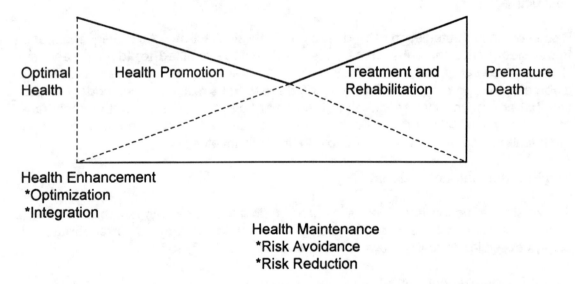

Figure 2-3. Health promotion: Conceptual integration. From M. S. Goodstadt, R. I. Simpson, and P. D. Loranger, "Health Promotion: A Conceptual Integration," *American Journal of Health Promotion*, 1(2), 1987, p. 62. Used by permission of the *American Journal of Health Promotion*.

CHAPTER SUMMARY

The goals of the health delivery systems of the future should include to a much greater extent the promotion of health and the prevention of disease. Health under this system is not viewed as the mere absence of disease but as the ability of the individual to control his or her life and to perform crucial social roles such as citizen, worker, spouse, and parent. The health goals employed vary for each individual with the objective of having each person achieve the fullest level of health possible depending on age, physical condition, and life circumstances, that is, high-level wellness.

A specific example can be used to illustrate this high-level wellness principle. If, with the necessary and appropriate support services, an elderly person has the capacity to participate in the community and to follow a pattern of living marked by enjoyment, it would violate health goals to place this individual in a nursing home. A health system that places elderly adults in nursing homes where they cannot fulfill their lives fails in its essential purposes. The operationalization of this high-level wellness principle requires the integration of health prevention and health promotion activities into existing services.

We can fully expect some resistance to the goals of health protection and health promotion from a number of health professionals. After all, our principal medical/public health territory is orderly, comprehensive, and manageable. The health promotion and health protection territory, represented by the wellness principles of social, emotional, philosophical, and spiritual dimensions, is disorderly and unmanageable (Carlyon, 1984). Some will argue that personal health habits are so deeply embedded in personal history that they are virtually impossible to modify. Others will contend that we have no right to tamper with people's way of life. Yet concerns about health care costs and changing definitions of health have forced health professionals to finally address themselves to personal health styles.

As depicted by the health promotion model described in this chapter, new knowledge, skills, and understanding about health are needed. It would be desirable that new kinds of personnel be developed who know a great deal about appropriate health habits for different age groups, ethnic cultures, and social-class backgrounds. Obviously, health promotion professionals will need to be equipped with the health education and interpersonal skill knowledge necessary to work with a diverse group of older adults. Some of them may employ health promotion skills in physicians' offices, senior centers, nursing homes, health centers, or as outreach workers who visit the homes of clients and families.

CHAPTER 3

HEALTH ASSESSMENT

Health professionals frequently make judgments that affect the health and quality of life of older adults. Many of the psychomotor, affective, and cognitive changes associated with the aging process make the older adult vulnerable to both primary and secondary disabilities. Yet small improvements in functional status can have a tremendous impact. Thus, the aim of rehabilitation programs is "to restore an individual to his or her former functional and environmental status, or alternatively, to maintain or maximize remaining function" (Williams, 1984, p. xiii). The objectives of restoring, maintaining, and/or maximizing remaining "function" places health assessment at the heart of health promotion programs.

In Chapter 3 we address the role of health assessment by presenting a conceptual framework for assessing the functional status of the elderly. The broad assessment model presented encompasses the areas of physical, mental, social, psychological, economic, and functional assessment. Our purpose is to illustrate a comprehensive view of health assessment. The role of health promotion within this overall framework will be emphasized.

HEALTH ASSESSMENT: A CONCEPTUAL FRAMEWORK

Most professional health organizations advocate and employ an assessment of some kind before initiating an action of change. The closer health promotion programs parallel such models of assessment, the easier it will be for their products to be accepted in the health community. Figure 3-1 schematically illustrates a comprehensive health assessment model relevant to the health promotion profession. The model has been sequenced algorithmically to assure an in-depth and orderly assessment. Information obtained includes:

- Health problems requiring immediate attention and treatment;
- Health conditions that are contraindications to participating in further testing;
- Lifestyle habits, values, and attitudes that influence the current health of a client and the way the client is reacting to the health promotion program; and
- Health risk factors compiled into a client profile to describe their impact on basic and daily living skills.

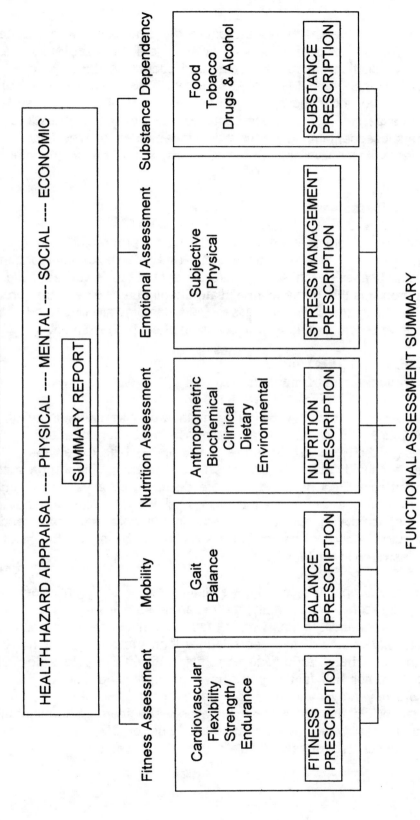

GENERAL HEALTH ASSESSMENT

HEALTH HAZARD APPRAISAL --- PHYSICAL --- MENTAL --- SOCIAL --- ECONOMIC

SUMMARY REPORT

Fitness Assessment

Cardiovascular
Flexibility
Strength/
Endurance

FITNESS
PRESCRIPTION

Mobility

Gait
Balance

BALANCE
PRESCRIPTION

Nutrition Assessment

Anthropometric
Biochemical
Clinical
Dietary
Environmental

NUTRITION
PRESCRIPTION

Emotional Assessment

Subjective
Physical

STRESS MANAGEMENT
PRESCRIPTION

Substance Dependency

Food
Tobacco
Drugs & Alcohol

SUBSTANCE
PRESCRIPTION

FUNCTIONAL ASSESSMENT SUMMARY

Activity Daily Living Skills
Instrumental Activity
Daily Living Skills

Figure 3-1. Health assessment model.

The schematic flow of the health assessment model commences with a General Health Assessment. This assessment is followed by specific health assessments for physical fitness, mobility, nutrition, emotional stress, and substance dependency. A summary report drawn from the General Health Assessment phase is used to delimit tests that are to be performed under the specific health assessment phase. Test results from specific health assessment phases are compiled into a descriptive health profile of the client and the subsequent impact on functional independence. The final report is used for constructing a prescriptive health promotion program that is uniquely tailored to the client.

General Health Assessment

A clear, complete problem-oriented health assessment program lists functional as well as undefined health problems, organizes them, and establishes intervention priorities. The assessment phases described in Figure 3-1 should be viewed as "building blocks" for selecting problems that demand immediate attention as well as other problems that may receive attention gradually. Five assessment domains are illustrated as part of the General Health Assessment phase. A discussion of each phase follows.

Health Risk Appraisal (HRA) and
Lifestyle Improvement Instruments (LII)

The HRA has become the most widely used method of assessment in health promotion programs. Actuarial and mortality data in response to a battery of questions concerning age, race, sex, and lifestyle practices are used to project life expectancy. The use of HRAs, however, should not be considered an exact science. Different results between HRA instruments are likely because they are designed by a variety of organizations using different questions with different assigned risk weights. Although the accuracy of HRAs may be somewhat suspicious, these instruments are not intended to be predictive of future individual health but are estimates based on the health of other people who answered in similar ways.

Most HRA computer printouts contrast the client's actual age (chronological age) with an appraised age score. For example, a 60-year-old female whose biological, environmental, and behavioral risk factors were all favorable might have an appraised age of 55, with a life expectancy of five years longer than the average of her 60-year-old peers. On the other hand, a 60-year-old female with unfavorable biological, environmental, and behavior risk factors may have an appraised age of 65, with a life expectancy of five years less than her 60-year-old peers. However, the appraised 65-year-old female would also be given an achievable age score. She might also be told that she could possibly achieve an appraised age of 55 if she adopted specific behaviors that offset each of several risk factors. Thus, she could add 10 years to her present life.

The Public Health Service's Office of Disease Prevention and Health Promotion classified HRAs in three categories: (1) the self-scored questionnaire, (2) the microcomputer questionnaire for use with personal computers, and (3) computer-scored questionnaires that are processed at a central computer facility. Self-scored questionnaires are simple instruments that pertain to health behavior areas, such as nutrition, smoking, and medical history. The respondent answers questions and then adds up points assigned to each answer to receive an overall score. Micro-computer instruments are more complex and can take different forms. For example, the respondent's data can be either entered from hard copy questionnaires, or the individual can enter the data directly. This latter format is considered an interactive program. Microcomputer HRAs may be used to provide both an individual health profile or an organizational profile. Computer-scored HRAs are considered to be the Cadillac of HRAs. These instruments may consist of 200 to 300 multiple-choice questions. The respondents answer these questions which are batch-scored for central processing units. Detailed, personalized reports on the impact of an individual's medical history and lifestyle habits on health risks are produced.

Lifestyle Inventory Instrument (LII). Despite the popularity of HRA instruments, some health professionals are advocating the use of LII as more useful for certain age categories, especially youths and older adults. Table 3-1 provides a comparison of the HRA and LII. Essentially, HRAs have three principal disadvantages. First, the health information collected is rather negative and contradictory to the positive balanced state expressed under a wellness philosophy. To offset these disadvantages, some organizations use "wellness inventories" to collect information that is not based on mortality and morbidity estimates (e.g., occupational and spiritual data). Second, many of the risks identified in a standard HRA that contribute to lowered life-expectancy may not be under the client's control (e.g., a predisposition to genetic disease). Third, and most important to the elderly, data used to construct health risk profiles are terribly complex and easily misinterpreted. For example, the mortality curve rises with age. Thus an increase in risk for an individual at one age can result in a very different impact for an individual at another age.

A good example of an instrument that draws from both the HRA and LII is the Lifestyle Assessment Questionnaire (LAQ) published by the National Wellness Institute. The LAQ provides an assessment of a respondent's current lifestyle under three appraisal sections: (1) Wellness Inventory–six dimensions of wellness and their subcategories, (2) Health Risk Appraisal–potential consequences of faulty lifestyle practices, and (3) topics for personal growth. An LAQ Results Interpretation Guide is provided to the respondent for assistance in understanding the meaning of LAQ results.

HRAs and LII as Catalysts. The use of HRAs and LIIs as motivational tools for behavioral change should be judicious. Health behavior change is a process that requires a variety of teaching and learning opportunities that affect knowledge, attitudes, and behavioral skills. The initial step requires motivation by the participant for change. This initial step is often initiated by the question, "What's in it for me?"

Table 3-1. Comparison of the HRA and the LII.

Health Risk Appraisals	Lifestyle Improvement Instruments
Identifies health risks	Identifies strengths and problems
Results state problems to avoid	Provides specific recommendations for improvement
Results provide a composite score (health age versus actual age)	Evaluates each health behavior separately and provides several, but not composite, scores
Reliability and validity has been questioned	Development of tools allows for validity and reliability studies to be done; good initial results
Most accurate for middle age and not the elderly or youth	Norms are established for different subpopulations
Additional information is needed to complete a lifestyle contract	Partially completed lifestyle to contract is included (assesses motivation to change, support systems, etc., for contracting)
Assumes that life can be extended	Focus is on the quality of life

Terry (1987) illustrates the motivational process and the role of HRAs and LIIs (Figure 3-2). Feedback from the HRA or LII can be used to create a perception of an unsatisfied health need by demonstrating susceptibility to disease. Theoretically, this perception will lead to tension and efforts to search for new health knowledge and skills to rectify health status. Through educational and/or intervention programs health risk data can be used to reinforce attainment of a satisfied health need. Tension, in turn, is reduced. Terry (1987), in Figure 3-3, illustrates this process for a smoking cessation program.

Prescreening by HRAs and LIIs is valuable for identifying groups of older adults that may benefit from more specific health-screening procedures. The assumption behind these instruments is that an individual's response to health threats largely depends on how he or she feels physically and not on a rational calculation of health benefits and risks. Zeman (1990) found that the use of HRAs for Milwaukee residents age 60 years or older could reduce health risk by 32%. To be valuable, however, HRAs and LIIs need to include not only health habits (e.g., nutrition, exercise, smoking, substance abuse, medication use) but sensory deficits, presence of chronic diseases, safety, and possibly, mental status.

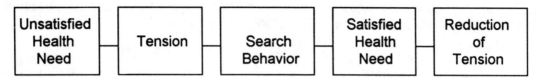

Figure 3-2. The motivation process. Developed by P. E. Terry, The Role of Health Risk Appraisal in the Workplace: Assessment Versus Behavioral Change. *American Journal of Health Promotion*, 2, 2, 1987, p. 20. Used by permission of the *American Journal of Health Promotion.*

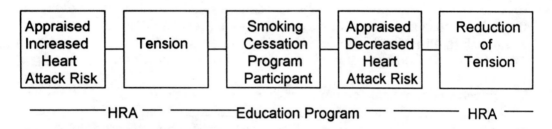

Figure 3-3. The HRA abetted motivation process. Developed by P. E. Terry. The Role of Health Risk Appraisal in the Workplace: Assessment Versus Behavioral Change. *American Journal of Health Promotion*, 2, 2, 1987, p. 20. Used by permission of the *American Journal of Health Promotion.*

Choosing HRA/LII Instruments. The design and implementation of HRAs and LIIs greatly influence their value as assessment tools for behavioral change. Instruments that focus on specific lifestyle habits that are modifiable, relevant to clinical measures and sensitive to small behavioral changes, and that provide personalized recommendations are more likely to be effective. Results that are easy to interpret and well illustrated and that provide personalized texts are especially valuable. Appendix B provides an overview of similarities and differences between HRAs and LIIs. Opatz (1985), in Table 3-2, provides five suggested guidelines for selecting instruments.

Physical Assessment

The health risk assessment, and social, psychological, and economic assessment phases under General Health Assessment lie outside the traditional medical model evaluation. Physical assessments have permeated the medical field. Generally, the physical examination of the older adult is no different than evaluations conducted for younger adults. The greater incidence of chronic disease and illness in the elderly, however, requires vigilance by the examiner to discover abnormalities (separating pathologic processes from "aging" processes) and to judge the relevance of abnormalities to the life of a particular patient. Gallo, Reichel, and Anderson (1988) add the following:

Table 3-2. Choosing a health hazard appraisal instrument.

(1) The instrument chosen should include more than just the basic health risk appraisal. Wellness inventories and other positive information should be included in the selected instrument.

(2) Confidentiality of results for individuals must be maintained. The procedures to assure this confidentiality should be provided to individual participants.

(3) Where appropriate, summary data describing the total group of participants should be obtainable.

(4) Group interpretations are the best method for helping participants understand their results. If this is not possible, some procedure must be provided whereby individuals can obtain answers to questions about their results. Also, on occasion there are inaccurate results due to poorly completed answer sheets or computer error. Therefore, procedures to correct these errors should be provided.

(5) The health risk appraisal and wellness inventory should be used as just one part of a larger program. Since the health risk appraisal at best can be a motivational and educational tool, it is necessary that opportunities be provided to assist the individual in making the desired behavioral changes. Weight reduction, fitness, stress management, breast self-exams, career programs, and the like, are examples of educational opportunities that can be linked to results obtained on HRA.

From Joseph Opatz, *A Primer of Health Promotion,* 1985, Oryn Publications, Inc., Washington, DC. Reprinted by permission of Joseph Opatz.

> This process is complicated because the presenting symptom in the elder may be a red herring, that is, a nonspecific signal that something is amiss somewhere but not necessarily in the system expected. Dysfunction in any organ system may only manifest as deteriorating mental status, for example, so that pneumonia (respiratory), appendicitis (gastrointestinal), or congestive heart failure (cardiac) cause confusion (central nervous system). The physical examination of the older person therefore needs to be as complete and systematic as possible. (pp. 35, 36)

The geriatric physician's review of the older adult is presented in Table 3-3. Multi-phasic testing employing physiometric measurements is often used to help the physician identify chronic diseases that may have an asymptomatic phase. Lab tests are employed for measuring blood pressure and blood serum levels. Glaucoma examinations, rectal examinations, Papanicolaou tests, chest x-rays, eight-lead electrocardiograms, visual acuity tests, and pulmonary functioning tests may also be conducted. Information gathered from the multi-phasic tests may suggest more exhaustive follow-up examination measures.

Table 3-3. The geriatric review of systems.

General	Weight change
	Fatigue
	Falls
	Anorexia
	Anemia
	Poor nutrition
Special Senses	Visual changes
	Cataract
	Hearing changes
	Imbalance
	Vertigo
Mouth and Teeth	Dentures
	Denture discomfort
	Dry mouth
Respiratory	Cough
	Hemotypsis
	Dyspnea
Cardiovascular	Chest pain on exertion
	Orthopnea
	Ankle edema
	Claudication
Gastrointestinal	Dysphagia
	Melena
	Change in stool caliber
	Laxative use
	Constipation
Genitourinary	Incontinence
	Dysuria
	Nocturia
	Hematuria
	Sexual functioning
Musculoskeletal	Morning stiffness
	Joint pain
	Joint swelling
	Limitation of movement
Neurology	Memory problems
	Headaches
	Syncope
	Gait
	Sensory function
	Sleep disorders
	Transient focal symptoms
	Voice changes
Psychiatric	Depression
	Alcoholism
	Anxiety

From J. Gallo, et al. *Handbook of Geriatric Assessment,* c 1988, Aspen Publishers, Inc. Reprinted by permission.

Physical Assessment Recommendation. On the surface, the notion of multi-phasic testing as part of comprehensive physical examinations appears to be wise and prudent, because of the potential for early detection of disease symptoms that may otherwise go undetected. However, growing evidence suggests that many of the multi-phasic tests are not cost effective and may actually cause more problems than they alleviate. Moreover, the reader is reminded that in the elderly the normal range of many values changes with age; cholesterol levels in middle age, for example, are considered high at 240 mg/dl but in the later years are increased to 260 mg/dl.

Physical assessment screening for older adults should be performed annually to detect diseases at an early and preventable stage. Such measures as height, weight, blood pressure, and cholesterol levels are generally useful because they can predict, with some degree of accuracy, the probability of a healthy person becoming ill. Other multi-phasic tests should be used more selectively.

Mental Health Assessment

In this section, the assessment of mental status is broadened to include both the older adult's mental status and screening for depressive illness. The routine screening for mental status is encouraged as a means to detect unsuspected mental impairment and to provide a more accurate medical or social history for the older adult. Our discussion of mental health assessment will focus on the (1) rationale for mental health assessment, (2) preliminary mental assessment, (3) clinical mental assessment, and (4) assessment for depression.

Rationale for Mental Health Assessment. In a study completed by Scogin and Rohling (1989) a battery of cognitive tests was administered to a group of community-dwelling older adults. Cognitive function, memory function, and mental health status were assessed. An additional set of questionnaires was given to people who knew the older adults. The study findings report that the older adults "were more attuned to mental functioning while others familiar with the older participants were more accurate in appraising the frequency of occurrence of memory and cognitive problems experienced by the older adult" (1989, p. 518). The findings from Scogin and Rohling are consistent with past empirical studies suggesting that older adults with either minor or no problems with memory experience some difficulty in subjectively assessing their own cognitive performance.

The Scogin and Rohling study suggests that assessments by caregivers or those people familiar with the older adult can be a valuable resource for providing a more accurate picture of mental health status. But many older adults with cognitive dysfunction or impairments can mask their problems to family members and practitioners. Gallo et al. (1988) underscore the importance of mental health testing to detect unsuspected mental function that may be masked by an older adult:

> Most practitioners who deal with elderly patients have had the experience of treating an elder who is seen by the casual observer to be able

to carry on a reasonably coherent conversation but in whom mental status testing reveals significant difficulties. The patient may be able to perform well in a job that has been held for many years as long as the routine is not interrupted. In novel situations, the extent of the deficit may only then become painfully evident to family or co-workers. Perhaps the family is not even aware that behavioral changes are secondary to subtle intellectual deterioration. As the patient has mounting difficulty in demanding situations, it is not uncommon that he or she "strikes out" against others or becomes depressed. (p. 11)

Health professionals estimate that approximately 25% of older adults have some sort of mental impairment. As older adults experience difficulty in subjectively evaluating their mental health and also have a tendency to mask symptoms, one would expect that routine screening for mental health would be a normal part of medical procedures and records. Unfortunately, this is not the case. Gallo et al. (1988) note that 37 to 80% of demented elders identified by a screening examination as mentally impaired were not diagnosed as such by the patient's physician. Psychiatrists diagnosed only 27% of patients with mental impairments prior to discharge from medical or surgical wards. Yet 62% of these patients were believed to have moderate or severe impairments.

The increased frequency and severity of mental impairment with increasing age is of major concern. Failure of physicians to provide routine mental health screening is unfortunate because it is the physician who is likely to have rapport with the older adult patient. It is difficult for other health consultants to provide an accurate mental health evaluation of an older adult without the rapport that normally exists between the older adult and his or her physician. A periodic mental health evaluation as an ongoing part of the older adult's medical record can be an invaluable assessment tool.

Preliminary Mental Assessment. Shorter versions of screening instruments are used as an attempt to provide a general impression of intellectual function. The intellectual functions assessed are cited in Table 3-4. Instruments consist of one or two questions under each of the intellectual components. Detection of mental problems under the preliminary assessment will usually lead to more extensive clinical assessment.

The components for mental status examination referenced in Table 3-4 include an assessment of level of consciousness, attention, language, memory, proverb interpretation, similarities, analogies, and questions. These components are used to evaluate higher orders of intellectual function. Calculations, writing, and constructional ability are also used as measures of more abstract intellectual functions. The reader is encouraged to consult Gallo et al. (1988) and Strub and Black (1985) for excellent discussions of the mental status components cited in Table 3-4.

Clinical Mental Assessment. Clinical mental assessment instruments are used to detect dementia, a global intellectual deficit characterized by loss of intellectual capacity in memory and cognition, language, visuospatial skills, and personality. Each of the

Table 3-4. Components of the mental status examination.
Level of consciousness

Attention

Language
  Fluency
  Comprehension
  Repetition

Memory
  Short-term memory
  Remote memory

Proverb interpretation

Similarities

Calculations

Writing

Constructional ability

From R. L. Strub and F. W. Black, *The Mental Status Examination in Neurology.* Copyright c 1980 F. A. Davis Company, Philadelphia, PA. Reprinted by permission.

five evaluated intellectual components do not need to be impaired for diagnosing dementia. Moreover, normal aging does not involve confusion, hallucination, delusions, or gross intellectual deficits. Thus the presence of these symptoms leads to diagnosis of organic or acute brain syndrome. The following instruments are examples of short, clinical mental assessment instruments used for diagnostic purposes.

- *Short Portable Mental Status Questionnaire (SPMSQ).* This short, easy to use ten-question assessment covers orientation, remote memory and calculations. However, it does not assess short-term memory or in-depth cognitive functioning. This assess-ment could be used in conjunction with other types of written assessments and more thorough assessments for detecting severe dementia. (Klein, Rola, & McArthur et al., 1985)
- *Folstein Mini-Mental (FMM).* The FMM is a mental function test with two parts: (1) verbal-assessment of orientation, memory, and atten-tion, and (2) written-assessment of sentence writing, drawing complex designs, naming objects, and responding to verbal and written commands. The common complaints with these two test parts are the fact that they rely heavily on questions of orientation, which may miss many older adults who may have mental impairment. (Folstein, Folstein, & McHugh, 1975)

- *The Kokmen Short Test of Mental Status(KSTMS).* The KSTMS is a short test which is easy to administer. It also incorporates "abstraction" as part of its test for assessing higher levels of intellectual function. (Gallo et al., 1988)

Regardless of the type of instrument used, the importance of performing some type of mental assessment on all elderly patients cannot be overemphasized. Mental assessment provides the practitioner with a tool, to be used in combination with other assessments, for evaluating a patient's overall cognitive performance. Thorough neuropsychological testing is a vital part of the older adult's treatment in diagnosing forms of neurologic damage and in delineating the patient's functional capacity. However, the time for administration and the cost incurred may be a deterrent for many patients. The reader is encouraged to consult Gallo et al. (1988) for a more thorough review of clinical mental assessment instruments.

Depression. Approximately 15 to 20% of older adults have some form of depression. Yet depression frequently goes unrecognized in the diagnostic process. Older adults suffering from depression frequently do not display overt symptoms, but may present depression by simply decreasing activity or social contact, or exhibiting sleeping problems and eating disturbances. Many health care professionals "write off" the subtle symptoms of depression as normal characteristics of aging. Some older adults exhibit symptoms of depression by visiting their physician more frequently simply because they feel ill. Instead of telling the physician they are "saddened" or "blue," the older adult may run a gambit of hypochondriachal complaints and passively wait for the physician to diagnose the condition as depression. Unfortunately, much of the time depression is never diagnosed. Despite this drawback, a number of assessment instruments have been devised for depression.

Symptoms described in the fourth edition of the Diagnostic and Statistical Manual of Mental Disorders (DSM-IV) are used by examining psychiatrists for diagnosing depression. To aid in the screening process, the following three short questionnaires have been commonly used with older adults:

- *Popoff Index of Depression (PID).* The PID was specifically designed for use in primary care practice. The instrument contains 15 groups of statements requiring the respondent to express feelings. The PID score is the total of overt and covert responses. (Popoff, 1969)
- *Geriatric Depression Scale (GDS).* The GDS is a 30-item instrument requiring yes or no responses to questions involving somatic symptoms, anxiety and insomnia, social dysfunction, and depression. A shorter version of 15 questions is also available. (Gallo et al., 1988)
- *Beck Depression Inventory (BDI).* The BDI consists of 21 questions that characterize depression; e.g., mood, pessimism, sense of failure, lack of satisfaction, guilty feelings, sense of punishment,

self-hate, self-accusations, self-punitive wishes, crying spells, irritability. The BDI may be administered by an interviewer or self-administered. (Beck, Ward, & Mendelson et al., 1961)

Assessment of older adults for depression may be difficult for two reasons. First, it is not clear as to how to evaluate a depressed person's response to mental assessment instruments. The person may answer assessment questions with either silence or "I don't know" responses, but usually errors are incurred more from no response rather than incorrect responses. Second, older adults access mental health services at a much lower rate than younger persons. Thus the administration of assessment tests falls on the shoulder of the physician who is already likely to be understaffed and pressed for time.

Mental Assessment Recommendation. The various mental assessment instruments discussed in this section are invaluable for providing an overall picture of intellectual function, dementia, and affective illness such as depression. But the screening instruments are tools to supplement, not replace, more detailed clinical assessment. The important point underlying the use of standardized mental assessment instruments is the uniform collection of data. Moreover, most of these instruments are brief enough to be administered at intervals for assessing changes in an older adult's condition.

Social Assessment

Assessment of the older adult's functional status by activities of daily living skills (ADL) and instrumental activity daily living skills (IADL) is certainly important. But social assessment plays an equally important role. A clear and concise picture of an older adult's functional status cannot be understood without an analysis of the social environment. The older adult's family or primary caregiver, as well as the support provided by social service agencies, churches, and neighborhood groups, included in social assessment. It is also important to realize that the elderly person's support system may be comprised of children who may be aged themselves or employed in the labor force. Gallo et al. (1988) add, "Since more people are living to old age, the average woman in 1980 might expect to spend more years caring for an elderly parent than could her counterpart in 1900" (p. 93).

Social Support Levels. The assessment of the social environment is vital for deter-mining the appropriate social service and/or health service agency who may respond to the special needs of the elderly client. This assessment should minimally include three support levels: (1) informal support, (2) semi-formal support, and (3) formal support levels.

The informal support environment is comprised of family and friends. Empirical evidence has consistently recognized the presence of a caregiver as the most important factor for disposition of elderly patients from the hospital to the community (Gallo et al., 1988). If an elderly patient is incapacitated for even a short period of time, his or her chance of being able to successfully return to the home environment is very slim without the support of some sort of caregiver. Family members and long-term friends often assume the caregiver role, through phone calls, visits, and transportation to the pharmacy and grocery store. Yet there are also other people who may provide informal support that the older adult may take for granted–a neighbor trimming the hedge, or someone picking up the mail in inclement weather. All of these informal support resources need to be assessed as they impact the functional independence of the older adult. Additionally, health professionals should realize that some family members living in close proximity do not perform an active caregiver role.

Church groups, clubs, and senior center activities are just a few examples of the semi-support system. These semi-formal organizations provide a strong sense of belonging and of life meaningfulness. One of this book's authors has served as the developer and director of Shepherd's Center in Wichita, Kansas, and has personally witnessed how semi-formal support systems can counter social isolation by providing valuable opportunities for socialization and, in essence, a reason for getting up in the morning.

The formal support system consists of such bureaucratic entities as Social Security, county health departments, and community mental health centers. These agencies play a key role in providing needed services and finances to dependent older adults. Accessing formal support organizations can often be difficult. Failure to successfully access the formal support system leads to even more heavy reliance on the informal and semi-formal support systems.

- *Social Assessment Instruments*. Stressful life events play a key role in determining health. Older adults without informal and semi-formal support ties are at high risk for increased functional dependence. This is especially true for the older adult who has lost a spouse. Thus health professionals need to assess all social support levels available to older adults. Four social assessment instruments that have been popularly used for this purpose are the (1) Older Americans Resources and Services (OARS) Multidimensional Functional Assessment Questionnaire, Social Resources, (2) Social Dysfunction Rating Scale (SDRS), (3) Family or Friends APGAR, and (4) Zarit Burden Interview (ZBI).
- *OARS, Social Resources*. The OARS instrument is invaluable for assessing the economic and physical health status components referenced in Figure 3-2. The social resources section includes questions that encompass such items as marital status, frequency of visitors, satisfaction with social contacts, loneliness, and availability of both informal and semi-formal persons for assistance. The respondents' answers to the questions are graded on a social functioning judgment ranging from a scale of 1 (unimpaired) to 6 (impaired).
- *Social Dysfunction Rating Scale (SDRS)*. Questions in the SDRS are graded on a subjective Likert scale that ranges from 1 (not present) to 6 (very severe). Questions pertain to such affective

areas as self-esteem, interpersonal relations, and self-perform-ance. The skills of the interviewer play a key role in the validity and reliability of this instrument due to its subjective nature. Despite this drawback, Gallo et al. (1988) report that the SDRS correctly categorized 92% of patients when applied to a group of 80 psychiatric and nonpsychiatric outpatients as compared to clinician judgments who were not aware of the scale.

- *Family or Friends APGAR*. The Family APGAR instrument was not developed to be exclusively used with older adults. But this short screening instrument has been used for social assessment purposes. Gallo et al. (1988) note that the APGAR instrument may be more appropriate for use with older adults who have more intimate social relationships with friends than family. Smilkstein, Ashworth, and Montano (1982) recommend employment of the Family APGAR instrument in four situations: (1) a new patient, (2) a person who will be caring for a chronically ill family member, (3) following an adverse event such as death of a spouse, and (4) when the client's history suggests that a dysfunctional family is the root cause of the problem. The five components of the APGAR instrument include adaptation, partnership, growth, affection, and resolve. Scoring of the instrument ranges from 0 (hardly ever) to 2 (always).

- *Zarit Burden Interview (ZBI)*. Because the caregiver, or one who is the primary caring support for the patient, is such an integral part of the entire social assessment, a separate assessment of that caregiver can be a vital link to a continuum of care for the client. This assessment should include the entire functional health status of the caregiver--mental, social, physical, and economical. The ZBI may be used for this purpose. (Zarit & Orr, 1984)

Caregiver tasks can range from simple assistance with daily living skills for the older adult to intensive assistance that requires round-the-clock care. Some of the specific problem areas that the caregivers personally encounter include loss of social support if the caregiver is caring for someone in their home, loss of personal career opportunities, and physical and mental health problems that occur due to caregiver stress. The ZBI focuses on the caregiver by identifying those feelings that contribute to "burden." The perception of burden by the caregiver is not well correlated with the symptoms exhibited by the person receiving caregiver support, that is, reported minority and behavioral problems, and deficits in mental status testing. Gallo et al. (1988) add, "Feelings of burden seemed more related to the social support available to the caregiver, how the caregiver interprets and responds to the patient's symptoms, and the nature of the premorbid relationship of the caregiver to the patient" (p. 105). Symptoms, such as depression, are labeled as "danger signals" to highlight the caregiver's need for respite and special assistance from support groups, self-help agencies, or health professionals.

Social Assessment Recommendation. The assessment of an older adult's social environment is essential for designing health promotion intervention programs. Gallo et al. (1988) write, "In all clinical situations, the social milieu must be kept in mind, but perhaps nowhere is this more important than in geriatric medicine" (p. 107). The assessment should include all three support levels, informal, semi-formal and formal. Assessment of the caregiver's health and support needs should also be determined. The Social Resources Section of the OARS questionnaire is an excellent example of a comprehensive social assessment instrument directed toward older adults.

Economic Assessment

Inquiry into economic security of the older adult is usually not a detailed inquiry by the health professional. However, the professional should not lose sight of the fact that the older adult may not be able to adhere to a prescriptive regimen (e.g., drug dosage level, nutritional diet) due to insufficient economic resources. Most definitions of comprehensive health assessment programs do not include the evaluation of financial factors (Applegate, 1987).

The economic picture of today's older adult is much brighter than the pictures of the 1950s to 1970s. In 1959, almost 35% of all persons 85 and older were in poverty, whereas in 1989 only 12% were defined at poverty level. Poverty levels are likely to be higher for those who live alone or who are not married. Persons of advanced age are especially vulnerable. For example, one-third of adults over the age of 80 have income below the poverty line.

Economic Assessment Recommendation. Assessment of economic resources can certainly include subjective observations of the older adult. For example, the health professional may make note of clothing conditions or make home visits that detail living conditions. One formal instrument for evaluating economic conditions, however, is the economic resources section of the OARS questionnaire. The economic resources section estimates the financial resources of the older adult.

The economic items contained in the OARS instrument focus on employment status, income sources, annual income, home ownership, and subjective estimates of financial adequacy. Many older adults who need financial assistance fail to receive help simply because they do not know where to go or how to proceed. Health professionals prescribing programs should be aware of whether such prescriptive plans are likely to be hindered by insufficient economic resources. The "Economic Resource" section of the OARS instrument is an excellent example of an extensive questionnaire that can serve this purpose.

SPECIFIC ASSESSMENT PHASE

A summary report is drawn up at the completion of the General Health Assessment phase. The reports from the health hazard appraisal, physical assessment, mental assessment, social assessment, and economic assessment become part of the lifestyle prescription and are used to delimit health assessments that fall under the specific phase. The assessments included are fitness, mobility, nutrition, emotional stress, and substance dependency.

Physical Fitness Assessment

Assessment of the older adult's physical fitness level is a critical initial component before introducing fitness programs. This assessment is necessary for establishing an effective and safe prescription level. The condition of the individual is divided into two separate but related categories: (1) medical condition and (2) physical condition. Qualified physicians assess the medical condition on a regular interval basis. The physiometric measures in the General Health Assessment phase are employed for this purpose. Physical condition is usually determined by an exercise physiologist or an acceptable, licensed health practitioner. Our focus in this section will be on physical condition.

Selection of Fitness Parameters. Physical fitness cannot be measured as a single quantity. Thus a comprehensive set of parameters is used. Unfortunately, most fitness parameters have been developed for younger populations and health promotion professionals should be aware of the population base used for norm data and fitness protocols. Additional factors that complicate the selection of fitness parameters are the sub-population heterogenity for older adults, modifications that influence results, and psychological factors that prevent maximal exercise test performance. Although these factors impact the assessment process for all age groups, they are especially pertinent to testing older adults. Health promotion professionals must use caution when collecting and interpreting fitness assessment data for older adults.

Prior Testing Procedures. Older adults should be advised not to eat within one to two hours prior to the testing session. Professionals should also help the older adult ease apprehension or anxiety that may accompany the fitness assessment process. A reasonably extensive personal health and exercise history is also strongly advisable. Osness (1989) summarized the historical information as follows:

> (1) A family history of heart attacks, high blood pressure, strokes, diabetes, blood lipids, heart surgery, premature death, and other conditions related to specific testing involved. (2) Past personal history relating to rheumatic fever, heart murmurs, high blood pressure, general cardiac conditions, abnormal blood chemistry, cardiac or pulmonary surgery, chest discomfort, heart palpitations, diabetes, gout, vascular diseases, surgery, muscular diseases, unusual fatigue, or other medical problems that have been treated during the last five years. (3) Medications that are being taken which would include the type of medication, the dosage of the medication, timing of the dosage, and the length of time this medication has been used. Common medications can simply be listed and checked if the response of the individual is affirmative. (4) A physical activity history that includes occupational

activity, recreational activity, the frequency of the activity, the duration of the activity, the intensity of the activity, and the type of physical activity involved. (p. 76)

The medical and fitness history should be reviewed by a qualified physician for determining whether fitness assessment should be done at all or whether specific restrictions may apply to testing protocols. The American College of Sportsmedicine (ACSM) recommends that, when prescribing exercise for the elderly, exercise testing for the purpose of assessing cardiovascular disorders and physical fitness levels should be performed "as appropriate." This recommendation is based on the assumption that the health professional prescribing the exercise program is thoroughly familiar with the participant's health history, current health status, physical activity level, and both absolute and relative contraindications for exercise testing. Shepard (1984) recommends the use of simple checklists such as the PAR-Q (see Appendix C) questionnaire and the Cornell Medical Index as useful preliminary screening devices to identify individuals with particular health or exercise contraindication problems that may demand more detailed clinical evaluation.

ACSM Guidelines for Max Stress Tests. Chronological aging is an unmodified factor that increases an individual's risk in exercise. As people become older, higher incidences of incapacitating conditions such as cardiovascular disease, cerebral atrophy, diabetes, orthopedic problems, arthritis, and neuromuscular disorders are more likely. The increased incidence of these conditions may severely limit the capacity of the elderly to exercise safely. Many of these disorders will not manifest themselves as serious clinical symptoms during daily routine activities typically performed by an older adult. But such symptoms can become evident when the elderly are engaged in light to moderate steady-state exercise.

Landin, Linnemeier, and Rothbaum et al. (1985) suggest that because of the high incidence of cardiovascular disease in the elderly, a thorough cardiovascular evaluation is necessary before embarking on a physical fitness program. This evaluation should include a careful health history, a cardiovascular evaluation with an electrocardiogram (ECG), and an exercise test. The American Alliance for Health, Physical Education, Recreation, and Dance (AAHPERD) and the American Heart Association (AHA) support the Landin et al. recommendation. For example, the American College of Sports Medicine (ACSM) recommends exercise stress assessment tests for the following individuals starting an exercise program:

- All apparently healthy individuals at or above age 45.
- All individuals at or above age 35 with at least one of the following coronary risk factors: history of high blood pressure (above 145/95); elevated total cholesterol/high density lipoprotein cholesterol ratio (about 5); cigarette smoking; abnormal resting electrocardiogram; family history of coronary or other atherosclerotic disease prior to age 50; and diabetes mellitus.

- Individuals at any age with known cardiovascular, pulmonary, or metabolic disease. (Franklin, 1986, p. 8)

These recommendations are in contrast to earlier ACSM recommendations published in 1980, which suggested maximal exercise stress tests for inactive, asymptomatic persons age 35 years or older without coronary risk factors. Table 3-5 summarizes the ACSM recommendations.

The ACSM recommendation for an exercise stress assessment is certainly prudent for exercise programs that include a progression to vigorous large muscle activities. However, an older adult embarking on a program that will not go beyond intensity levels of normal daily activities may not require a stress test but still should obtain the approval of a physician before starting. Many of the fitness programs designed for the elderly center around flexibility, calisthenics, and chair-supported exercises. Often these exercises do not go beyond the two to four MET level and thus are activities that closely approximate daily activities in terms of intensity level.[1]

Table 3.5. Guidelines for exercise testing.

	Apparently Healthy		High Risk			Any Age
	Below 45	45 and Above	Below 35 No Symptoms	35 and Above No Symptoms	Symptoms	
Max-Exercise Test Recommended Prior to Exercise Program	No	Yes	No	Yes	Yes	Yes
Physician Attendance Recommended for Max. Testing (under 35)	No	Yes	Yes	Yes	Yes	Yes
Physician Attendance Recommended for Sub-Max. Testing	No	No	No	Yes	Yes	Yes

From the American College of Sports Medicine, *Guidelines for Exercise Testing and Prescription,* 4th edition. Copyright 1991 Lea & Febiger. Reprinted by permission of Williams and Wilkins, a Waverly Company.

---

[1]A MET is equal to 3.5 MLxKg1$_6$xMin -1$_6$ of oxygen consumption and represents a person's resting metabolic rate. METs are used to measure the difficulty of work tasks. For instance, moderate work is described as eliciting an oxygen consumption (or energy expenditure) of up to three times the resting requirement (i.e., 3x3.5). Hard work requires three to eight times the resting requirement. If an activity is measured at six METs, it demands six times the energy of the resting state and is considered hard work.

The fitness level of elderly participants can vary greatly and can range from 2.5 METs for institutionalized elderly to 12 to 14 METs for elderly competitive athletes (Smith, 1984). If health promotion professionals are to prescribe fitness programs with confidence, it is logical to assume that the prescription would be preceded by a preliminary formal evaluation. The decision whether an exercise test is necessary is undoubtedly best made as a result of informed discussion between the elderly participant and his or her personal physician. This informed discussion should include the participant's past and present health status, goals of the suggested fitness program, and how those goals are to be attained.

Parameters to be Evaluated. Fitness assessment evaluations should minimally include cardiopulmonary capacity, flexibility, and muscle strength and endurance. Balance is tested under the mobility domain and body composition as part of the nutritional assessment domain. Appropriate testing cooldown and an explanation of the assessment results should be provided to the older adult. A brief explanation of popular fitness parameters follows.

Cardiopulmonary Capacity. The prescription of exercise programs rests largely on stress tests that evaluate cardiopulmonary capacity, that is, the ability of the heart to pump blood, of the lungs to breathe volumes of air, and of muscle cells to extract and utilize oxygen. Thus, cardiopulmonary stress tests are employed for three principal reasons: (1) to confirm the presence or absence of heart disease, (2) to identify exercise contraindications, and (3) to establish a safe and effective level of exercise. Two types of stress tests are used to accomplish these objectives: single-stage tests and multi-stage tests.

In a single-stage test, the physical work (stress) is kept constant throughout the exercise. Single-stage tests cannot be used for confirming the presence or absence of heart disease. They are valuable, however, for detecting exercise contraindications and program prescription. Three of the more popular single-stage tests are the Master Two-Step Test, Kasch Pulse Recovery Test, and the Twelve-Minute Run/Walk Test.

The Master Two-Step Test and Kasch Pulse Recovery Test consist of stepping onto or over a bench. The variations in these tests include bench height, intensity level, duration, and scoring methods. The heart rate is measured to approximate the oxygen consumption and fitness level of the participant. The Cooper Field Test is often used as a 12-minute open run/walk. Distance covered during this time is used to measure oxygen consumption and fitness level. A variation of the Cooper test is a one and one-half mile run/walk. The amount of time taken to complete this distance is then used to assess the participant's fitness level.

The Master-Two Step Test and the Kasch Pulse Recovery Test are considered sub-maximal tests (i.e., the individual does not approach his or her maximal functional capacity because exercise is limited to 75% to 85% of the individual's age-adjusted maximal heart rate). The open run and the one and one-half mile run/walk have the potential of being maximal tests. Maximal tests, without proper physician supervision, are inadvisable for the elderly because cerebrovascular arteries tend to lose their elasticity with age.

Maximal tests employ an isometric function that significantly impedes the flow of blood through the arteries during a maximal exertion. At the completion of the maximal exertion, the held-back blood rushes through the artery. The loss of elasticity, in tandem with the rushing blood, may cause artery rupture leading to stroke. For that reason, maximal tests are not advisable for individuals above age 40 unless proper physician supervision is maintained (American College of Sports Medicine, 1980).

Step testing probably offers the best submaximal exercise tolerance test for the elderly. Step testing is a reasonably familiar activity that requires minimum learning and minimum monetary investment in equipment, and provides proper supervision to assure that the participant does not exceed a safe exercise tolerance level. Nagle, Balke, and Naughton (1965) and the Canadian Home Fitness Test (Campbell, Mangeon et al., 1976) are step-test protocols that can be conveniently adjusted for elderly participants.

Despite the popularity of step tests, major problems include taking blood pressure while the participant is stepping onto and down from the bench and progressive loss of balance as the participant becomes fatigued. Use of a handrail to stabilize the participant is advisable for older subjects but negates accurate prediction of workload due to modified efficiency (Serfass, Agre, & Smith, 1985). Smith and Gilligan (1983) have attempted to solve this dilemma by developing a step test that is performed while seated in a straight-backed chair. The Smith and Gilligan protocol is especially well suited for elderly participants with low fitness levels.

Multi-stage tests employ successively increasing levels of physical work and are used for detecting cardiovascular disease, exercise contraindications, and program prescription. The multi-stage tests are considered maximal functional capacity tests for maximal, volitional fatigue, or presence of an untoward physiological response. Although a symptom-limited test for measuring maximal functional capacity will provide substantially more information relative to eventual abnormal cardiovascular responses to increasing exercise levels, most recommendations for exercise tests for the elderly favor the submaximal end-points of 75% to 85% of age-adjusted maximal heart rate. For a discussion of the controversy that surrounds maximal stress testing for the elderly, the reader is encouraged to consult Sefass et al. (1985).

In multi-stage testing, participants exercise at a low-intensity effort level and then progress to high levels of effort. The participant stays at each level of physical work long enough for his or her body to attain an equilibrium or steady response to that level of exercise. Equilibrium is that point at which the heart rate stabilizes and does not continue to increase or decrease. Multi-staging can be continuous, going from one level to the next without stopping, or intermittent, with a period of rest after equilibrium at each level of activity achieved. Today, most multi-stage testing is continuous (Solomon, 1984). Cycle ergometers and treadmills are the devices usually employed.

Electrocardiogram (ECG) measurements are used to monitor the heart's response to the exercise levels.

Serfass et al. (1985) reference major advantages of the cycle ergnometer. The cycle ergnometer is weight supportive, counters many of the participant's balance problems due to the use of handle bars, is relatively inexpensive, and can be stopped by the participant without signalling the tester. Disadvantages of the cycle are that many elderly subjects may not be familiar with cycling skills; or the quadricep muscle may fatigue and force the subject to cease the test before attaining maximal functional capacity, and thus the cycle will systematically underestimate the true maximal oxygen consumption. The reader may consult Smith (1984) for cycle ergnometer protocol testing for the elderly.

There are several treadmill protocol tests available for multi-stage testing. The most common protocol was developed by Bruce, Kusumi, and Hosmer (1973). Unfortunately, the testing increments used in the Bruce et al. protocol are too large to be comfortably tolerated by most elderly subjects. Smith (1984) recommends the Modified Balke Treadmill test (Balke & Ware, 1959) as the most adaptable protocol for the majority of elderly participants. Although treadmill walking is the most familiar skill for exercise testing, it is not without problems. Serfass et al. (1985) reference balance, pain in joints and muscles due to weight-bearing exercise, and levels of anxiety associated with motorized treadmill testing as special problems.

Flexibility. Flexibility is particular to each joint or to a combination of joints. For example, it is common to be flexible in the legs but not in the shoulders. Because flexibility is specific to each joint, there is not a general test that indicates total body flexibility. Thus, indirect methods are used to measure flexion for a variety of body areas. Table 3-6 provides a battery of indirect flexibility tests.

The assessment method used depends on the purpose for gathering flexibility data. The indirect methods specified in Table 3-6 are generally acceptable when determining gross measurement and not precise estimates. For therapeutic purposes, more precise techniques are required such as the mechanical goniometer and Leighton flexometer. The reader is encouraged to consult Piscopo (1985) for an excellent discussion of therapeutic techniques.

Muscle Strength and Endurance. Similar to flexibility, muscle strength and endurance are particular to each muscle area. For example, indirect methods measuring muscle strength and endurance of the back, abdomen, legs, shoulder, and chest are important for posture and mobility. Three categories of strength and endurance testing are used: (1) calisthenics, (2) gymnasium equipment, and (3) force against equal and variable resistance.

Calisthenics. Calisthenics are the most popular fitness tests used to assess strength and endurance. This popularity is based on low cost (no equipment required) and familiarity of calisthenics to the participant. Such tests usually determine the maximal

Table 3-6. Flexibility assessment.

Type	Muscle Group	General Instructions
Sit & Reach	Lower Back (D)* Hamstrings (D) Upper Back (I)* Shoulders (I)	Sit on floor, heels 5 inches apart. Yardstick placed by heel at 15-inch mark. Individual reaches forward 3 times (don't jerk). Measure point on yardstick at third movement.
Sternum to Floor	Lower Back (D) Groin (D) Hamstrings (I)	Sit on floor with legs straight and spread as far as possible. Lean forward toward floor with back straight. Distance between sternum and floor measured.
Shoulder Hypertension	Shoulders (D)	Lie on floor face down, holding a dowel with hands shoulder length apart. Raise dowel as high as possible. Distance from dowel to floor measured.
Trunk Hypertension	Trunk (D) Lower Back if arms not used (I) Buttocks (I)	Lie on stomach with hands under shoulders, arch back, eyes forward. Use arms and back muscles to raise head as high as possible. Distance between tip of nose and floor measured.
Knee to Chest	Lower Back (D)	Lie on back flat on floor. Pull one knee to chest. Measure bottom of breastbone to top of kneecap. Measure other knee by same process. The fewer inches, the more flexibility.
Spread Leg	Groin (D)	Sit on floor. Spread legs as far as possible. Measure between inside kneecaps.
Hip Flexor	Hip Muscles (D)	Lie face down with pelvis flat to floor. Lift knee off floor as far as possible without lifting pelvis off floor. Measure from ground to top of kneecap. Perform for each leg.

*D is a direct flexibility measurement for a muscle group and I is an indirect flexibility measurement for a muscle group.

number of exercise repetitions completed within a specified period of time (strength) or the total number of repetitions completed without time restriction (endurance). Common calisthenic exercises completed include sit-ups, push-ups, and torso-raises. Sit-ups, however, should not be used with participants who have lower back problems. Norms are then used to classify the fitness level of the participant.

Endurance testing is particularly important for older adults. The modified Kraus-Weber test, a minimum endurance test, has often been employed with older adults for this purpose. Failure to pass the Kraus-Weber test is an indication of endangered body health. Modified push-ups and bent-knee sit-ups are the principal endurance exercises assessed. Norms for the modified version of these exercises are not yet available.

Gymnasium. A more accurate estimate of strength for isolated muscle groups may be attained through maximal lifts on gymnasium equipment (free weights, weight machines). However, as cited earlier, maximal tests are inadvisable for older adults. Muscle endurance can be assessed on gymnasium equipment. Common exercise tests involving free weights include bench press, military press, arm curl, leg extension, leg curl, leg pull, and upright rowing. These tests are less accurate for novice lifters. Norms do not exist for endurance tests on free weights and contained gymnasium equipment (e.g., Nautilus, Universal).

Force/Resistance. Force against equal and variable resistance is conducted on an apparatus that exerts an equal and opposite force against the force of the muscle (O'Donnell & Ainsworth, 1984). Such tests avoid the fatigue error inherent in the repeated trials of calisthenics or gymnasium equipment. The grip-strength test has been commonly used as the best measure of overall body strength (Golding, Myers, & Sinning, 1973). A handgrip dynometer or manuometer is employed. The instrument is held in the hands and squeezed. Montoye and Lamphiear (1977) provide norms for the dynometer test. These norms are applied only up to age 59 and, therefore, should be lowered by approximately 5% for each decade past age 60.

Fitness Assessment Recommendation. The purposes of fitness assessment are to determine program baseline data that serve the objectives of program prescription and evaluation, to detect asymptomatic cardiovascular disease, to provide a motivational dimension for participants, to prevent exercise contraindications, and to protect the organization against litigation due to improper assessment or fitness programming. A variety of instruments or equipment may be used for measuring the discussed fitness components. The health promotion professional should base the selection of appropriate instruments and equipment on the following criterion: (1) instrument validity and reliability, (2) cost and maintenance, (3) instrument intrusion, (4) storage and portability, (5) simplicity for operation and measurement, (6) available instrument norms, (7) relevancy to older adults, and (8) program purpose (O'Donnell & Ainsworth, 1985). Maud and Foster (1995) provide an overview of physiological assessment techniques.

Mobility Assessment

Dysmobility is defined as any problem that may interfere with getting from one place to another, for example, getting in and out of bed, transferring from bed to bath, or walking up or down stairs. The mobility spectrum is marked by degrees of optimal functioning or dependence in bed mobility, sitting, standing, transfers, ambulating, and balancing. Balance is a common thread throughout the mobility spectrum. Cardiopulmonary, musculoskeletal, neurological, sensory, and psychological factors greatly influence each of the aspects represented in the Lewis mobility spectrum.

The goal for health professionals is to assist the older adult in attaining maximal enjoyment at any level of the mobility spectrum. Lewis's example of assisting an older adult getting into and out of a wheelchair independently without fear emphasizes this point. In the past, rehabilitation efforts have been too narrow, focusing only on walking or gait movement. Lewis (1989) adds,

> Dysmobility risks for older persons arise throughout the mobility spectrum. Older persons at the very extreme ends of the mobility spectrum have the greatest risk for falling; those people who transfer from bed to wheelchair are at very high risk, and those who walk a great deal are also at high risk. The greater the person's activity the greater the person's chance of falling. Therefore, health care professionals may want to use just this one piece of data to begin investigating the ends of the spectrum for improving older persons' mobility. (p. 3)

Approximately 15% of adults age 65 and older have some type of mobility problem. Eighty-five percent of people confined to nursing homes have major mobility problems. These statistics are rather startling when one considers that older adults tend to underreport mobility problems (Lewis, 1989). Musculoskeletal disorders (e.g., arthritis, osteoporosis), age-related changes in the musculoskeletal system (cross-linkages of collagen), sedentary lifestyle, neurological changes (e.g., decreased reaction time), neurological conditions (e.g., stroke, Parkinson's disease), cardiopulmonary problems (e.g., atherosclerosis, arteriosclerosis), sensory factors (e.g., presbyopia, presbycusis) and psychological factors (e.g., depression) all seriously compromise mobility.

Health professionals are initially challenged to determine the causes of dysmobility. The previously discussed General Health Assessment phase plays a key role in this effort. The health professional should inquire as to the activities the client has performed in the past, activities the client would like to do but can no longer perform, the length of time the client has had the problem, and environmental adaptations that the client may have initiated to compensate for dysmobility. Based upon this review, the health professional may assess two mobility areas: (1) evaluation of gait and (2) evaluation of balance.

Evaluation of Gait. The discussion of the three tests that follows is largely drawn from Lewis (1989). Gait is the loss and recovery of balance, the body's ability to use inertia to attain efficient, effortless walking. Problems in gait mobility for the elderly primarily originate from their inability to maximize inertia and use gravity effectively. Three basic walking tasks are associated with gait: (1) weight acceptance, (2) simple limb support, and (3) limb advancement (Lewis, 1989). Weight acceptance incurs great impact and requires control. The four groups of muscles most involved in weight acceptance are the hip extensors, hip abductors, quadriceps, and plantar flexors. The normal older adult experiences a 28% decrease in quadricep strength, and 38% in the abductor muscles. Compensations to weakening muscle strength include decreasing stride length, leaning forward from the hips, and decreasing plantar flexion.

The hip abductors are largely responsible for single limb support. These muscles keep the pelvis level and hold up the hip and leg. Weak hip abductors will cause the body trunk to shift to the weak side. Limb advancement requires both flexibility and strength by the quadricep muscles, abductor muscles, and plantar flexors. Weak plantar flexors will decrease the stride length and produce inefficient gait pattern.

Older adults experience an overall decrease in the range of motion. For example, there is a 5° decrease in the motion of the hips, knees, and ankles. This reduction in range of motion alters the efficiency of the musculoskeletal system. Because of inefficient gait pattern, the actual task of walking for the elderly requires more energy. Lewis (1989) reported that the normal energy requirement for walking is 0.16 ml O_2/kg/min. Expenditure for healthy older adults is 0.23 ml O_2/kg/min. Although this is not a significant difference, older adults compromised by other health disorders may be seriously affected.

Numerous techniques are available for evaluating gait. These techniques may range from sophisticated electronic equipment to subjective measures. The assessment of gait includes the three stages of gait as well as the following gait components: (1) heel strike, (2) toe off, (3) terminal extension of the knee, (4) hip flexion and extension, (5) trunk rotation, and (6) automatic movements. Two popular objective instruments for evaluating gait stages are Nelson's Functional Ambulation Profile (FAP), and Tinneti's Performance-Oriented Assessment of Mobility. The reader is encouraged to consult Nelson (1974) and Tinneti (1986) for a thorough discussion of these instruments.

Evaluation of Balance. Balance has been defined as "the harmonious adjustments of parts and performance of functions" (Dorland's Illustrated Medical Dictionary, 1965, p. 178). The components of balance involve all systems of the body. Potential balance problems may occur due to weak muscles that lead to alignment problems and changes in the neurologic system, sensory system, cardiovascular system, and the psychological system. For this reason, assessment of balance begins with a thorough medical screening and then is followed by use of a series of balance assessment instruments for measuring static and dynamic balance.

Balance or equilibrium is not a general characteristic. It is a quality that consists of specific abilities including stationary and dynamic balance. These categories of balance may be further subordinated into inverted and upright balance. Inverted balance, however, is not a major objective for older adults. Unfortunately, standardized balance tests for the well-elderly are generally not available. Medical tests to diagnose pathological conditions (e.g., vertigo) are sometimes used. To assess balance, therefore, the professional must adapt tests that were designed for younger populations. Four promising balance tests adapted for the elderly include: (1) One-Foot Balance Stand, (2) Modified Dynamic Beam Balance Test, (3) Performance-Oriented Balance Evaluation, and (4) Balance Actuator.

One-Foot Balance Stand. The objective of the one-foot balance stand test is to assess upright stationary balance of the participant. The participant stands on his or her preferred leg within a prescribed area 15 inches by 15 inches. Eyes are kept open and arms raised to the side. The arms serve as a balance pole to assist in stability. To provide visual reference, the eyes are focused on a particular point on an opposite wall. At a given signal, the participant attempts to balance on one foot for 15 seconds without moving or falling. A subjective checklist is then used to determine the participant's balance stability (e.g., steadiness, form).

Modified Dynamic Beam Balance Test. Dynamic balance requires gross changes in posture dependent upon the nature of the motor skill, for example, walking and jumping. The Springfield Balance Beam Walking Test and the Bass Stepping Stone Test (Piscopo, 1985) are often used to assess dynamic balance. The Springfield test involves walking nine beams of equal length and height. The beams vary, however, in widths from four to one-fourth inches. The objective is to walk 10 steps on each of the progressively narrower beams in a heal-to-toe fashion. The hands are kept on the hips. Developed by Ruth Bass, the Stepping Stone Test assesses the ability to jump from one designated position to another in a zig-zag fashion using one leg and then leaping on the opposite leg to a designated circle target that serves as a landing area.

The Springfield Balance Beam Test is probably the most appropriate for measuring dynamic balance for older adults. However, this technique should be slightly modified. One narrow beam 10 feet long, 4 inches wide and 4 inches high should be used. The older adult should be instructed to walk along the beam with eyes focused at the end of the beam. Arms should be raised sideward to serve as a balance force. A heel-to-toe walking fashion should be employed. Based on these modifications, Piscopo (1985, p. 401) provides a subjective checklist for evaluating upright dynamic balance.

Performance-Oriented Balance Evaluation. Tinetti (1986) provides a mobility assessment instrument that evaluates balance and gait. Impaired mobility and falls, like most geriatric problems, are over-lapping and multifactorial. Mobility, the ability to get around in one's environment, is a complicated function that consists of multiple component maneuvers. The component maneuvers, in turn, depend on psychologic, cognitive, and physical characteristics. The Tinetti assessment tests identifies (1) components of mobility a person is likely to have trouble with during daily activities, (2) potential reasons for difficulty with particular maneuvers, (3) other problems (e.g., falling) besides mobility a person is likely to experience, (4) potential medical or rehabilitation interventions that may improve mobility, and (5) potential environmental manipulations that may prevent problems and aid individuals in adapting to mobility problems.

Balance Actuator. This instrument requires the client to balance on a board while the actuator automatically measures shifts in weight and balance changes. The balance actuator measures the number of seconds a client touches on one side and the number of weight shifts.

Mobility Assessment Recommendation. Many older adults experience a decline in mobility. Changes associated with psychomotor organs and multiple chronic diseases and disabilities are responsible for this decline. The Canadian Task Force on the Periodic Health Examination concluded that assessing physical, social, and psychologic functions as they affect progressive incapacity with aging was the most important assessment for clients over the age of 75 (Tinetti,1986). Locomotor, sensory, and cognitive functions are intricately related to balance. Assessment of mobility for gait and balance plays a key role in this prevention challenge.

Nutritional Assessment

Nutritional assessment may be defined as the evaluation of an individual's state of health resulting from the intake and utilization of nutrients (Frankel & Owen, 1978). General health, body composition, dietary intake, eating and lifestyle habits, and metabolic disorders are but a few dimensions that influence nutritional health. The objective of nutritional assessment is to identify principal nutrition risk factors that may be lessened or eliminated through nutritional intervention programs (e.g., cholesterol levels, balanced nutrients). Thus nutritional assessment is used to screen individuals for selection into appropriate intervention programs, to monitor progress and evaluate the program (MacNeil & Teague, 1987).

The information obtained from nutritional assessments includes food intake and eating patterns, health history, home and work environments, personal and family situations, stress coping mechanisms, and physical activity patterns. This information is used to identify the participant's attitudes, values, and beliefs that shape health behavior. O'Donnell and Ainsworth (1984) cite five nutritional assessment techniques that are used to gather this information: (1) anthropometric assessment, (2) biochemical assessment, (3) clinical assessment, (4) dietary assessment, and (5) environmental assessment.

Anthropometric Assessment. Anthropometric assessments are physical measurements and estimation of body fat composition. The techniques used are the skinfold caliper and circumference techniques discussed earlier. The information gained from anthropometric assessment reveals important details about nutritional status, such as, under-nutrition, over-nutrition, or muscle development.

To assess body composition, it is important to differentiate between the terms "overweight" and "obesity." Overweight means too much weight according to the standard height-weight charts. Obesity refers to an excess of body fat. The intent of body composition testing is to measure the relative percentage of fat body weight to lean body (muscle and bone) weight. Two principal body composition techniques are used: (1) hydrostatic weighing and (2) skinfold techniques.

Hydrostatic weighing is the most accurate measure but is terribly expensive and complex and is generally not used in the clinical setting or for mass testing. Various height-weight ratios are often used to evaluate body fatness. However, research has shown that skinfold techniques yield more accurate estimates of hydrostatically measured body density than height-weight ratios (Katch & McArdle, 1983). The two skinfold techniques commonly employed are skin-caliper and circumference testing.

Skin-Caliper. Approximately one-half of the body's total fat content is located directly beneath the skin. Skin-calipers are used to measure this fat content. Three principal body areas are generally measured: posterior arm, abdomen, and scapula. A fourth area, the chest, is also often used with male subjects. The caliper technique involves lifting a skinfold with the thumb and index finger. The skinfold is held while the caliper is applied approximately 1 cm away.

Skinfold measurements can be evaluated in two ways. First, the sum of the body site measurements may be used to estimate body fat percentage. Nomograms, according to age and sex, are then used to approximate fat coat. Second, a series of mathematical formulas that estimate body fat percentages may be used. These formulas were determined by norm testing for different ages, sexes, physiques, and other characteristics. The skinfold caliper technique does not measure intramuscular fat, that is, lean body mass. It is advisable to use the mathematical formula approach to improve accuracy.

Fatfold measurement comparisons with norms should be matched with similar population age groups and sex because of the variability through the lifespan (Piscopo, 1985). Katch and McArdle (1983) estimate that the skinfold caliper technique is within 3 to 5% of the estimates of hydrostatic weighing. The skinfold caliper technique, however, is not recommended for extremely obese individuals. Although the use of the skinfold caliper requires careful training, the accuracy, economy, and convenience of this technique make it highly practical for health promotion programs. Yet the reader is cautioned that the validity of anthropometric measures is less accurate beyond the age of 60 years. To offset this problem, multiple formulas are used with averages calculated.

Circumference Testing. Body circumference measures are also used for predicting body fat content. The measurement positions for older women are the abdomen, right thigh, and right forearm. Older men are measured on the buttocks, abdomen, and right arm. Mathematical formulas based on the circumference measurements are then employed to estimate body fat content. The circumference technique is estimated to be within 3 to 5% of the hydrostatic technique estimates (Katch & McArdle, 1983). Circumference testing is very practical as it is inexpensive, easy to use, and fairly accurate. This technique, however, is not suitable for the obese or very thin individual.

Biochemical Assessment. Biochemical assessment is an analysis of the levels of nutrients or metabolic by-products found in the blood and urine. The purpose of this assessment is to identify nutritional inadequacies, marginal nutrient deficiencies, and nutrient excesses. Pender (1982) references laboratory tests as including cholesterol, triglycerides, glucose, and high-density lipoproteins. Additional information is gathered concerning protein (creatine index, serum protein, serum albumin, total lymphocyte count, blood urea nitrogen, uric acid), serum or plasma vitamin levels (water soluble, fat soluble), and minerals (calcium, sodium, chloride, potassium, iron, phosphorus, magnesium). Thus biochemical assessments identify nutrition-related problems that can be managed by health promotion programs, as well as track the physiological changes that result from intervention programs.

Clinical Assessment. Clinical assessments examine the body for the signs and symptoms of poor nutrition that are related to health disorders and dental problems. The methods employed are subjective and include an evaluation of physical appearance and medical history. The overall object is to detect signs and symptoms that indicate nutritional inadequacies and to determine factors that influence nutritional health.

Dietary Assessment. Dietary assessment is an evaluation and monitoring of the participant's diet. Nutrient intake, diet quality, eating patterns, and eating habits are assessed. The most commonly employed dietary assessment techniques are the 24-hour recall, food frequency record, food diary, and nutrition history. The overall intent is to construct a profile of nutritional status as affected by increased requirements due to illness, stress, increased activity level, food or drug interactions, or abnormalities in nutrient absorption and excretion. Emotional, psychological, cultural, and economic condition factors are also considered.

Environmental Assessment. Environmental assessment analyzes lifestyle, social, cultural, and economic conditions–the individual's personal environment that affect eating habits. Food availability, eating patterns, attitudes, and general nutritional health are the dimensions of interest. The health hazard appraisals and wellness inventories cited in the general health assessment are often used to collect much of the information under environmental assessment.

Nutrition Assessment: A Special Problem. Osteoporosis in elderly individuals can compress the spinal column and thus cause a gradual decline in height. It is not beyond reason to see decrements in height from 5 to 8 inches over a two-decade span. As York (1985) contends,

> It is not difficult to assess what is an appropriate body weight in a woman whose spinal column is compressed and so she is shorter, or her spine is bent because of a development of a dowager's hump. Her height is now five inches lower, her body weight may have stayed the same but in terms of comparing her to charts we have available, she is going to look more overweight than she did ten years before though nothing has really changed. (p. 80)

To offset this problem, some health professionals are now looking at the possibility of using arm length to structure body weight tables which keep skeleton frame size constant.

Other nutrition assessment dimensions that need to be taken into consideration are decrements in cardiac output, basal metabolic rate, and kidney function. These decrements alter the individual's need for nutrients. The kidney may cease to save nutrients as well as in the past, or it may handle the nutrients differently. The gastrointestinal tract is less efficient in absorption and metabolism as an individual becomes older and thus affects nutrient status in ways that have not yet been quantified. In sum, it is difficult to incorporate biochemical assessment results into nutrient needs for the elderly (York, 1985).

Nutrition Assessment Recommendation. In most cases, the comprehensive use of nutrition assessment techniques is neither financially feasible nor desirable. The two tests that provide most of the necessary nutrition information are the anthropometric and biochemical assessments. These two assessments identify obese persons, high cardiac risk persons, and individuals who are experiencing serious nutritional problems. Dietary assessment may also be used for counseling and designing nutritional programs.

It is important to note that a comprehensive health promotion assessment program provides much of the biochemical assessment information on its health hazard appraisal. If a comprehensive health assessment program is not used, a biochemical analysis and dietary analysis may cost approximately $10 if performed in bulk quantity. The information collected from nutrition assessment is obviously technical and complex. Because standards for nutrition assessment are critical for quality assurance, O'Donnell and Ainsworth (1984) recommend that the services of a registered dietician be employed.

One very promising assessment development has been the Nutrition Screening Initiative, a five-year multifaceted effort focusing on routine nutrition screening and care. The initial focus of this effort is on older adults. Leading professional organizations such as

The American Academy of Family Physicians, The American Diabetic Association, and the National Council on Aging are sponsoring the nutrition screening program. An advisory committee consisting of 30 key organizations and professionals plays an important planning role. For more information, the reader is encouraged to contact The Nutrition Screening Initiative, 2626 Pennsylvania Avenue, N.W., Suite 301, Washington, DC 20037.

Stress Assessment

Stress assessment instruments are not well developed for use in health promotion programs. Deficiencies in the development of stress assessment instruments include (1) limits in current understanding of the stress concept; (2) validation of many stress instruments have been based on emotionally ill people; (3) interpretations of stress assessment data are subjective and thus difficult to use for stress purposes; (4) competency of practitioners to use and interpret many of the specialized instruments is questionable; and (5) the honest response of participants to stress instruments may also be questioned (O'Donnell & Ainsworth, 1984). Nevertheless, stress management programs are very popular and thus demand some type of stress assessment.

Subjective Measures of Stress. Stress management intervention programs attempt to eliminate stressors, increase the ability of the individual to manage stress, and/or limit the effects of stress by-products (serum cholesterol, hydrochloric acid). Ability to manage stress is determined by assessing the personality traits and physical health that indicate stress resiliency. These dimensions are measured by inquiring about strain symptoms (physiological, emotional, psychological), causes and exposure to stress, and stress coping techniques employed.

Stress management programs essentially attempt to teach individuals three types of activity. First is a self awareness process that asks the participant to critically assess why he or she is doing certain things and what effects these actions bring. The second activity is self-renewal or an inner exploration of the effects of one's behavior on his or her body and psyche. Finally, individuals are taught self-management skills for responding to daily pressures. Hundreds of instruments exist that can be used during these three activity processes. These instruments are not used for prescriptive program purposes but as awareness devices for enabling the individual to personally manage stressful situations.

Measuring Physical Reactivity to Stress. Health promotion professionals may find a physical reactivity measure of stress insightful both for program prescription and client motivation. Blood pressure may be checked at rest and then under mild stress conditions to assess stress physical reactivity. Eliot and Breo (1984) identify individuals as either "hot stress reactors" or "cold stress reactors" based on a continuum measure of blood pressure. This measure provides the client with some idea of how he or she is responding to stress in terms of emotions, behavior, and ultimately the cardiovascular system.

Blood pressure is the force with which blood pushes against the walls of the blood vessels. Systolic pressure is the peak at which the heart beats and pumps blood into the arteries. Diastolic pressure is when the heart relaxes between beats. On a continuum of possible readings, 120/85 mm Hg is average for adults and readings above 140/90 mm Hg are abnormally high and carry increased risk for cardiovascular disease.

Eliot and Breo (1984) have used both a treadmill test and a cold pressor test (ice water) to measure an individual's response to a physical stress condition.[2] During the "cold pressor" test, for example, if a client's blood pressure goes up beyond 164/106 mm Hg, the client is paying a physiological price for a moderate physical demand. Eliot and Breo also have clients play a simple video game like Atari's "Breakout." Some people playing Breakout raised their resting blood pressure from 130/80 to 220/130.

Moreover, most of these game players had absolutely no awareness of what was physiologically happening to them. Approximately one out of five Americans overreacts physiologically to mental stress, and it is this unsuspected overreactivity that dramatically impairs the heart.

It can be determined if an elderly client is a "hot stress reactor" or "cold stress reactor" by taking the individual's blood pressure at rest and then under mild stress conditions. Blood pressure kits (pressure cuff and stethoscope) are only about $35. However, for optimal ease and reliability, Eliot and Breo (1984) recommend an electronic kit or a digit readout kit (cost ranges between $60 and $175). If the client has heart trouble or any concern about the ability of his or her heart to tolerate any type of stress testing, the client's physician should be consulted. Moreover, if during stress testing the client develops symptoms of any kind (e.g., chest pains, palpitations, lightheadedness), the test should be terminated immediately and the client should consult his or her physician.

The resting blood pressure should be taken after the client has had at least 10 minutes of relaxation. Dim lights and soothing music may help create the proper environment. The blood pressure should be taken twice, the second reading a few minutes after the initial reading. The second blood pressure reading is recorded. Physical and mental stress conditions are then employed. Stress conditions developed by Eliot and Breo include a cold pressor test, mental arithmetic test, video games, and a daily life stress test.

---

[2]In the cold pressor test, the individual places his or her hand in a bucket of ice water for 70 seconds. The difference between resting and stress demand blood pressure is then measured.

Blood pressure falls within a wide range of normality, but there is a gray zone toward the high end of the continuum. Generally, a physician is concerned when blood pressure readings are 140/90 or higher. Similarly, Eliot and Breo define a hot stress reactor as an individual whose systolic blood pressure rises above 160 mm Hg on the stress tests. Diastolic pressure that increases to 95 mm Hg after the mental arithmetic, video game, or daily life stress test, or to 105 mm Hg after the cold pressor test are likely to be hot stress reactors.

Three caveats are suggested for using a physical reactivity measure of stress. First, accurate readings must be taken during or immediately after the stress test. Second, blood pressure readings over a period of two weeks should be taken and the results should be averaged. Third, potential drug interactions that could affect test results should be considered.

Stress Assessment Recommendation. Stress assessment instruments differ widely by format (questionnaire, observation, interview) and focus (symptoms, exposures, coping). O'Donnell and Ainsworth (1984) provide criteria that may assist the health promotion professional in selecting appropriate stress assessment instruments. They are (1) breadth of range of test focus, (2) applicability to the available intervention program, (3) who the tests were designed for, (4) variables measured by the test, (5) conditions under which the tests are administered, and (6) methods for interpreting, explaining, and applying the test results.

Substance Dependency

There is little agreement among theorists regarding the causes of substance dependency and even less agreement among practitioners on clinical assessment. The field of substance dependency is in a preparadigm stage of development (Shaffer & Kauffman, 1985). Although there are a variety of preparadigm perspectives explaining addictive behavior (e.g., moral turpitude, social deprivation, intrapsychic defense), practitioners continue to apply their own ideas about addiction, treatment strategies, and assessment. This confusing state of affairs is principally aggravated by the plethora of drugs involved in substance dependency. Thus accurate assessment of abuse and addiction requires a wide range of informational and observational skills.

Addiction Patterns. The term dependency means that one is excessively vulnerable to or at risk of becoming addicted to a variety of substances, such as alcohol, illegal drugs, or pharmaceutical drugs. Patterns of addiction for substance dependency are very difficult to pin down because so many factors enter into the formula. The distinction between "habit" and "addiction" is fragile, but there are some signs that can help differentiate these conditions. Many health professionals, for this reason, tend to employ subjective assessments that look at patterns of substance usage. These assessment instruments are based on the following behavioral predictors.

- The addictive behavior starts to dominate the person's life; he begins to neglect other facets of his life (even basic ones, such as cleanliness).
- The person's usual behavior patterns or day-to-day patterns of living have become seriously disrupted.
- The abrupt discontinuation of the addictive behavior after continued or prolonged manifestation results in a state of extreme anxiety, a hypnotic trance, or, in some cases, an actual physical "withdrawal" illness (such as that seen among drug or alcohol addicts).
- The person cannot seem to get enough of the addictive behavior or substance--or, after getting enough, he still can't stop.
- The person has lost the ability to make choices about the addictive behavior--he can't rationally determine whether it is an appropriate time or setting for the behavior and act accordingly. In simple terms, he is forced into the behavior, regardless of his own feelings or circumstances at the time.
- The person continues the addictive behavior even after it has lost some of its excitement or appeal to him; even though it isn't as pleasant as it once was, he continues on a regular basis. A person who once got a real thrill out of betting on horses may continue to do so even when he is ridiculed or nagged, loses continually, or no longer feels the same "thrill."
- The person no longer does something because he wants to progress and improve; he does it because he wants to be left alone, because he fears he can't progress, or because he needs to get away from a stressful situation. He may not find joy or pleasure at all in the addictive behavior, but it may indeed help him erase other things in his life that he dreads. (Hafen & Frandsen, 1985, p. 3-4)

These behaviors underscore the differences between substance use, substance misuse, and substance abuse. The best way to assess whether an individual is abusing a substance is the use of a health diary and some of the many standardized self-tests.

Health Diary. Older adults may be asked to construct a health diary for self-assessing drug behavior. The diary is usually kept for one month whereby the individual notes any situations in which the individual uses drugs, talks about drugs, or is around others who use drugs. Behavioral antecedents and consequences of drug use are also kept. For example, the older adult may note usage of a specific drug, how the drug was obtained, drug cost, and sensations before and after drug usage.

The diagnostic standard for alcohol dependency or abuse in DSM IV requires a detailed interview that is too cumbersome for use in routine clinical screening. A variety of short screening questionnaires have been developed that are more practical for routine screening.

- Michigan Alcoholism Screening Test (MAST). The Mast is a 25-item questionnaire that is relatively sensitive (84–100%) and specific (87–95%) for DSM IV-diagnosed alcohol abuse. An abbreviated 10- and 13-item versions are also available but are less sensitive (66–78%) and specific (80%) for routine screening. (Barry & Fleming 1993)
- CAGE. The 4-item CAGE questionnaire is the most popular screening instrument used in primary care settings. The CAGE sensitivity is 74–99% and specificity is 79–95% diagnosing alcohol abuse or dependence. (Chan, Pristach, & Welte, 1994)
- Alcohol Use Disorders Identification Test (AUDIT). AUDIT is a 10-item screening instrument developed by the World Health Organization (WHO). This instrument includes questions about drinking quantity, frequency, and binge behavior. Consequences of drinking are also addressed. Validation studies for the AUDIT have varied but present research suggests that the AUDIT is less sensitive (61%) and specific (90%) for current drinking problems but more effective than the MAST 13-item questionnaire. (Barry & Fleming, 1993)

Substance Dependency Recommendation. Presently, a multitude of popular assessment models that apply to substance dependency: behavioral, cognitive-behavioral, multimodal, psychoanalytic, biologic, psycho-social, and biosocial. Assessment protocols within each of these models are overwhelming and confusing. However, these theoretical orientations and paradigms are still responsible for determining (1) the focus of the assessing clinician, (2) data considered to be relevant and important, and (3) the system of organization that will be implemented to organize the data for treatment strategies (Shaffer & Kauffman, 1985). The reader interested in the subjective symptoms associated with addiction should consult Hafen and Frandsen (1985). For a more clinical perspective of assessment, the reader is encouraged to consult Shaffer and Kauffman (1985).

FUNCTIONAL ASSESSMENT AND THE ELDERLY

The homeostatic mechanism of most older persons is in a very delicate state of balance. This delicate state makes the older person vulnerable to disability from a variety of perspectives--physical, psychological, economic, and social. The rehabilitation emphasis on restoration and maintenance requires an assessment process that emphasizes an impact on independent functioning in society or the home with some assistance. The constellation of medical diseases or medical problems of an individual patient as part of health assessment are not sufficient to assess the older person's functional capacity. Gallo et al. (1988) write,

Disturbance of homeostasis in the previously compensated organ system by a disguise process will be expressed in the most vulnerable, delicately balanced system. For example, congestive heart failure may present only acute confusion (or, more subtly, as worsening of a preexisting dementia) in a patient in whom the central nervous system is the most vulnerable to insult, for example, because of atherosclerotic disease. Unlike in the young, illness in the elderly may present not as a single, specific symptomatic complaint that helps to localize the source of the trouble but rather as a nonspecific disability. Examples include the following: urinary incontinence, dizziness, confusion, or not eating or drinking. (p. 5)

A seemingly clear indication of a poorly managed disease is the deterioration of functional independence. Corrections of minor health problems can greatly enhance the older person's quality of life in regard to functional independence. The purpose of functional assessment, in relationship to functional independence, is to help the health professional focus on the client's capabilities and to distribute appropriate resources when functional change is apparent. The multitude of physical, social and psychological changes associated with aging can easily overwhelm the health professional. Yet corrections of minor health problems can greatly enhance the older person's quality of life. Functional assessment, used in concert with a physician's examination, can help the health professional delimit specific problems that interfere with the important activities of daily living. Unfortunately, the elderly and health professionals too often write off many health problems as the inevitable consequences of long life. This narrow view of aging seriously impairs the health assessment process.

Functional Disability and Geriatric Rehabilitation

Functional independence, not disease eradication, is gaining acceptance as the principal focus of health care for the aged. Consequently, health promotion professionals need to implement a comprehensive assessment of functional status that is fully analagous and complementary to the careful, disease-oriented diagnostic assessments that precede treatment decisions. The following statistics support this need:

- Of the total noninstitutionalized adult population, those 18 and over, of whom there are just over 153 million, 4.9 million need the help of another person in performing everyday activities. Of those needing help, the majority, 2.8 million are 65 years of age and over. At all ages some adults need help, but as age increases the percentage needing help increased dramatically, almost doubling with each succeeding decade between age 45 and 84, and then nearly tripling. Of community residents over age 85, 44% were found to need help. (Fillenbaum, 1985, p. 698)
- Individuals over the age of 65 carry a disproportionate burden of disability. Fifty percent of those living at home have functional limitations in performing activities of daily living and 80% have one

or more chronic illness. For those 75 and over, 15% are homebound and 20% of those over the age of 80 are homebound.
(Besdine, 1983, p. 652)

The aging process involves two basic gerontological principles. First, specific age-related changes are expected to occur at various levels--biological, psychological, and social. From a biological perspective, gradual decline in physiological reserves of major organ systems commences during the fourth decade. Moreover, there is an increasing probability of specific age-related disease processes that accelerate the loss of physiologic reserve. Within the psychological component, age-associated alterations in cognitive and perceptual abilities occur that can be exacerbated by concomitant disease processes. From a social perspective, the elderly may face different social attitudes and are confronted by a decline in family and social support networks. (Becker & Cohen, 1984). Despite the progression of senescence from a biological, psychological, and social perspective, the aforementioned changes are not universal.

A second basic gerontological principle suggests heterogeneity rather than homogeneity in the elderly population. From a clinical perspective, the progression of age-related changes becomes important when those changes break through the clinical threshold and impair functional status. In other words, the accumulation of chronic diseases by the elderly does not necessarily lead to a severe functional disability. Many of the elderly afflicted by numerous health problems are functioning independently (Besdine, 1983). The focus of a comprehensive health assessment, therefore, must recognize the interrelationship between declining functional status and its impact on the daily and basic living skills of the elderly.

Functional Assessment Categories

Although 66% of adults age 65 and older have one or more chronic conditions, only 35% experience major activity restrictions (Gallo et al., 1988). As noted earlier in this book, older adults on the average experience 39 days of restricted activity annually. The Year 2000 health goal for older adults is to reduce the number of restricted activity days by 20%. Measurement for attaining this objective is based on a systematic assessment of both activity daily living skills (ADL) and instrumental activity daily living skills (IADL). ADL skills are those functions fundamental to independent living such as eating, toileting, transferring from bed to chair, dressing, and continence. IADL skills include more complex activities such as traveling, meal preparation, shopping, house-work, and handling personal finances. Both ADL and IADL assessments provide quali-tative data on health in the later years. Several empirical studies link independence in ADLs and IADLs with longer life. Gallo et al. (1988) note that:

the ability to perform tasks such as traveling, shopping, meal preparation, housework and handling of money is correlated to mortality.
Patients who were able to perform all five tasks had a death rate of 2%
in comparison to the overall death rate of 5%, those incapable of
performing any of the activities had a death rate of 27%. (p. 66)

ADL Instruments. ADL instruments evaluate one's ability to live independently in the community. Two popular instruments for this purpose are (1) Katz ADL and (2) the modified Barthel Index. Included in the Katz Index (Katz, Ford, & Moskowitz, et al., 1963) for ADL are bathing, dressing, toileting, transfer, continence, and feeding. This index uses a three-tiered scale response instead of a four or more response scale in order to improve instrument validity. Assessment of the respondent's ability to live independently is made to ensure maximum independence. For example, a person experiencing meal preparation difficulty, but still capable of independence in other functional life areas, may be introduced to an inhome meals program.

The Barthel Index (Mahoney & Barthel, 1965) is used to assess the respondent's ability for self-care. This index includes items that are weighted to account for the amount of physical assistance needed to function independently in the community and can be used as an evaluation tool for documenting program impacts on functional status. A modified Barthel index was constructed to assess the respondent's need for home health services. This instrument was correlated to the actual number of activities the respondent could perform independently. The reader is encouraged to consult Gallo et al. (1988) for a review of the modified Barthel Index instrument.

IADL Instruments. Five IADL skills are assessed as a simple assessment screen for determining whether a more exhaustive assessment is necessary. They are travel, shopping, meal preparation, housework, and handling personal finances. The five IADL skills can be arranged in order or placed along a Guttman Scale. Thus, if a person can perform a particular task when the items are arranged vertically and in order, he or she can also perform the tasks arranged below the reference point. If they are not capable of performing a particular task, then those tasks below the reference point cannot be performed. In other words, the Guttman scale ranges the five IADL tasks from most difficult to least difficult. The difficulty of the five tasks consistently falls in the following order: housework (most difficulty), travel, shopping, finances, and cooking (Gallo et al., 1988).

The main concern for IADL assessment is to distinguish functional dependence from functional independence, the activities that a person can or cannot perform. Administration of IADL instruments may be made on a quarterly or yearly basis to demonstrate change in functional independence. The Multidimensional Functional Assessment Questionnaire, developed by the Duke University Center for the Study of Aging and Human Development, is an especially valuable IADL instrument for this purpose. However, two other IADL instruments that have received special attention for community and acute care hospital use are the Older Americans Resources and Services (OARS) instrument and the Comprehensive Functional Assessment (CFA) instrument.

  OARS. The Multidimensional Educational Assessment Questionnaire (MFAQ) consists of both IADL and PADL (Physical Activities of Daily Living) sections. This section of the OARS instrument can be self-administered or given by a trained interviewer. As time and personnel are often limited, a briefer version was established. The OARS IADL adaptation consists of seven items: telephone use, travel, shopping, meal preparation, housework, taking own medication, and handling personal finances. The outcomes of the questionnaire can be related to current mental and physical health functioning as they affect one's performance. This adapted version can also be used algorithmically as IADL tasks are more complex than PADL tasks and can have a broader impact on the person's over-all functional status. Employment of the MFAQ is used to target older adults who need more extensive assessment or to facilitate their entrance into a health service program that may assist functional independence.

CFA. Besdine (1983) discussed the applicability of the CFA to both acute care hospitals and long-term care facilities. Acute care hospitals have been reluctant to implement comprehensive functional assessments for two primary reasons. First, acute care hospitals primarily focus on catastrophic and rapid-evolving illness and not on chronic diseases. Secondly, hospital administrators perceive that a comprehensive assessment is too time consuming (average is 45 to 60 minutes) and would overburden an already pressured staff. Despite this reluctance, Besdine provides a strong rationale for using the CFA in long-term care facilities and acute care hospitals.

Functional Assessment Recommendation

Functional assessment focuses not just on disease and declining biological, psychological, and social components inherent in aging but on their consequences. Client deficits as well as their remaining capabilities and assets are identified. Consequently, health promotion assessments that include functional status provide more systematic and comprehensive information that can be used for preventive and rehabilitation objectives. As Becker and Cohen (1984) conclude:

> Since the aging process is characterized by the acquisition of multiple age--and disease--related deficits, primary care providers need to appropriately detect functional impairments through multi-dimensional assessment and orchestrate compensatory responses in an effort to restore, maximize, and maintain functional status and independence for as long as possible. (p. 923)

CHAPTER SUMMARY

The general applicability of a comprehensive health assessment that includes functional status is not restricted exclusively to the care of the elderly. A comparable approach can be taken toward persons of any age who are prone to acute and chronic illness. However, due to increased probability of acquiring age- and disease-related deficits associated with the aging process, the elderly are most likely to benefit from a comprehensive approach to health assessment; such an approach would include an assessment of physical, psychological, emotional, social, and economic components.

Because the health problems of the elderly are multidimensional, Becker and Cohen (1984) emphasize the need for a variety of health-related disciplines to participate in assessment programs. The team approach allows the division of time, labor, and expertise among several key health professions. Dividing multidimensional health assessment into several components facilitates data collection and interpretation. By emphasizing functional status, the basic continuum and integration of health promotion services to meet the interests and needs of the elderly may be maintained.

CHAPTER 4

PRESCRIPTIVE PHYSICAL FITNESS FOR OLDER ADULTS

The attainment of physical fitness has been glorified today through exercise centers, racquetball clubs, and a myriad of celebrity aerobic exercise programs. Advertisements depicting sleek, physically trim bodies running or swimming make physical fitness look simple. However, these misleading images cause the novice to acquire unrealistic expectations. Disparity between the image of physical fitness and the reality of exercise leads to exhaustion, pain, and finally withdrawal. Although persons of any age can significantly increase their habitual levels of physical fitness safely, it is imperative that guidance be provided for assuring they exercise safely.

Proper fitness guidance is especially important for older adults. Due to declining responses to homeostatic displacements with aging, vigorous exercise programs for older adults should be prescribed in the same manner drugs are prescribed. This chapter addresses prescriptive exercise programs by focusing on: (1) the human machine and the energy system, (2) basic components of well-balanced fitness programs, (3) safety considerations, and (4) conceptual design of physical fitness programs.

THE HUMAN MACHINE AND THE ENERGY SYSTEM

The human body is a complex, sophisticated and extraordinarily versatile machine. Similar to any machine, its performance on the outside is dependent on what goes on inside. The process of generating energy and putting it to work is the most important internal bodily function. Basically, the amount of work one can perform is determined by the working condition of a number of vital parts in the human machine; i.e., the lungs, blood, heart, blood vessels, and the muscle cells. These vital parts are directly affected by fitness, particularly those parts involved in the energy-generating process.

Reduced Human Machine Efficiency

All bodies require approximately the same amount of oxygen to meet minimal existence requirements. However, the key is not how much oxygen the human system requires at any one time but rather the ease and efficiency with which it is able to meet that requirement. The more fit the human system, the less effort it will take to receive, process, distribute, and utilize the required oxygen. Probably the clearest indicator of how hard the human system is working is the heart rate. The average heart rate of a fit person generally ranges from 55 to 65 beats per minute.

An unfit human machine normally has to work 20 to 30% harder just to meet the minimal existence requirements of everyday life. In a day, that totals 28,000 more heart beats for the unfit heart compared to the fit heart. In one year, the unfit heart has experienced approximately 10,512,000 extra beats of unnecessary workload. This increased tax on the heart leads to a loss of efficiency in the machinery network of the human system.

- The lungs transfer less oxygen in the blood.
- The oxygen-carrying capacity is reduced by up to 20%.
- The heart muscle becomes weak and flabby and requires more beats to perform its basic functions.
- The blood vessels become less elastic and clogged with sediment. Fewer vessels are in service for delivering oxygen-laden blood. Those vessels still in service are less efficient due to inelasticity and impeded blood flow.

The inefficiency of the human machine has many detrimental effects on everyday performance. An unfit person feels less energetic, sluggish, and tires easily. But, reduced efficiency is only one-half of the picture. Reduced total capacity is the second half.

Reduced Total Capacity

Even in modern sedentary life, the human system is called on to do something extra. This "extra" demand may require access to large quantities of oxygen. For many older adults, simply climbing a flight of stairs or carrying groceries from the car to the front doorstep can create a sudden demand for oxygen. In response to an increased energy demand, performing muscles accelerate the energy-generating process. Oxygen is burned at a more rapid rate and a call to the cardio-respiratory system is placed to replenish the oxygen supply. Immediately, the lungs commence breathing faster, the heart pumps harder, and the oxygen extracting system between the blood and the working muscles is more efficient. Whether or not the human machine can cope with the increased demand for oxygen is dependent on how well-prepared it is to meet these functions.

The unfit body goes through the same motions as the fit body, albeit with different results. The lungs breathe more and more in a valiant attempt to keep up with energy demands. The heart beats harder and harder in an attempt to deliver oxygen-laden blood. But the blood vessels strain under the volume of blood being forced through inelastic channels. No matter how hard the unfit human system works, the unfit system still may not be able to meet the oxygen demand. As a whole, the unfit human system is suffering from a reduced total capacity. Eventually, oxygen deficit builds up and the human system shuts off. This experienced energy crisis of the human machine can happen even to the Olympic-caliber athlete. The salient point, however, is that the energy crisis happens sooner and more frequently to the unfit human machine. In the unfit body, a casual stroll can be too taxing.

Homeostasis and Organ Reserve

The human body may be viewed as an assembly of components functioning at various levels of organization. Homeostasis, in turn, has been defined as the regulation of bodily functions within precise limits. But, homeostasis is an ideal concept; regulatory mechanisms do not always return bodily functions to their original state. Health, therefore, may be viewed as corresponding to the situation in which the organism responds adaptively and restores its original integrity. The important point is that with age there is a decline in the ability to respond to disturbances. Fries and Crapo (1981) describe this declining vitality to the human machine using an automobile analogy:

> . . . given the human age of puberty, one might speculate that most individuals should live 70 years or so without serious malfunction. As in our automobile analogy, the body seems designed to outlast the warranty period (puberty) and the period of initial ownership (parenthood), with enough reserve to ensure that most individuals will survive these stages without a serious breakdown. After that, both you and your automobile are on linear lines of decay of performance of components, and on exponential lines of likelihood of total breakdown. (p. 39)

Admittedly, the declining human machine is a normal process of wear and tear. But, the human machine is not inherently fallible to decline and decay. Although intrinsic limitations may be imposed by normal aging, physical activity is a vital factor in establishing the boundaries of these limitations. For example, one of the clearest predictors of life expectancies is called "vital capacity" which is basically the exhalation volume and force from the lungs. In those people who engage in regular moderate activity, the level of vital capacity does not taper off as fast as in those people who don't exercise (Bortz, 1992).

Summary — Effects of Exercise on the Aging Process

This section explored the human machine as an energy system. The reduction of total capacity and the principle of organ reserve were addressed. Essentially, as the organism ages one expects losses in functional capacity at the tissue level, organ level, and the system level of organization. It is not a major revelation to claim that functional decrements can, and often do, affect physical and mental health. Yet, there is evidence that carefully planned physical activity programs can help prevent or diminish the severity of many chronic health conditions affecting the elderly.

A detailed discussion of the role that physical activity plays for enhancing physiological and psychological biomarkers is beyond the scope of this book. However, the reader is encouraged to consult Bortz (1992) and deVries (1982) for such a discussion. Fossel (1996) reviews physical changes associated with aging and includes exercise impacts.

Six Keys to Physical Fitness

Fitness programs must be balanced to incorporate five key components. They are: (1) aerobic training, (2) strength and endurance, (3) flexibility, (4) balance, (5) body composition, and (6) range of motion (ROM). The author's discussion of these components is not meant to be a blueprint for every conceivable guideline for working with older adults; older people are too diverse for that.[1] Instead, we will focus on the basic goals and principles for each of the fitness dimensions and include pertinent resource references for further exploration.

Key 1: Aerobic Training. The more oxygen we can supply to our working muscles determines our cardiorespiratory fitness. And through exercise the body can be conditioned to use oxygen more efficiently. A body that does little work becomes deconditioned and is inefficient in extracting oxygen for muscle use. Thomas Cureton, an exercise physiologist, notes: "the human body is the only machine that breaks down when not used. Moreover, it's also the only mechanism that functions better and more healthfully the more it is used" (Shepherd, 1984, p. 94). However, aerobic training programs, for older adults, must be designed with the utmost care. Crash programs that attempt to do too much too soon result in injuries and program attrition. Prescriptive aerobic training, therefore, must pay particular attention to (1) the type of aerobic activity, (2) the intensity level of the activity, (3) duration of the activity, (4) frequency of the activity, and (5) progression of fitness levels.

Type of Activity. The intent of an exercise program should be to increase or maintain the participant's functional capacity. Aerobic exercise accomplishes this goal. Muscles work by converting fuel (nutrients) to energy. They do this by two different processes: (1) Anaerobic and (2) Aerobic. Anaerobic activity involves chemical processes in the muscles that release energy without oxygen. Aerobic activity requires oxygen and is dependent upon the cardio-respiratory system muscles and oxygen to function, and the need for oxygen increases dramatically during work performance.

Aerobic exercise is generally defined as steady state exercise that demands an uninterrupted output from working muscles over a 12 minute period. Aerobic endurance activities are generally classified into two groups. Group I exercises require sustained exercise intensity with little variability in heart rate response. Group II exercises do not maintain continuous exercise intensity (see Table 4-1).

---

[1]When the older adult has identified medical problems or diagnosed disease, the exercise prescription must be modified to enable the participant to attain the best physiologic and psychologic adjustment to the physical activity program. The reader interested in such modifications for older adults should consult the American College of Sports Medicine (1980) and Piscopo (1985).

Table 4-1. Aerobic classification.

Group I Steady-State	Group II Stop and Go
Cross-Country Skiing	Tennis
Jumping Rope	Downhill Skiing
Running in Place	Football
Cycling Outdoors	Calisthenics
Stationary Bicycle	Handball
Rowing	Racquetball
Mini-Trampoline	

The main criteria of aerobic exercises are that they are continuous and steady. Intermittent exercises can be used for aerobic benefits but usually take longer in order to achieve the necessary cardio-respiratory goal. Although both Group I and Group II physical activities are valuable, there are a few guidelines that should be considered when prescribing such exercises for older adults.

Working with older adults requires particular concern about increased blood pressure. Muscle contractions that squeeze down blood vessels within the muscle tissue create significant and undesirable pressure elevations. Higher pressure becomes necessary for blood flow in this muscle area. Such localized blood pressure can reset the "central mechanism" and cause an increase in total blood pressure. Isometric exercises, muscle contractions maintained in a stationary position for prolonged periods, cause the greatest elevations.

According to deVries (1982), crawling and cycling exercises produce isometric tension. Activities requiring the least cardiac effort, which do not cause elevated blood pressure, are muscle contraction activities followed by relaxation. Walking and jogging fit this criteria since they are rhythmic activities using large muscles which minimize the high activation of small muscle masses. In other words, there isn't time during the period of contraction for blood pressure to build.

Group I activities should be used in the early stages of a conditioning or rehabilitation program. Group II activities are valuable for directing the participant's attention away from exercises and boredom and, yet, can be used for obtaining aerobic training. Competitive games and sports should not be used until participants obtain a minimum exercise intensity of 5 METs and an exercise specialist becomes familiar with the psychologic and physiologic responses of the participant. If used, competitive activities for C-H participants (Table 4-2) should be modified for sedentary or multiple risk participants. Asymptomatic sedentary participants (C-E) may usually be included in recreational games and sports activities after a six to ten week conditioning period.

Intensity of Exercise. How hard should a person exercise? A certain level of vigor in exercise is necessary to condition the cardio-respiratory system. Finding the proper intensity is not easy. Let's say you pick running as an exercise. If you run too slowly, it may take forever to receive the desired effect. If you run too fast, you'll tire too quickly

Table 4-2. Classification by age and health status of participants for exercise testing.
Category

A	Asymptomatic, physically active persons of any age without CHD risk factors or disease.	
B	Asymptomatic, physically inactive persons less than 35 years of age without CHD risk factors or disease.	
C	Asymptomatic, physically inactive persons 35 years and older without CHD risk factors or disease.	
D	Asymptomatic, physically active or inactive persons of any age with CHD risk factors but no known disease.	
E	Asymptomatic persons of any age with known disease.	
F	Symptomatic, physically active persons clinically stable for 6 months or longer.	
G	Symptomatic, physically inactive persons clinically stable for 6 months or longer.	
H	Symptomatic persons with recent onset of CHD or a change in disease status (Example: Recent myocardial infarction, unstable angina, coronary artery bypass surgery).	
I	Persons for whom exercise is contraindicated (see Table 3, Contraindications for Exercise and Exercise Testing).	

From The American College of Sports Medicine, *Guidelines for Graded Exercise Testing and Exercise Prescription, 2nd edition.* Copyright 1982 Lea & Febiger. Reprinted by permission of Williams and Wilkins, a Waverly Company.

and get nowhere. There is an in-between point at which you are working your muscles hard enough for maximum benefit but not overdoing it. The key for using aerobic programs is the intensity and vigorous levels of exercise which do not exceed safe training limits. Zohman (1974) describes the ideal exertion level as a target zone of between 60 to 80% of maximal aerobic power (i.e., functional capacity).

> The concept of maximal aerobic power . . . is merely the technical description of the fact that there is a point for each of us where, despite our best efforts, the heart and circulation cannot deliver any more oxygen to the tissues and we cannot exercise much longer or harder without approaching exhaustion. At this point, the tissues are making oxygen available to the bloodstream but that oxygen cannot be transported by the blood to the muscles fast enough to create energy

for exercise. Almost simultaneously with reaching this limitation of
oxygen supply, the heart becomes unable to beat any faster.
(Zohman, 1974, p. 11)

The recommended conditioning for asymptomatic adults is between 60 to 80% of their
functional capacity. Exercise prescriptions for older adults should never exceed 85% of
their functional capacity. Participants, including cardiac patients, who have a low
functional capacity may initiate their physiologic conditioning between 40 and 60% and
increase the duration of the physical activity. Thus it is important to evaluate a particular physical activity in terms of the stress it places on the participant's cardiorespiratory
system. Oxygen consumption and pulse rate methods are employed for this purpose.

Oxygen Consumption. The actual oxygen consumption during exercise, termed
maximal volume of oxygen uptake (VO_2 MAX), is determined. Stress tests are used for
determining the difference between oxygen content of inhaled and exhaled air during a
maximal exertion. For example, if jogging at five miles per hour requires an oxygen
consumption of 30 ml/kg min. and if the jogger's maximum oxygen consumption is 60
ml/kg min., this particular exercise would represent an aerobic stress of 50% of the
maximal aerobic capacity. For another person with a lower aerobic capacity of 50 ml/kg
min., jogging at five miles per hour would still approximate 30 ml/kg min., but this
person would be exercising at 60% maximum. Thus the strenuousness of any physical
activity is relative and depends on the present level of physiologic conditioning
(Neiman, 1990).

Once the participant's health status and functional capacity are known, the exercise
intensity can be defined. Graded exercise tests are generally used to establish the
boundaries for conditioning intensity. Peak and average intensity of exercise are
determined by taking a prescribed percentage of the individual's functional capacity.
According to deVries (1982), peak conditioning should be set no higher than 90%.
Average conditioning would approximate 70% of the individual's functional capacity.
For example, peak conditioning for a person with a maximal functional capacity of
8 METs would receive an exercise prescription of 7.2 METs (.90 x 8). The reader is
cautioned that exercising people at peak intensity levels can be hazardous, especially
for older adults, and thus should be approached with extreme caution. As a general
rule of thumb, until the participant becomes accustomed to exercise, an intensity level
of one MET lower than estimated should be utilized. Once the physical activity director
has determined the prescribed fitness intensity level in METs, the next step is to select
an activity that can obtain the desired physiologic conditioning level. Physical activities,
such as walking, jogging, and the bicycle ergometer are directly related to the speed of
movement, measurable resistance, or mass lifted. However, these activities may be
complicated by changes in the environment; e.g., snow, wind. Prescription and maintenance of safe exercise intensity levels for complex individual sports (e.g., tennis,
swimming) are much more difficult. If complex individual sports are used, however, the
reader is encouraged to consult Howley and Franks (1992).

Pulse-Rate Monitoring. Although the assessment of exercise intensity by direct measurement of oxygen consumption is quite accurate, it is impractical to complete such measurement without a fairly extensive exercise physiology laboratory. Fortunately, the problem of exercising at a prescribed conditioning level, regardless of the physical activity used and/or most environmental conditions, is simplified by using pulse-rate monitors as a measure of exercise intensity. In general, a linear relationship exists between the individual's exercise heart rate and the exercise intensity in either METs or oxygen uptake. The VO_2 maximum corresponds closely to the maximal heart rate in most normal individuals. The reader should key in on the word "normal." Many older adults may suffer from physical limitations requiring precise measurement of the maximum oxygen uptake.

Similar to a physician's specific prescription for a given illness, there are recommended prescriptions for developing physical fitness. The minimal prescription is called the "threshold level" and is that intensity level below which a conditioning effect will not occur. Most prescriptive levels are between 60% and 85% of your maximum heart rate. The range between 60% and 85% is called the target heart rate. Three methods are popularly used for calculating the target heart range: (a) maximum heart rate formula; (b) resting heart rate formula; and (c) maximal/ minimum heart rate correction formula (MHR Range Formula).

The maximum heart rate formula attempts to develop a threshold level represented by minimal and maximal heart rate for optimal training performance. Exercise intensity below the threshold level will not attain an optimal conditioning effect. Exercise intensity above the threshold level is too intense and dangerous for the participant's health. Figure 4-1 illustrates the "training sensitivity zone" that represents the lower threshold level of 70% and the upper level of 85% of maximum heart rate for each age group.

A second method for calculating the target heart rate is determined by multiplying the difference between the maximum and resting heart rates by the same percentage used to determine the exercise prescription in METs. This value is then added to the resting heart rate. For example:

Maximum Heart Rates (beats per minute) =	150
	- 70
Resting Heart Rate	80
	x 70%
Conditioning Intensity	56
Resting Heart Rate	+ 70
Minimum Training Heart Rate	126

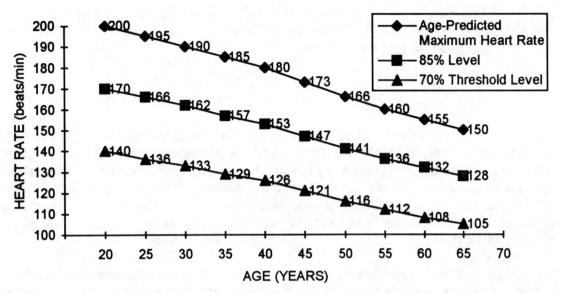

Figure 4-1. Training sensitivity zone for maximal heart rate for use in aerobic exercise programs.

Although one should be concerned about attaining the minimum heart rate performance required to attain optimal aerobic impact, an even more vital concern is that the participant does not exercise him or herself into a stroke or heart attack. The MHR Range formula, the third pulse rate method, is a more conservative approach to prescribing exercise and is highly recommended by the author. Three steps are used in calculating the MHR Range:

- Step 1. Determine your resting heart rate (RHR). During one week take your RHR several times during the day and average them. For example, let's assume your daily RHR averages were 70, 68, 72, 72, 68, 66, 74. The average for these seven daily RHRs is 70 RHR.
- Step 2. Determine your maximum heart rate (MHR) by subtracting your age from the number 220 and for accuracy (+) and (-) 10%. For example, an age 40 participant's MHR would be 220 - 40 = 180. Then for accuracy: 180 + (.10) x (180) = 198 and 180 - (.10) x (180) = 162. 198 and 162 are the limits of your MHR.
- Step 3. Decide on the intensity level you will use during your aerobic exercise. This intensity level should depend on your present fitness level, program goals, and personal interests. If you selected an intensity level of 70%, then your THR Range would be calculated as follows:

$$[(MHR - RHR) \times .7] + RHR = \text{Target HR}$$

This calculation should be done using 198 and 162 as the MHR in separate calculations. Using the MHR Range formula, the intensity exercise heart range would be:

(a) Maximum Range: [(198 - 70) x .7] + 70 = 199.6 MHR
(b) Minimum Range: [(162 - 70) x .7] + 70 = 134.4 MHR

Table 4-3 summarizes the exercise heart rates that would be calculated using the 70% and 85% intensity exercise level for the three pulse-rate monitoring systems. The MHR formula has been found to commonly underestimate the target heart rate for a given MET level by approximately 15%. For that reason, some exercise enthusiasts recommend that the MHR formula automatically be adjusted by adding 15% to the target heart rate calculated. Thus the training heart range for our 40-year-old specimen using the MHR formula would be 145 (70% intensity) and 165 (85% intensity).

One urgent caution: I would like you to look at Figure 4-1 again. The maximum advised intensity of 85% for a 65-year-old adult suggests a heart rate not to exceed 128 heart beats per minute. It is important that exercise participants learn to pulse monitor their exercise so as not to exercise themselves into a heart attack. Employed by the participant and the instructor, pulse rates can be used to determine whether the individual is exerting enough or too much. As an indicator of how much blood the heart is pumping, pulse rate is related to how much oxygen is being delivered to the working muscles.

Taking the pulse from the radial artery, carotid artery or temporal artery have been used objectively to measure the heart rate. As one becomes familiar with the feeling of the appropriate intensity of aerobic exercise, the need for an objective measure of intensity declines. "Perceived exertion" can then be used as a subjective monitor of intensity. Borg's perceived exertion scale is an excellent monitor for this purpose. Subjective exertion symptoms are discussed later in this chapter.

Duration of Training. Generally, exercise conditioning periods will vary between 15 to 60 minutes. This length of time is necessary in order to improve functional capacity. The duration of the activity will be inversely related to the exercise intensity; i.e., the more intense, the shorter the duration. Persons with higher functional capacities, compared to people with lower functional capacities, may maintain a higher intensity level for a longer duration. The conditioning response is a result of the interaction between the exercise intensity and duration.

Table 4-3. Technique for pulse rate estimates.

Technique	70 percent	85 percent
MHR Formula	145	176
RHR Formula	147.0	163.5
MHR Range	134.4- 159.6	148.2- 178.8

It is possible to achieve significant cardiovascular improvements by exercising for only five to ten minutes at a 90% intensity level of functional capacity. However, this practice is not advisable for older adults. For older adults, deVries (1982) recommends a duration of 30 minutes at about a 60% intensity level for continuous training physical activities. This can be done by walking, jogging, swimming, cycling, and rope skipping type activities. By their very nature, continuous activities used for physiologic conditioning are submaximum and can be engaged in for considerable periods of time. The American College of Sports Medicine provides more precise recommenda-tions for sedentary, asymptomatic, and symptomatic participants (Table 4-2, Categories C-H); i.e., moderate duration (20 to 30 minutes) and moderate intensity (70 to 80%). Changes in the exercise prescription may then be applied as the individual's functional capacity increases and as physiological adaptation to exercise occurs.

Frequency of Training. In general, it is necessary to exercise at least twice a week in order to obtain adaptation changes in the cardio-respiratory system. The ideal frequency for training is three times per week. Interestingly, several studies suggest that running four or five times per week was either no greater or only slightly greater than when the same exercise was performed three times per week (Katch & McArdle, 1983). If weight control is a main concern, strong consideration should be given to exercising five or six times per week. After the age of 40, however, participants exercising five or six times per week should switch exercises from day to day. The reason is that muscles can't repair as quickly after use as we get older. Additional time is needed for recuperation.

The frequency of exercise, in part, will depend on the duration and intensity of the exercise session and session objective. For individuals with a functional capacity of 3 METs or less, sessions of five minutes several times daily would be desirable. Fifteen-minute sessions twice daily would be advisable for participants with three to five METs capacity. Participants with five to eight METs should exercise three times a week for 20 to 30 minutes.

Training Progression. Fitness programs must take into account training progression. The salient point is that in order to ensure continued improvement in cardio-respiratory capacity during training, the relative degree of exercise overload must keep pace with the adaptive changes that occur both in performance and physiology (Katch & McArdle, 1983). Thus exercise leaders need to adjust the level of activity in order to obtain the maximum fitness impact. Three steps of progression are employed: (1) initial conditioning, (2) improvement, and (3) maintenance.

Initial Conditioning. Included in the initial conditioning stage are stretching, light calisthenics and low-level aerobic activities which should be accompanied by a minimum of muscle soreness and discomfort. The point is to avoid debilitating injury and program attrition. It is advisable to start your exercise regimen one MET lower than the estimated 70 to 80% of functional capacity. With physiologic conditioning, the heart rate will decrease for a constant exercise intensity. Thus, the heart rate is a good indicator of activity progression from one level to another. Progression should be determined through consultation between the physical activity director and a physician. Both objective and subjective factors should be used in the progression decision.

The initial phase of the aerobic program should be at least 12 minutes duration and then, gradually increased. Frequency depends on the initial functional capacity and cardio-respiratory level. The initial conditioning activities will usually last from four to six weeks, but this duration is dependent on the adaptation of the participant to the program. For example, a participant ranked "fair" may reside in the initial program for six to ten weeks, while the participant marked "good" or "high" may be exempted from the initial program or remain in this program for a short period of time. However, health status must also be considered in progression decisions. For example, a patient with symptoms of exertional angina may only be able to tolerate a workout of 40 to 50% of functional capacity.

Improvement Conditioning Stage. The improvement stage differs from the initial conditioning stage since the participant is progressed at a more rapid rate. During this stage, the older adult is advanced to the peak conditioning rate of 70% of functional capacity and the duration is increased rather consistently every two or three weeks. The ability of the participant to adapt to the current level of conditioning will dictate the frequency and magnitude of the progression. As a general rule, the adaptation to conditioning takes approximately 40% longer, or an additional week, for each decade of life after age 30. Cardiac patients and less fit individuals will require more adaptation time. It is also recommended that symptom limited participants initially use discontinuous aerobic exercises and progress toward more continuous exercise. Duration of exercise should be increased before increasing the intensity.

Maintenance Conditioning Stage. After the first six to eight months of training, the maintenance stage of exercise prescription begins. During this stage, the participant has obtained a satisfactory level of cardio-respiratory fitness and is no longer interested in increasing the conditioning load. Although further fitness improvement may be minimal, continuing the same fitness level workout enables one to maintain fitness. It is at this point that the fitness objectives and goals should be reviewed. To maintain fitness (i.e., prevent deconditioning), a program similar to caloric cost to the initial program should be combined with the needs of the participant over a long span. Enjoyment becomes paramount. In other words, more enjoyable activities may be substituted in place of walking or jogging. This is not to say that walking and jogging are not enjoyable. The point is that participation in activities that are enjoyed are more likely to be continued.

Recommendation. Almost any aerobic activity that is rhythmic, sustained for at least 12 minutes, and rigorous in that it maintains a 60% intensity level (perhaps a little less for obese participants) is good for developing cardiopulmonary fitness. The type of prescriptive activity, intensity, frequency, duration and progression plan are all critical considerations. Probably the safest aerobic activities for the elderly are progressive walking, jogging, and swimming. For aerobic programs, deVries (1982) Vigor Regained, and Corbin and Corbin's (1983) Reach For It, and Yanker's (1983) Exercise Walking are highly recommended. Shepherd (1994) provides a science foundation for aerobic conditioning and health.

Key 2: Muscular Strength and Endurance. Strength is the capacity of the muscle to exert force against a resistance. Endurance is the capacity of the muscle to exert force repeatedly over a period of time, or to apply and sustain strength. It is beneficial for the older adult to be conditioned not only to apply force (strength) or apply strength with speed (power) but also to sustain such force over a prolonged period (endurance). Fatigued muscles provide less force and become less efficient and less effective. Muscles can become fatigued, however, without significant physical exertion. For example, long hours of standing can fatigue back muscles. In other words, muscles in poor condition fatigue more readily. Well-conditioned muscles are able to perform more work and still call in less muscle fibers. Thus, a well-designed muscle strength and endurance program can enable older adults to have more energy for normal daily activities and enough extra money to pursue new and different leisure interests.

Strength Training. Isotonic and isometric represent the two basic muscular contractions. Isotonic (dynamic) contractions shorten the muscles with a resulting motion; e.g., bending your arms to pick up a bag of groceries. Isometric (static) contractions apply muscular force but muscle length does not change and the movement does not occur; e.g., pushing against an immovable object such as a wall (Getchell, 1983). Recently, isokinetic exercises have been employed as a method to combine the advantages of both isotonic and isometric movements. Isokinetics involve the use of specialized apparatus to provide a maximal resistance to the muscles (isometrics) throughout their full range of motion (isotonics).

Isotonic, isometric, and isokinetic exercises have been shown to increase strength and endurance by focusing on two fitness principles, overload and specificity. A muscle must be overloaded to be strengthened. Strength is accrued through an increase in muscle fiber (muscle bulk) rather than from an increase in muscle fiber number. This strength development accrues only to the actual muscle(s) exercised. Overloading can be applied by (1) increasing the magnitude of the load (weight), (2) increasing the number of repetitions, and/or (3) changing the body position to favor or unfavor mechanical leverage position of the movement performed (Piscopo, 1985). Mechanical leverage requires some knowledge of basic kinesiology principles. For example, a sit-up is more difficult to execute with hands behind the head than along the thighs— changes the center of gravity to one's chest. Strength development occurs through any of these three methods provided greater tension is placed on the muscle fibers.

In structuring strength development programs for older adults, we must remember that overload is a relative term. Excessive resistance type exercises for the younger athlete is quite different than an overload regimen for an older adult. Although faster gains in muscular strength accrue through the use of heavier loads or mechanical leverages, older adults should not be exposed to heavy overload practices. For example, in weight lifting, lighter weights and increased repetitions should be employed. Due to biological changes, excessive overload poses potential injury to an older adult's cardiovascular and musculoskeletal systems. Isometric exercises have also, historically, been disfavored by the medical profession for older adults due to blood pressure concerns.

Despite the concern over isometric activities, it is unrealistic to suggest that isometric work is not part of the everyday pursuits of the older adult. Lifting, holding, or moving an arm or leg involves some muscle static contraction. Moreover, recent research suggests that both dynamic and static contractions increase systemic blood pressure. The magnitude of this pressure increase is dependent upon the degree of tension exertion on the muscle, as well as other factors; e.g., using big muscles of the trunk and legs versus arm exercises (Piscopo, 1985).

Recommendation. Three types of resistive training programs have been very popular: (1) free weights and weight machines (Universal gym apparatus), (2) Nautilus System, and (3) isokinetic systems. Free weights and nautilus systems are commonly found in community recreation centers and YMCAs. Nautilus clubs are a form of commercial recreation and their fees may be prohibitive. Isokinetic systems are terribly expensive and are usually housed only in hospitals and/or university research centers. Therefore, free weights and strength resistance exercises appear to offer the most potential for community agencies working with older adults. As long as older adults know the proper techniques for strength training, are careful about pulse-rate monitoring, avoid breath-holding during isometric maneuvers, and are generally sensible in training protocol, there is no reason why older adults can't benefit relatively as much from strength training as younger individuals. The reader is encouraged to consult Piscopo (1985) for resistance type exercises for older adults. Rosenberg and Evans (1991), Williams (1994) and Zatsiovsky (1995) are excellent resources.

In addition, isometric training can and should be employed through light weight lifting or low-level isometric activities. The valsalva effect can be avoided provided free breathing is utilized during muscular contraction without breath holding. This procedure keeps the windpipe open and serves to counteract interthoracic pressure. However, the use of resistive or isometric exercises for older adults should be pursued only after medical clearance has been received. The following protocol, developed by Spackman, should also be employed for isometric activities:

- Slowly ease the contraction. Slowly beginning to push or pull as hard as you can without pain, holding for 6 seconds.
- As you ease the contraction, begin counting aloud: 1000-and-one, 1000-and-two, for 6 seconds.
- Ease the contraction off slowly at the end of 6 seconds.
- Relax for 6 seconds.
- Repeat the exercise three times holding for 6 seconds each. Breathe normally!!
- Always count aloud during each exercise.
- Should you have any pain, ease the contraction off and only push as hard as you can without pain.

- As your strength increases, all pain should disappear.
- If pain persists, stop the exercise and see your physician.
  (Spackman, 1981, pp. 12-14)

Key 3: Flexibility. If you were to gaze into the distant horizon and note a short, stopped figure, walking with slow, short steps, you may readily conclude that this person is old. Why does aging contort so many people in this way? The problem is prolonged non-use of muscles and joints through full ranges of motion, and so the muscles shorten. Until our muscles ache, we ignore them and lose some of their potential. With age, the ligaments, tendons and muscle fasciae (sheaths covering muscles) become less extensible. Unless we make efforts to maintain flexibility as we age, we literally fold up. Our hinge joints contract and the trunk tilts forward as the angle between the trunk and hip closes. The knees bend and ankle tendons shorten. The result is a folded, tottering, unstable stance.

To improve flexibility, the goal is not just to lengthen the muscles but to lengthen the tendons and connective tissue. Muscle fibers are held together by fibrous connective tissue between the fibers. The network of connective tissue and fasciae connect together into dense connective tissue that attaches to bones. The joints are commonly encased in a fibrous capsule which is also connective tissue. Connective tissue is composed of elastic fibers and protein fibers called collagen. Collagen has a chemical composition that is elastic in quality and substances that are more plastic which behave like putty. Stretching for flexibility depends upon this plastic characteristic and is directed toward permanent lengthening of muscle structures as opposed to the stretch-snapback character of the elastic substance.

Fasciae are the easiest muscle structures to stretch and tendons the most difficult. But, failure to stretch these components shortens the fasciae and places undue pressure on nerve pathways. Many of the muscle aches and pains we experience are due to this blockage of nerve impulses. As we experience aches and pains, we tend to shy away from further use. Eventually, calcium salt deposits in the joints and the process of complete, irreversible immobilization takes place.

Muscles are not the only body components that fall toll to disuse. Bones suffering from inactivity lose minerals, soften and shrink. Osteoporosis, bone softening, is a common affliction associated with inactivity or immobilization. As the bones dissolve they become more fragile, and even a slight fall can lead to a serious fracture. For example, three-fourths of hip fractures in older persons are related to osteoporosis. Although the cause of osteoporosis is not known, it is known that its prevention includes the old adage, "use it or lose it." Stretching and strength exercises maintaining the full range of joint and body motion have been shown to prevent osteoporosis (Wiswell, 1980). Once bone has become damaged, however, it is also imperative to learn how to do things easily. The inclusion of proper stretching and strength exercises will go a long way in preventing the crippling deformities and complications of osteoporosis.

Planning a Flexibility Program. Medical and fitness experts concur that stretching is the single most important part of an exercise program designed to prevent injuries, reduce muscle tension and promote flexibility. For stretching serves not just as a preface (warm-up) and epilogue (cooldown) to exercise programs, it is a vital workout component in itself. However, stretching done incorrectly can cause more harm than good. Thus it is important to understand the right stretching techniques and progress gradually. Exercise for stretching can be performed in any of four popular ways: (1) ballistically (active), (2) statistically, (3) passively, and (4) hold-relax.

Ballistic Stretching. Ballistic stretching consists of a series of bouncing movements designed to increase the range of muscle motion. For example, many of the calisthenic exercises we all experience in our scholastic physical education courses employed ballistic stretching; e.g., toe touches. Ballistic stretching is not recommended, at any age, as they pose injury risk to muscles and joints.

Static Stretching. Static stretching increases the length of the muscle but without a bouncing or forcing movement. It simply involves moving until you feel tightness in the muscle and then holding that position for a set period of time. Commonly associated with yoga, muscles are stretched for a period of 30 to 60 seconds for maximum benefit. After the participant has held the stretch for this period of time, the muscle tension will seem to decrease and thus allow further stretching without pain. Static stretching lengthens the muscle and surrounding tissue, reducing the risk of injury. Jean Couch, author of the Runner's World Yoga Book, adds that the slowness of this approach gives greater control and positioning of the muscle.

Passive Stretching. Passive stretching uses partner to apply enough pressure to cause stretching beyond what an individual can do himself or herself. If a person can totally relax his/her muscle fibers, another person's applying of pressure can avoid the problem of partial contraction of muscle fibers. Physical therapists often employ this device. There is a danger, however, of forcing a stretch beyond the point of normal relaxation of the muscles and tendons causing tear and injury. Passive stretches, therefore, should be limited to supervised medical situations and for older adults who cannot move under their own volition.

Hold-Relax. A more sophisticated stretching program is the hold-relax method. Hold-relax stretching is based on Herman Kabat's Proprioceptive Neuromuscular Facilitation (PNF). PNF is a popular stretching program, largely focusing on range of motion and strength, prescribed by surgeons for injury rehabilitation. Many experts consider the hold-relax method the most effective technique for increasing the range of motion of muscles and connective tissue. The muscle is not stretched directly but is contracted or "held" for five seconds against a resistance. Then, as the muscle is "relaxed" for five seconds, the opposing antagonistic muscles will move the stretched muscle gently into a new and broader range of motion (Tyne & Mitchell, 1983).

Recommendation. Static, passive, PNF and hold-relax stretching programs are all valuable techniques for older adults. Ballistic stretches are to be avoided. Piscopo (1985) provides an exhaustive list of exercises for static and passive flexibility methods. Tyne and Mitchell (1983) and McAtee (1996) should be consulted for both static and hold-relax stretching exercises. Special concerns for older adults include stretching programs directed toward low back pain, maintaining good posture and escaping muscle spasm and injury. However, it is worthwhile to remember that flexibility operates under the principle of specificity. If a senior adult is seeking better athletic performance in a selected sport, the flexibility program should parallel the movements required by that sport. Alter (1996) provides an excellent foundation for flexibility and stretching programs.

Key 4: Balance. Motion and stability rely on that silent sense we call balance. Balance empowers us to dance, to walk, to run, to catch a ball and even to think straight. It is the first discipline of human economy. Without balance, our bodily energies would be depleted and our psychological states disturbed by a minimal ripple in habit or expectations. Despite its place in overall fitness, most of us are precariously out of balance in at least one of the three bodily planes: (1) left to right, (2) top to bottom, and (3) front to back. Unbalance in these planes is not caused by our fault alone; cultural bias leads us to be knocked off center (Jones, 1984).

Though these three balance preferences are subtle, chronic posture imbalances bend and stretch our bodies in harmful ways. Slight crookedness can lead to impairment of the circulation system, asymmetry of skeletal and muscular systems, added tension on joints and bones and tension pools in muscles that must constantly counter gravity to maintain us upright. In final,, we feel uncomfortable, confined and drained of energy. But, such feelings need not be a part of our lives. Good balance can conserve energy.

Balance Programs for Older Adults. Our relationship to gravity is regulated by the vestibular apparatus. This apparatus consists of an array of tiny fluid-filled sacs and tubes suspended in the bony labyrinth behind the middle ear on either side of the head. The vestibular apparatus, our innermost sensory organ, operates both physically and metaphorically. Although yielding no direct sensations, it is a silent sense orienting us to our environment. Thus, the vestibular apparatus provides the grid for all other sensory elaboration.

Similar to other bodily dimensions discussed in this book, the vestibular system operates under the adage "use it or lose it." A vestibular system that is only partially stimulated during development will result in less sensory integration and an overall decrease in function potential. For example, children between the ages of three and twelve with various sorts of developmental problems can be helped by a series of vestibular exercises that operate in concert with other sensory systems; e.g., transferring marbles from one container to another while swinging face down in a net. In other words, vestibular training heeds us to pay attention to our urges to walk on a curb, ride a roller coaster or ferris wheel (Jones, 1984).

The important point is that balance, vestibular training, is not confined to the early years. Balance can be enhanced at any age through static and dynamic balance training. Static balance is largely a property of centeredness by keeping the body aligned on the gravitational axis; e.g., the diver's poise as he or she prepares to dive. Dynamic balance is the ability to maintain balance during a balance movement; e.g., a pole vaulter rising toward the cross-bar. A subordinate category of dynamic balance is upright (walking upright) and inverted (walking on hands) balance. Upright and inverted balance also applies to static positions.

The commonest practice form for static balance is to diminish the accustomed base of support. For example, balancing on one leg as you put on your socks and shoes refines your sense of "groundedness." Dynamic balance also responds to practice. However, the balance objective is not to retain equilibrium but to regain it. Research by NASA on space sickness has added significantly to our understanding of dynamic balance. Both motion sickness and space sickness may occur from a sensory mismatch among vision, touch, proprioceptive and vestibular sensory systems. To date, it is a puzzle how the brain accommodates the incongruity between these sensory systems. The solution to this puzzle, however, is significant not only to space sickness but to correcting vestibular deficits that affect the elderly (Jones, 1984).

Recommendation. Fitness commences through a balanced and centered stance. Balanced implies that body weight is evenly distributed, right and left, forward and back, head and toe. Centeredness means that body awareness is concentrated in the center of the abdomen. There are many ways to practice balance and centeredness. Piscopo (1985) provides an excellent series of exercises for static and dynamic balance, using balance beams, calisthenics and aquatic activities, based upon the following principles:

- Maintain an adequate *base of support*; e.g., keep feet slightly apart when standing.
- *Lower the center of gravity* when greater stability is needed; e.g., crouch rather than stand on toes when faced with a fall situation.
- Keep the *line of gravity within the base of support*; stand and sit with proper body alignment so that the line of gravity falls near or on its base of support.
- Widen the base of support in the *direction of the force* or movement; e.g., leaning into the wind with feet apart and one foot forward.
- *Increase friction between the body and supporting surface* for better stability; e.g., wearing rubber soles and appropriate footwear to increase gripping action of the shoe.
- *Maintain adequate strength* to provide the force necessary to regain balance after an unexpected loss; e.g., develop strength of legs to counter the effects of tripping or falling.
- *Focus vision on a stationary object* rather than moving items; e.g., walking a narrow path or plank, focus eyes on a fixed point ahead of your body.

Balance programs for older adults may also draw from the Eastern martial arts practice of centeredness. The practice of centeredness training teaches one to concentrate awareness on different parts of the body; particularly the abdomen. For example, Leonard Energy Training (LET) is a mind-body discipline derived from the sophisticated Japanese martial art of akido and from Western psychology and physical therapy (Leonard, 1984).

Key 5: Exercise and Weight Control. The medical literature well establishes that chronic disease is more prevalent in obese people than individuals with normal body fat levels. It is not clear the degree to which obesity causes specific medical problems since the obese condition is usually intimately related to a number of other indicators that directly affect the risk of medical considerations. Katch and McArdle (1983, p. 135) have summarized the plight of the obese individual as follows: (1) hypertension and increased risk of stroke, (2) renal disease, (3) gallbladder disease, (4) pulmonary disease, (5) osteoarthritis and gout, (6) complications with anesthesia during surgery, (7) breast and endometrial cancer, (8) abnormal lipoprotein and blood plasma concentrations, (9) diabetes mellitus, (10) impairment of cardiac function, (11) psychological traumas, (12) flat feet and intertriginous dermatitis, (13) organ compression by adipose tissue, and (14) impaired heat tolerance.

To get older adults to exercise for weight control, and for that matter all of us, requires that we educated them on the role that exercise plays in weight control. The goal is fat content loss and not weight loss. Exercise and controlled dieting that seeks to gradually alter the energy balance equation offers the best opportunity. Our tendency to add on adipose tissue and reduce our metabolic rate as we age, makes it imperative that we move in this direction.

Theory of Exercise and Weight Control. Until a plan is developed for establishing normal body composition, the rationale underlying the energy balance equation will be utilized. The equation states that body weight will remain constant as long as calorie intake is equal to calorie output (expenditure). Any imbalance in this equation will result in weight loss or weight gain. When more calories are consumed than expended, the excess calories are stored as fat in the adipose tissue depots. An "extra" 3500 KCAL on either the input or output side of the equation equals approximately one pound of stored fat.

Three ways exist for unbalancing the energy equation: (1) reduced caloric intake below daily energy requirements (diets), (2) maintain regular food intake and increase caloric output through additional physical activity above daily energy requirements, and (3) combine the methods of (1) and (2) by decreased food intake and increasing daily energy expenditure through exercise. To illustrate how sensitive this energy balance equation is, a caloric input that exceeds the output by 100 KCAL per day (e.g., one banana) would result in a 10.4 pound gain of fat in one year (365 days x 100 KCAL or -36,500 KCAL = 10.4 pounds).

Weight conscious people, in their attempts to unbalance the energy balance equation, have tended to rely on dietary strategies. Little attention has been paid to exercise. The author's intent is not to review the extensive literature that criticizes an exclusive diet approach to weight control.[2] Yet, Exercise has proven to be an effective weight lowering strategy since it affects our basal metabolic rate by enabling us to burn more calories at rest, burn more calories while we exercise, burn more calories as we become more fit, and is effective in over-coming our body set points for weight control. Despite the effectiveness of exercise for weight control, most people will still choose dieting. Part of the answer may be that it takes no real effort to diet. Exercise, on the other hand, takes effort. Dieting also offers rapid reinforcement as measured in weight loss on a scale. A person would have to walk up and down stairs for four solid hours – time enough to scale the Empire State Building – to lose one pound. Jogging a half mile burns the equivalent of only one apple. As you can see, some people will mistakenly assume that it is easier not to jog, skip the apple and watch TV.

Aerobic Activities — The Key to Weight Control. Richard Simmons, through a very popular daytime television show and a best-selling book entitled *Never-Say-Diet Book*, has become evangelical in emphasizing exercise over faddish dieting. Unfortunately, his zeal has also encouraged millions of viewers and readers to forget aerobic exercise and to engage in spot-reducing regimens through body correcting exercises. Bennett and Gubin (1982) extract the following from Simmons' book, "If you exercise but continue to eat like a horse ... the fat surrounding your muscles will just become firm and solid" ... and that deep breathing is essential to weight loss because "carbon dioxide lives in all those cute little fat cells you're trying to get rid of and just helps them puff up and fill out." These statements might be excused by an exercise physiologist as not dangerous if it were not for Simmons' continued irrationalities. Bennett et al., (1982) continue with Simmons' appeal:

> Unfortunately, walking and related strategies don't do a great deal for many other body areas that need alteration.... The hips, the double chins, the saggy arms don't benefit from all that huffing and puffing...walking, running, jogging are partial exercises, not complete ones. (p. 260)

The Simmons' regimen of body correcting exercises for fat thighs, fat buttocks, bags under the eyes and bulging stomachs is just another pitch for spot-reducing exercises. Weight does tend to be removed from the largest deposits more than the small deposit areas. However, spot exercises do not cause such reduction. Spot-reduction is a myth (Katch & McArdle, 1983; Bennett et al., 1982). The best form of exercise for weight reduction is the very form that Simmons dismissed – aerobic. Why this occurs is due to the fuel used during aerobic exercise and its effect on the cardiovascular system.

---

[2]The reader may wish to consult Katch and McArdle (1983), Bennett and Gurin (1982), Brodie (1982), and Bailey (1978) for such a critique. Essentially, many "fad" diets (e.g., low carbohydrate) have been proven to be detrimental to health and lead to water loss and lean body mass loss and not fat loss.

Fat contains, per gram, about twice as many calories as protein and carbohydrates. The activity that burns fat is aerobic. Muscles rely on two different kinds of power fuel: (1) sugar for short-bursts and (2) fatty acids for sustained activities. Short-term burst activities draw glycogen, a form of stored sugar in the muscle which is continually replenished from the bloodstream. Fatty acids are drawn from adipose tissue and combine with oxygen to derive a standby supply of power or energy. Because this second process consumes oxygen, it is referred to as aerobic.

Although this dual system can supply a great deal of energy, glycogen is bulky and difficult to store. Fat, on the other hand, is stored in a very compact way, and muscles can readily metabolize it during aerobic effort. Thus, aerobic activities using fatty acids can continue for a long time. Aerobic exercises are those that can push muscles to work moderately for a long enough time to shift them from a heavy reliance on glycogen to predominant dependence on fatty acids (Bennett and Gurin, 1982).

In addition to the difference in the kinds of fuels burned, aerobic and anaerobic exercises have different consequences over the long time. Repeatedly pushing a muscle to its near maximum capacity leads to additional contractile tissue (anaerobic activity). This anaerobic activity increases muscle strength but has minimal effect on the rest of the body. Adding a minimal amount of contractile protein to the muscle, aerobic exercise markedly increases the number of muscles required for energy metabolism. By stimulating the local circulation system, aerobic exercise strengthens the heart muscle and produces body-wide conditioning changes. Fat stores are thus reduced more effectively throughout the body (Katch & McArdle, 1983).

Recommendation. Fitness programs for obese older adults should involve the physician, the fitness specialist and, if possible, a dietitian. Moreover, prescriptive programs for the generally overweight (excessive fat content) and obese older adults should involve three principal ingredients. They are: (1) understanding of obesity and its impact on health, (2) the role that exercise plays in reducing body fat content, and (3) inclusion of fitness activities that efficiently burn calories and/or improve physical appearance. Baseline measurements of fat content should be determined before embarking on actual fitness programs.

Individualized fitness programs are then utilized over an extended period of time to reduce weight by no more than two pounds per week. Bear in mind, that as one reduces fat content he or she may actually experience a slight gain in weight. Lean muscle weighs more than fat muscle but is healthier. Two principles should govern the implementation of the fitness programs: (1) aerobic activities should be the heart of the program and (2) activity intensity must be carefully designed in accordance with the participants' physical capacity and health limitations. Excellent aerobic activities include brisk walking, swimming, stationary bicycles, dancing and calisthenics. Postural-type exercises for physical appearance should be concentrated on the chest region, abdomen and waist, pelvic and gluteal regions and the shoulder girdle. Baechle and Groves (1994) provide a resource for weight training intervention.

Summary: Six Keys

The importance of physical activity and its impact on the aging process has not gone unnoticed. Program directors from community park and recreation departments, nursing homes, YMCAs and a myriad of other social service agencies have been actively engaged in soliciting and developing sound resource material for the purpose of establishing physical activity programs for older adults. An increasing number of professionals, in concert with professional organizations like the American College of Sports Medicine, the American Alliance for Health, Physical Education and Recreation, the President's Council on Physical Fitness and Sports, and the National Recreation and Park Association, have generated a significant amount of interaction and public education devoted to stimulating intellectual curiosity and professional responsibility about aging and exercise science.

Whether or not this new found enthusiasm for the development and evaluation of exercise programs for the elderly will continue remains to be seen. In the face of an exploding fitness craze, leisure service professionals, and other health care providers, must respond with an organized effort for training personnel to direct programs for a rapid increase in the number of elderly citizens. Many of today's and tomorrow's elderly are and will be poorly motivated to initially participate and persist in a regular physical activity program. The majority will have substantially restricted incomes and, the older they are, the more likely they will suffer from debilitating conditions requiring adaptation of normal exercise regimen. In order to meet their needs, it will be incumbent upon the professional to tax his or her adaptive ingenuity for developing physical activity programs that are based on sound exercise principles and to design fitness programs that are economically feasible and motivationally attractive (Serfass, 1981). General fitness programs meeting this criterion for older adults include specialty programs in water aerobics and walking. Recommended resources include: Water aerobics (Sora, 1995; White, 1995 and Elder, 1995), and walking (Yanker, 1983; *Consumer Guide*, 1988).

Safety Considerations

Because of the phenomenal increase in fitness interest, several overuse and misuse injuries have become quite common. Although these injuries are generally not serious, they can become aggravated if ignored. Fitness injuries are usually the result of excessive repetitive movements or improper techniques, especially if there are already existing anatomical abnormalities in the musculoskeletal elements which are involved. Particularly important for avoiding injury is proper attention to (1) warm-up, (2) cooldown, and (3) symptoms of over-exertion.

Warm-Up. The organs of the human system must be alerted to the forthcoming exertion responsibility. Proper warm-up assists in maximizing the potential benefits of a workout and minimizing the potential for injuries. Preliminary warm-up serves to decrease muscle viscosity, susceptibility to injury, and the experiencing of electrocardiographic abnormalities that may be provoked by sudden strenuous exertion. Injury prevention is accomplished by elevating the pulse rate, raising the body temperature and allowing the muscle fibers to be slowly stretched in preparation for the vigorous phase of the workout. Stretching exercises increase the amount of oxygen-laden blood reaching the performance muscle sites. The key in warm-up is to break a sweat. Activities readily suggested for warm-up include light calisthenics, slow jogging or walking and light stretching of the specific muscles to be used in the activity. Skeletal muscle contracts more efficiently and more safely when it has been properly warmed up.

The stretching phase of the warm-up should emphasize a slow, gentle stretch. Rapid or ballistic stretches should be avoided since they have the greatest potential for injury to connective tissue and muscle fibers. The time devoted to warm-up will vary according to the environmental temperature and the intensity of the subsequent workout. Generally, five to ten minutes for warm-up is considered a minimum recommendation.

Cooldown. The principal intent of cooldown is to prevent blood-pooling and to rid the body of metabolic products of exercise. When you exercise, smooth muscle relaxation and vessel expansion allows blood to flow into the heavy demand (metabolically active) muscle areas. During exercise, the accumulation of blood in the heavy demand areas is avoided by a massaging action of the muscles on the veins. However, when exercise stops suddenly, the free flow of blood may continue unabated from the balanced effect of muscle action. The blood may then accumulate or pool in the extremities.

Pooling of blood in the extremities may temporarily disrupt or reduce the return of blood to the heart, momentarily depriving the heart and the brain of oxygen. Fainting or even a coronary abnormality may occur. By continuing in a tapered down or light activity for a cooldown effect, muscle massage will assist proper blood flow return while the blood vessels gradually return to their normal smaller diameter. The cooldown activity will also help remove metabolic by-products of exercise and decrease the possibility of post-exercise soreness and stiffness.

Similar to warm-up, the time devoted to cooldown is dependent upon environmental conditions and the exercise program intensity. A minimum of five to ten minutes should be devoted to cooldown. Mimicking the exercise at a slower pace, walking or light stretching combined with walking are excellent cooldown activities. In all cases, sitting down, standing in a stationary position and/or taking saunas or hot showers immediately after the main exercise program should be avoided.

Symptoms of Over-Exertion. If a participant experiences any of the following problems associated with an exercise program, he or she should consult his or her physician before exercising again: (1) pain or pressure in the left or mid-chest area, jaw, neck, left shoulder or left arm during or just after exercise; (2) sudden nausea, dizziness, cold sweat, fainting or a pallor look; and (3) abnormal heart beats such as pulse becoming irregular or fluttering, sudden rapid heart beats or a very slow pulse rate immediately after a rapid exercise pulse rate. Specific warnings that an exercise bout has been too intensive should also be observed. For example, Ebel, Sol, Bailey, and Schechter (1983) provide some valuable symptoms of over-exertion.

- During exercise, the program may be too intense if you experience any of the following:
    (1) The skin around your lips and fingernails turns blue.
    (2) Your skin is either pale or cherry-red.
    (3) A muscle or group of your muscles twitches involuntarily.
    (4) You develop a headache.
    (5) There is a tightness or pain in your chest, jaw, or along your arm.
    (6) You become nauseous or dizzy.
    (7) You sweat excessively.
    (8) You feel confused or disoriented.
- After exercise, your program was too intense if you experience any of the following:
    (1) You do not regain normal breathing within 10 minutes.
    (2) Your heart rate does not return to normal rate within 10 minutes.
    (3) You do not feel comfortable within 30 minutes after your exercising has ended.
    (4) You are unusually tired after a good night's rest (pp. 11, 12).

Summary: Health Warnings. Exercise is not without drawbacks. There is a dark side to the fitness boom, too. Fatigue, boredom, muscle pain and the potential for injury are present. But many times, these problems begin only if the participant fails to warm-up properly, over exercises or improperly cools down. The key for preventing exercise injuries is to follow sound exercise science principles and to teach the participant to be aware of general health warnings. The interested reader should consult Howley and Franks (1992) for an excellent discussion of safety principles and injury treatment.

Despite the potential for exercise injury, the health promotion professional needs to clearly convey that the lack of exercise may be more hazardous to the participant's health—socially, mentally, spiritually and physically. Most fitness injuries tend to be relatively innocuous, especially compared to the potential for ill health due to sedentary activity. Moreover, most fitness injuries can be prevented with a medium of proper planning, preparation and care.

Conceptual Design of Physical Fitness Programs

Exercise programs have been advocated for the prevention and treatment of a variety of chronic diseases. Appropriately, prescribed exercise programs have been shown to influence the cardio-pulmonary system and the musculoskeletal system. Yet, conventional exercise programs are oftentimes ineffective in achieving these changes due to inappropriate attention toward fitness education and participant motivation.

Figure 4-2 provides a conceptual flow for fitness programs. Preliminary screening is used to build program effectiveness and safety. Elderly participants are then channeled into appropriately balanced physical fitness programs. The actual compliance of participants, however, is largely determined by two major program objectives: (1) educating participants why and how they should be physically active, and (2) motivating them to follow a personally designed physical fitness program.

Physical Fitness Education. Exercise testing and exercise prescription are often emphasized more than the educational and motivational components of fitness programs. This unbalanced attention leads to negative variables outweighing the positive variables that contribute to sustained program interest and enthusiasm (see Table 4-4).

Educational components of physical fitness programs play an integral role. Substantive education information should include: body mechanics, energy expenditures, importance of warm-up and cooldown, exercise myths and misconceptions, recommendations for exercise clothing and equipment, exercise nutrition, symptoms of over-exertion, exercise interactions with drugs, and effects of ambient temperature and humidity on performance. Films, booklets, lectures, workshops, facility visitations, newsletters and bulletin boards are only a few of the programmatic variables
that can be used to facilitate the educational component.

Motivational Strategies. Motivation is a critical component for determining exercise program effectiveness, safety, and long-term compliance. The topic of motivation or program compliance as it applies generally to health promotion programs is the topic of Chapter VIII. Here, however, there are a few motivational strategies suggested by Franklin that have proven effective in sustaining participant interest and enthusiasm. They are:

- Moderate exercise prescription should be used to minimize musculoskeletal injuries. Excessive training frequency (>5 days/week) or duration (> 45 minutes/session) offer little aerobic gain in functional capacity. Moreover, the incidence of orthopedic injury increases substantially. Similarly, high intensity exercise (> 90% of VO_2 MAX) is associated with 50% increased injury rate while providing minimal cardio-pulmonary gain. Recommendation prescription guidelines for the elderly suggested in this chapter should be followed.
- Group participation should be strongly encouraged. Nine out of ten people prefer group exercise as opposed to individual exercise. Social support and social participation are the principal reasons behind this attitude.
- Variety and fun are essential components in the planning of physical fitness programs. Regimented calisthenics that are overly emphasized lead to monotony and boredom.

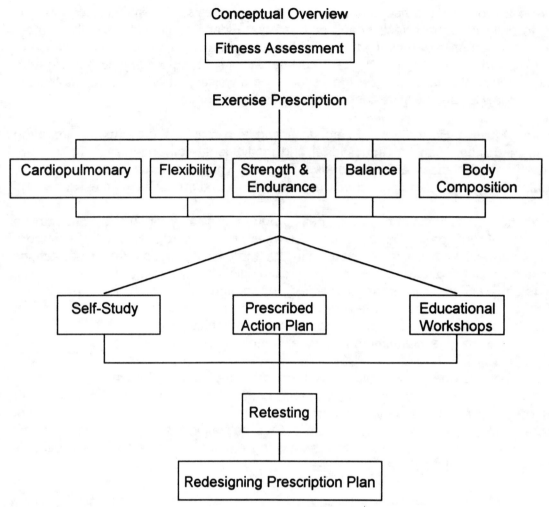

Figure 4-2. Flow of Participants Through a Fitness Program.

Table 4-4. Programmatic and Related Variables Affecting Long-Term Exercise.
Compliance

Negative Variables	Positive Variables
Inadequate Leadership	Instruction and Encouragement
Time Inconvenience	Regular Routine
Musculoskeletal Problems	Freedom from Injury
Exercise Boredom	Enjoyment-Fun-Variety
Individual Commitment	Group Camaraderie
Lack of Progress Awareness	Periodic Fitness Testing
Spouse and Peer Disapproval	Spouse and Peer Approval

From B. A. Franklin, "Clinical Components of a Successful Adult Fitness Program" in *American Journal of Health Promotion,* 1, 1-9, 1986. Michael P. O' Donnell Publishers, Rochester Hills, MI. Reprinted by permission.

- Effective behavioral and programmatic techniques for compliance are based on "personalized" program prescription and feedback. These techniques are discussed, in detail, in Chapter VIII.
- Fitness assessment should be conducted periodically to measure the elderly participant's fitness progress. For example, reduction of body weight, improved cardiopulmonary capacity, and decreased blood cholesterol are powerful motivators for continued enthusiasm.
- Spouse support should be promoted. Interpersonal influences and environmental support have a dramatic impact on program compliance. Program counseling and educational gatherings are likely to build and maintain positive fitness attitudes.
- Immediate positive feedback on program performance may be effectively used to reinforce health related behaviors. Progress charts detailing daily and cumulative exercise achievements are excellent immediate feedback tools; e.g., mileage walked.
- Music should be used to facilitate a positive exercise environment. Such music should be based, however, on the participants' musical interests and not the exercise leader's interests.
- Extrinsic rewards such as t-shirts, trophies, cups and certificates are possible motivators. These awards, however, should be based on exercise accomplishments and should be fairly inexpensive (1986, pp. 10–12).

Regardless of the motivational strategies employed, program compliance will largely be determined by the competency and enthusiasm of the exercise leader. Leaders who feel they must wear high-heeled boots and use whips to convert participant "savages" are likely to produce program attrition and injuries. Fun, pleasure, and repeated success must be employed to offset the pain and discomfort associated with many traditional exercise programs. Stretching, flexibility, strength, and aerobic objectives camouflaged as recreational games can be a program option. More specifically, the exercise leader may consider the behavioral strategies suggested in Table 4–5.

Summary: Staffing the Fitness Program. The size of a fitness program staff depends on the intensity, focus of the program and the number of participants. If the program is delimited to educational and awareness objectives, then the program could easily be managed by a part-time staff member. However, a prescriptive program that includes regular fitness activities will require a more extensive and knowledgeable staff. Staff members should be selected specifically for the responsibilities they will be charged to fulfill. Particularly, the fitness staff will need to be knowledgeable in exercise science, fitness assessment and individual and group leadership.

No single educational degree provides a staff member with all the knowledge required to perform these functions. For this reason, certification programs have been used as supplements to formal degrees, especially in clinical areas. Workshops, seminars, and

---

Table 4–5. Behavioral strategies of the good exercise leader.

1. Show a sincere interest in the participant.
2. Be enthusiastic in your instruction and guidance.
3. Develop a personal association and relationship with each participant and learn to know their names.
4. Consider the various reasons why adults exercise (i.e., health, recreation, weight loss, social, personal appearance) and allow for individual differences.
5. Initiate participant follow-up (e.g., written notes or telephone calls) when several unexplained absences occur in succession.
6. Participate in the exercise session yourself.
7. Honor special days (e.g., birthdays) or exercise accomplishments with extrinsic reward such as t-shirts, ribbons, or certificates.
8. Attend to orthopedic and musculoskeletal problems.
9. Counsel participants on proper foot apparel and exercise clothing.
10. Motivate participants to make a long-term exercise commitment.

From B. A. Franklin, "Clinical Components of a Successful Adult Fitness Program" in *American Journal of Health Promotion,* 1, 12, 1986. Michael P. O' Donnell Publishers, Rochester Hills, MI. Reprinted by permission.

selected courses on exercise principles are also used for attaining the proper background. Generally, the exercise test technologist must demonstrate competencies in graded exercise testing. Many of these tests were discussed in Chapter 3. The exercise specialist, in addition to the competencies of the exercise test technologist, must demonstrate competencies in exercise prescription and leadership. For a detailed outline of competencies required for each of the three fitness classifications, the reader is encouraged to consult Neiman (1990).

CHAPTER SUMMARY

Old age isn't necessarily a white beard, a decreasing leg, or an increasing belly. Nor is it a broken voice, double chin, or a body blasted with antiquity. Admittedly, there are gradual decrements in physiologic and psychologic functions which lead to increased susceptibility to disease. Biologically, the body loses its ability to renew itself. Various body organs and systems slow down and become less acute. Psychologically, the aging individual experiences changing sensory processes, i.e., perception, motor skills, problem-solving ability, and drives and motivations are frequently altered. Sociologically, the older adult encounters changing roles and definitions. Behaviorally, the aging individual will move slower and lose dexterity. The irony is that, through exercise, the ability to delay these changes is within the grasp of the individual.

The potential physical and emotional gains that participation in a "balanced" fitness program can provide for an older adult have been underestimated. Benefits of fitness are not contingent upon a youthful life filled with vigorous activities (deVries, 1982). Yet, for a long time, physicians and other health professionals were reluctant to prescribe exercise as an effective therapy for older adults. As Ryan (1975) "observed":

> Rather than encouraging the senior citizen to a life of vigorous activity, our society has tended to push them out of the mainstream and into the backwaters where they drift in a desultory fashion, lapsing into a gradual decline which leads inevitably to a hospital, a convalescent home and eventually to a death which may be untimely. They pay the price with their lives, and society pays in hundreds of millions of dollars for medical and ancillary care. (p. 61)

Ostrow (1984) suggests that there has been an excessive emphasis on moderation when discussing fitness programs for older adults, and an underestimation of what older people can achieve physically. It has only been in the last decade that we have come to understand that older adults are trainable, and that despite excessive years of inactivity, we can restore some of the vitality associated with youth. Yet, many of the present fitness programs that have been designed for older adults are unclear as to what specific components of fitness each activity is supposed to enhance. "It is almost as if the program leader hopes that a potpourri of physical activities will inevitably contribute to the fitness welfare (or at least the social welfare) of the older adult" (Ostrow, 1984, p. 143). If fitness programs are to gain credibility by policy decision-makers and acceptance by the older adult, they will need to be based on sound scientific principles and diverse enough to meet a variety of physical and mental needs.

CHAPTER 5

NUTRITION IN LATER YEARS

The task of providing elderly clients with the best available nutrition information is not without its obstacles. Nutritional information must be thoroughly examined, interpreted, and summarized for dissemination to clients. At the same time, the health promotion staff must evaluate nutritional advice provided by lay nutrition publications, vitamin and mineral advertisements, as well as promotional claims made by promoters of health foods and diet plans. Clearly this is a formidable task. In this chapter, we will review the *Healthy People 2000* report nutritional objectives for older Americans, discuss physical and psychosocial factors that will influence attainment of these objectives, discuss nutritional recommendations based on physical aging, and present a comprehensive nutritional model.

YEAR 2000 NUTRITION OBJECTIVES

The Public Health Service (PHS) has long maintained an interest in the relationship between nutritional practices and health. In the 1970s, the PHS focused on how dietary excesses and imbalances increased the risk for chronic disease. The 1989 release of the Surgeon General's Report on Nutrition and Health (U.S. Department of Health and Human Services, 1989) summarized several decades of research on the role of diet in health promotion and disease prevention. The findings in this report clearly established the importance of diet to health. Marion Nestle, managing editor for the report, testifies to its landmark status in her introductory remarks.

> The fact that this broad panel of experts was able to reach consensus on the implications of that evidence marks a milestone in the recent history of nutrition. The consensus demonstrates that there can no longer be any doubt that diet is important to health. It is now time to move beyond dietary advice and to take action to put it into practice. This report lays the foundation for such action and, in so doing, demonstrates the need for a new cultural environment for American eating habits--one that promotes healthier food choices. (Nestle, Housman, & Hurley, 1989, p. 1)

The *Surgeon General's Report on Nutrition and Health* was initiated in response to a policy priority shift from a focus on disease of malnutrition to a focus on chronic diseases. The early 1900 nutritional recommendations advised consumption of food from several dietary groups. High energy fat and sugar foods were specifically recommended. These early dietary recommendations did not distinguish between saturated and nonsaturated fat content and did not place a recommended limit on Kcal intake. The 1970s, however, were to bring about specific recommendations that were linked to chronic diseases.

Link to Chronic Diseases

Research in the 1970s linked chronic disease to diets that were too high in saturated fat, calories, salt, and alcohol. The five chronic diseases linked were coronary heart disease, certain types of cancer, strokes, diabetes, and atherosclerosis. The precise contribution of these dietary factors to chronic diseases is uncertain due to the interrelationship between multiple risk factors (e.g., genetics, exercise, smoking) and chronic disease. Despite this uncertainty, the Surgeon General considered the magnitude of diet-related problems as enough reason for requiring dietary changes. Nestle writes,

> The leading chronic diseases account for nearly three-quarters of all deaths annually in the United States. When the effects of obesity, high blood pressure, dental diseases, and osteoporosis are also considered, it becomes evident that diet-related diseases affect the vast majority of Americans, cause untold personal suffering, and account for astronomical health care costs. Even if dietary changes result in only a small reduction in disease risk, the health benefits to the nation would be substantial. (U.S. Department of Health and Human Services, 1989, p. 3)

This new perspective on dietary recommendations was presented in the 1977 Dietary Goals for the United States report (U.S. Department of Health and Human Services, 1989) released by the U.S. Senate Committee on Nutrition and Human Needs. Dietary recommendations included a reduction in total fat intake (especially saturated fat), cholesterol, calories, salt, and alcohol. Foods containing complex carbohydrates and fiber were highly recommended for increased consumption. The current dietary consumption patterns and recommended dietary goals are presented in Figure 5-1.

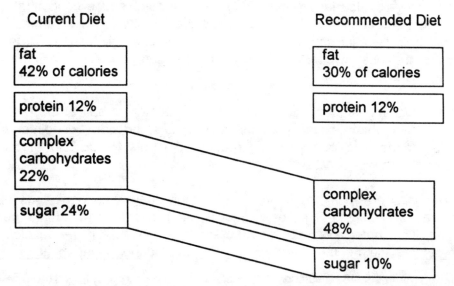

Figure 5-1. The current U.S. diet and the recommended diet, according to the *Dietary Goals*. Reprinted by permission from E. N. Hamilton, E. N. Whitney, & F. S. Sizer, *Nutrition: Concepts and controversies*. Copyright 1988 by West Publishing Company. All rights reserved, p. 45.

The initial set of recommendations for dietary goals prepared by the Senate Committee generated considerable political controversy. This controversy was fueled by a charge that the Senate Committee was making sweeping generalizations prematurely without sufficient research documentation linking dietary practices to chronic diseases. The diet recommendations presented in Figure 5-1 are actually a set of recommendations published in the 1980s by the U.S. Department of Agriculture and the U.S. Department of Health and Human Services. These goals were followed by specific recommendations on what we should and should not eat (Table 5-1).

Table 5-1. Dietary guidelines for Americans and suggestions for food choices.

1. *Eat a variety of foods daily.* Include these foods every day: fruits and vegetables; whole grain and enriched breads and cereals; milk and milk products; meats, fish, poultry, and eggs; dried peas and beans.

2. *Maintain ideal weight.* Increase physical activity; reduce calories by eating fewer fatty foods and sweets and less sugar, and by avoiding too much alcohol; lose weight gradually.

3. *Avoid too much fat, saturated fat, and cholesterol.* Choose low-fat protein sources such as lean meats, fish, poultry, dry peas and beans; use eggs and organ meats in moderation; limit intake of fats on and in foods; trim fats from meats; broil, bake, or boil—don't fry; read food labels for fat contents.

4. *Eat foods with adequate starch and fiber.* Substitute starches for fats and sugars; select whole-grain breads and cereal, fruits and vegetables, dried beans and peas, and nuts to increase fiber and starch intake.

5. *Avoid too much sugar.* Use less sugar, syrup, and honey; reduce concentrated sweets like candy, soft drinks, cookies, etc.; select fresh fruits or fruits canned in light syrup or their own juices; read food labels—sucrose, glucose, dextrose, maltose, lactose, fructose, syrups, and honey are all sugars; eat sugar less often to reduce dental caries.

6. *Avoid too much sodium.* Reduce salt in cooking; add little or no salt at the table; limit salty foods like potato chips, pretzels, salted nuts, popcorn, condiments, cheese, pickled foods, and cured meats; read food labels for sodium or salt contents, especially in processed and snack foods.

7. *If you drink alcohol, do so in moderation.* For individuals who drink—limit all alcoholic beverages (including wine, beer, liquors, etc.) to one or two drinks per day. Note: Use of alcoholic beverages during pregnancy can result in the development of birth defects and mental retardation called Fetal Alcohol Syndrome.

The 1990 Health Objectives for the Nation (U.S. Department of Health and Human Services, 1989) report was directed toward achieving the goals in Figure 5-1 and the specific recommendations in Table 5-1. In response to these objectives, a number of special nutrition programs were targeted to special population needs, such as the Federal Food Stamp Program, Meals on Wheels, and the National School Lunch Program. The mid- to late-1980s, however, saw a significant reduction in funding for many of these programs. Despite this reduction in funding, nutrition programs made advances toward attaining the nutrition objectives contained in the 1990 Health Objectives for the Nation report.

Summary: Year 2000 Nutrition Objectives and Older Adults

Nutrition objectives contained in the *Healthy People 2000* report are an extension of the 1990 objectives. Objectives that include older adults are presented in Table 5-2. Four foundations for attaining these objectives are specified: (1) maintenance and improvement of basic and applied nutrition research; (2) further development of the National Nutrition Monitoring System; (3) dramatic improvement in nutrition information and consumer education programs; and (4) development of a sustained program to implement and evaluate nutrition objectives.

The *Healthy People 2000* nutrition objectives, as they apply to older adults, are certainly worthwhile. But these objectives may be very difficult to achieve because of the unique needs and problems that accompany later life. For example, the older adult living alone and suffering from mobility problems has difficulty in shopping for groceries and preparing meals. Health promotion programs including a comprehensive nutrition program can help in overcoming the special hurdles facing older adults. The success of such programs, however, will depend on the health promotion professional's knowledge of physical and psychosocial factors that impact the nutritional needs and practices of older adults.

FACTORS AFFECTING NUTRITIONAL PRACTICES OF OLDER ADULTS

In college level health promotion courses, one of the most common nutrition questions asked by students revolves around the following: "I keep hearing exciting but conflicting news about nutrition. How can I tell what to believe?" The answer to this question involves building fundamental nutrition principles based on molecular biology and chemistry. Structuring sound nutritional principles for the elderly, in turn, requires a careful consideration of physical aging and psychosocial dimensions. Nutrition guidelines drawn from this discussion are presented later in this section.

Physical Aging and Nutrition

The process of aging includes physiological decline. This process, however, is not uniform; various organs and systems lose their functional capacity at different rates. The greatest change that occurs with aging is declining homeostasis. With aging, the

Table 5-2. Summary table of objectives to improve nutrition.
By the Year 2000 . . .

RISK REDUCTION

Reduce overweight among people ages 20 through 74 to a prevalence of no more than 20%. (Baseline: 25.7% in 1976-1980; 24.2% for men and 27.1% for women)

Special Population Targets
  Among low-income women: 25% (37% in 1976-1980)

  Among black women: 30% (43.5% in 1976-1980)

  Among Hispanic women: 25% (39.1% for Mexican-American women; 34.1% for
    Cuban women; and 37.3% for Puerto Rican women in 1982-1984)

Increase to at least 75% the proportion of overweight people age 12 and older who have adopted sound dietary practices combined with physical activity to achieve weight reduction. (Baseline: 30% of overweight women and 25% of overweight men for people age 18 and older in 1985.)

Reduce average dietary fat intake to no more than 30% of calories and average saturated fat intake to no more than 10% of calories among people age 2 and older. (Baseline: 36.4% of calories from total fat and 13.2% from saturated fat in 1985.)

Increase to at least 50% the proportion of people age 12 and older who consume at least three servings daily of foods rich in calcium. (Baseline: 20% in 1985-86.)

Increase average intake of dietary fiber and complex carbohydrates in the diets of adults to five or more daily servings for vegetables and fruits and to six or more daily servings for grain products and legumes to provide between 20 and 30 grams of daily dietary fiber. (Baseline: 2 1/2 servings of vegetables and fruits and 3 servings of grain products and legumes for women ages 19 through 50 in 1985, data on men available in 1990; approximately 10 grams of dietary fiber in 1987, 11.5 grams for men and 8.8 grams for women.)

Reduce to less than 5% the proportion of people age 21 and older who consume more than two drinks of beverage alcohol per day. (Baseline: 9% in 1985.)

Increase to at least 50% the proportion of households purchasing foods low in sodium, preparing foods without adding salt, and not adding salt at the table. (Baseline: 20% of women ages 19 through 50 regularly purchased foods with reduced salt and sodium content, 46% who served as the main food planner or preparer used salt in food preparation, and 32% used salt at the table in 1985.)

Table 5-2. Summary table of objectives to improve nutrition.   (continued)

PUBLIC AWARENESS

Increase to at least 90% the proportion of people age 12 and older who can identify the principal dietary factors that are associated with heart disease, hypertension, cancer, and osteoporosis. (Baseline: 74% for fat and heart disease, 70% for cholesterol and heart disease, 64% for sodium and hypertension, 43% for calcium and osteoporosis, and 25% for fiber and cancer among adults in 1988.)

Increase at least 75% the proportion of people age 12 and older who can identify the major food sources of fat, saturated fat, cholesterol, calories, sodium, calcium, and fiber. (Baseline: 62% for saturated fats, 55% for polyunsaturated fats, and 3 to 46% for fiber, in 1988.)

Increase to at least 80% the proportion of people age 21 and older who use food labels to make food selections. (Baseline: 74% used labels to make nutritious food selections among people age 18 and older in 1988.)

From: *Promoting Health/Preventing Disease: Year 2000 Objectives for the Nation.* Public Health Service Department of Health and Human Services, 1989, pp. 1-3 to 1-5.

ability of an organ or system to respond to challenge is neither as rapid nor as effective as in the younger adult. This declining function in homeostasis has a dramatic impact on the nutritional needs of the elderly. Our discussion of declining function will focus on the basal metabolic rate, aging of cells and body organs, definition, skeletal structure, sensory function, and neuromuscular coordination.

Basal Metabolic Rate. Basal Metabolic Rate (BMR) is defined as the rate of energy expenditure at complete rest. A "resting" body is actually quite busy pumping blood, repairing tissue, digesting food, and regulating body temperature. On average, the human body uses about 1,450 calories per day for basal metabolism. BMR is highest in the growing years and tends to decrease about 2% per decade after age 25, or about 20% between the ages of 25 and 90. This means that if one's physical activity level remains the same, one's energy needs decline as one grows older, forming a reduced daily caloric requirement.

Aging of Cells and Body Organs. Cells appear to undergo both a built-in (genetic) aging process and a response to environmental forces. Environmental stresses that promote aging include extremes of cold and heat, disease, lack of nutrients, the wear and tear of physical labor, and lack of stimulation caused by disuse or atrophy. But even in the most pleasant environments, genetic aging will have a profound impact on the structure and function of the body's cells. Despite numerous biological theories of aging, all theories have one element in common. They agree that at some point the cells become incapable of replenishing their constituents. Cells are interdependent in the human body. When some cells die and lose their function, other cells dependent on the first ones suffer and eventually die. Thus whole bodily systems are affected (Whitney & Hamilton, 1984).

Pulmonary. Pulmonary capacity declines by approximately 40% with advancing age. This decline is the result of normal physiologic alteration and compromises super-imposed by acute illness and chronic disease. The principal impact on the older adult is the reduced efficiency in air expulsion. Exercise tolerance declines and breathless-ness increases. Both of these conditions lead to varying degrees of fatigue. But pulmonary function decline can be seriously aggravated by such variables as sinuses and smoking.

Cardiovascular System. Decreased functioning of the cardiovascular system occurs with advancing age. Hardening of the blood vessels occurs, with calcium salt and fat deposits being deposited and a loss of artery elasticity occurring. The changes respon-sible for this reduced cardiovascular efficiency include increased rigidity of the arterial walls, reduced contractility of the heart muscle, and reduced cardiac output. Changes in the pulmonary and cardiovascular system with age manifest as a longer time period for the rate of respiration and pulse to return to normal after exercise or exertion. Many of these changes may be related to life-long dietary habits. Because all organs and tis-sues depend on the circulation of nutrients and oxygen, degenerative changes in the pulmonary and cardiovascular systems have a profound effect on all other systems.

Renal Function. The decrease in blood flow through the kidneys makes them gradually less efficient for removing nitrogen and other waste from the blood and maintaining the correct amounts of glucose, salts, and other valuable nutrients in the body fluids (Whitney & Hamilton, 1985). From age 25 to 80, the glomerular filtration rate decreases by about 50% paralleling a decrease in the renal plasma flow. But as both the heart rate and blood volume pumped into the kidneys depend on the muscular activity of the person, this dispersive process can be retarded in aging. Moreover, the body loses its ability to regenerate nephrons after age 40. Nephrons are the functional unit of the kidney. A loss of nephrons results in a decreased ability of the aging kidney to form either a dilute or a concentrated urine. This loss is important during periods of excessive fluid loss (e.g., humid or hot weather) when dehydration may result or when fluid overload may cause congestive heart failure (Whitney & Hamilton, 1985).

Gastrointestinal Function. Digestive enzymes and the secretion by the stomach of hydrochloric acid decreases with age, as does the secretion of digestive juices by the pancreas and small intestine. The motility of the colon decreases which, when com-bined with a decline in physical activity, results in constipation. Weakening of gastrointestinal tract muscles causes pressure in the large intestine which leads to outpockets of diverticulosis. Motility is the involuntary folding and unfolding of the intestine which serves to move food through it. The decrease of movement causes food to remain in the intestines for a longer period of time, thus producing harder stools and constipation.

Liver. The liver is somewhat unique. Liver cells regenerate themselves throughout life, and thus the loss of liver cells is not a major problem. However, even with good nutrition practices, fat gradually infiltrates the liver and reduces its output. Although the response of the liver to moderate blood glucose level is not appreciably altered with age, the response to a large glucose level is reduced. Two reasons have been suggested for glucose tolerance loss. First, the pancreas cells may be less responsive to high blood glucose levels, and it may take more glucose to make them respond by producing insulin. Second, the body's cells become less resistant to insulin, so that it takes more insulin to make them respond (Whitney & Hamilton, 1985).

Definition. Painful deterioration of the gums and subsequent loss of teeth have obvious and traumatic changes on the digestive system. The 10-state survey (1968-70) estimates that 90% of the population age 65 to 74 have gum disease. The American Dental Association also estimates that 75% of individuals 70 years of age and older have lost all of their teeth. Moreover, 80% of those who have lost their teeth either do not replace them or replace them with poorly fitting dentures.

The loss of teeth, or the use of painful, ill-fitting dentures, may severely limit the food choices and nutritional intake of the elderly person. Chewing is difficult and inadequately masticated food is difficult to swallow. To offset these problems, many of the elderly avoid foods high in fiber such as fruits and vegetables. Constipation and the loss of Vitamin C (necessary for wound healing, tissue repair, and maintenance of cellular walls) become critical nutritional problems. Meat is also avoided since it is difficult to chew. The avoidance of meat greatly decreases the intake of protein. Protein is a readily available source for iron and Vitamin B. This shortage of protein, Vitamin B, and Vitamin C leads to lethargy, anemia, and susceptibility to infection.

Skeletal Structure. Human bones are remolded throughout life by the processes of absorption (loss of minerals from bone) and deposition (addition of minerals to bone). But by the third or fourth decade of life, the process of absorption becomes more rapid then deposition. The result is demineralization, the loss of bone, or negative calcium intake. Bone demineralization occurs in both sexes, although it is four times more prevalent in women than in men after age 50. An overall decrease in skeletal mass occurs as a result of bone demineralization. When the loss of skeletal mass is severe, it is termed osteoporosis--thinning and weakening of the bones so severe as to produce fractures in as many as one out of every three people over age 65 (Lutwak, 1969). Fractures of the wrist and femoral neck are the most common.

Several factors have been identified as causing or contributing to osteoporosis: (1) a too-low intake, reduced absorption, or increased excretion of calcium; (2) hormonal changes; (3) reduced physical activity or immobilization; and (4) reduced renal function (Whitney & Hamilton, 1985). Advanced osteoporosis is irreversible. However, a person who wants to prevent or retard bone demineralization should be aware of several factors. First, the minimum intake of calcium for most men is just above 400 milligrams, and for women after menopause, it is about 1,000 or more milligrams of calcium. Second, high fiber diets impair calcium absorption, and high intakes of protein promote urinary excretion. Due to these concerns, several nutritional authorities now recommend that older women need a daily intake of 1 to 1 1/2 grams of calcium, the amount available from 5 cups of milk per day (Gallagher & Riggs, 1978). Third, the reduction of estrogen in women after menopause accelerates bone demineralization. Estrogen replacement therapy may help prevent bone loss but cannot strengthen bones already weakened. Fourth, bones lose material at a dramatic rate when they are immobilized or inactive. Evidence is rapidly accumulating that bone loss can indeed be slowed, prevented, or even reversed by physical exercise (Aloia, 1981).

Arthritis, a painful swelling of the joints, is another skeletal problem that is critical to the elderly. During movement, the bones rub against each other at the joints. The ends are protected from wear by cartilage and small sacs of synovial fluid which acts as a lubricant. With advancing age, the ends of the bone become pitted or eroded as a result of wear. The cause of this erosion is unknown and thus has attracted a variety of quack nutritional remedies, for example, eat no meat, drink no milk, eat all food raw, avoid all additives, or eat only "natural" food. Although no known diet prevents arthritis, the recommendation is that the elderly be educated against quack remedies and that they maintain sound nutritional practices in accordance with contemporary standards.

Sensory Function. The ability to adapt to dim light decreases with age, as does the ability of the eye lens to focus at different distances (called presbyopia). Cataracts (clouding of the lens) are a frequent condition among the elderly. A slow, progressive decline in hearing acuity (presbycusis) often manifests itself as an inability to distinguish speech patterns from background noise and tones of high frequency. The number of taste buds present at age 30 decline by about one-third by age 70. In addition, the ability to discriminate flavors at low concentrations is lost; particularly for detecting sweets and salt. The reduction in olfactory sensitivity compounds the reduced ability to enjoy food. Some investigators claim that two-thirds of the sensation of taste depends on olfactory sensitivity. When combined, impaired vision, hearing, taste, and smell may lead to a general apathy of the elderly toward meals. Thus, the elderly may experience problems in food preparation, shopping, eating with others, and difficulty in communicating in a group (Whitney & Hamilton, 1985).

Neuromuscular Coordination. Fine neuromuscular coordination declines with age. This decline in coordination can make it difficult for the elderly to adequately manipulate eating utensils, causing embarrassment in the company of others. The lack of coordination can also be hazardous when boiling water and sharpening kitchen utensils. To avoid hazardous conditions, the elderly may choose foods that require little or no preparation. This limiting of food choices to those that require minimal preparation leads to food that is more expensive and less nutritious.

Psychological Aging and Nutrition

Adequate nutrition is a vital factor for health throughout life. Based on our discussion of physiological changes with aging, many older adults have a lower energy require-ment because of lower basal metabolic requirements and decreasing physical activity.

Caloric intake must be accordingly adjusted due to the physiological changes. Moreover, nutritionally inadequate diets may contribute to or exacerbate acute illness and chronic diseases. Many studies have documented the relatively poor nutritional status of today's older Americans. It is important to realize, however, that this poor nutritional status is not solely due to physiological changes with aging. Psychosocial factors seriously affect nutrition practices. Some of the more pertinent factors include: (1) social status and aging, (2) economic status, (3) living arrangements, (4) social isolation, (5) loss of mobility, (6) chronic illness, (7) drugs, (8) cultural and ethnic factors, (9) food habits, and (10) foods and special diets.

Social Status and Aging. Old age, unlike youth, has not been viewed as a period of prestige, status, power, or influence. Sociologists and psychologists studying affective dimensions and aging suggest that life adjustments to loss of societal status or prestige may dampen self-esteem. In turn, food and eating are generally viewed as a social activity. Thus feelings of lost status or lower self-esteem may lead to less healthy food and eating patterns; i.e., food practices may become an outlet for negative emotions.

Economic Status. Economic status is the most important environmental factor influencing the nutritional practices of older Americans. The reduced income in late life and the eroding purchasing power during inflation may force older adults to purchase foods that satiate hunger but provide empty calories. Consumption food patterns of older adults are similar to low income groups of all ages. Breakfast tends to include slightly higher nutrients, but the evening meal is slightly lower. Snacks represent almost half of daily nutrients. Some older Americans may exist on only one meal per day. In addition to empty calorie consumption, older adults on fixed and low incomes tend to purchase "quick sale" food items that are less fresh (e.g., day-old bread). Fresh fruit and vegetables may be avoided due to cost.

Living Arrangements. The many combinations of living arrangements common to older Americans are likely to affect food shopping, preparation, and intake. For example, the 1971-74 National Health and Nutrition Examination Survey found that living alone can lead to less healthy dietary practices (Davis, Randall, Forthofer et al., 1984). The presence of a spouse, especially for men, was an especially important dietary factor.

Social Isolation. Social isolation is obviously closely related to the effect of living arrangements on eating patterns of older adults. Sociologists have popularly used the term "isolates" and "desolates" to describe social isolation. Isolates are people living alone by choice, and desolates are people who live alone but not by choice. More older women than older men tend to be social isolates. Men and blacks beyond the age of 75 are at a much greater risk of being social desolates. Desolate older adults tend to cling to the past and suffer more from grieving and depression. The loneliness associated with "desolate" behavior leads to faulty food preparation, reduced caloric intake, empty calorie consumption, and lack of proper nutrient intake.

Loss of Mobility. Loss of mobility hinders both shopping and food preparation. Driving automobiles, reading food labels, and fear for personal safety are but a few of the consequences associated with the loss of mobility. Lack of public transportation, lack of local large supermarkets, and loss of "mom and pop" food stores aggravate the problems associated with declining mobility. Schlenker (1984) reported that 70% of older adults have problems with food shopping. Reliance on small local grocery stores is especially troublesome for low income older adults because prices are higher. Infrequent shopping trips limit the elderly person's ability to purchase and store such available items as dairy foods, fruits, vegetables, and meats. Dehydrated foods and packaged mixes may be used as replacements for fresh food.

Chronic Illness. The prevalence of chronic illness in later life was documented in earlier chapters. The physical and social problems associated with chronic conditions indicate a vital need for proper nutritional counseling. For example, common chronic illness disorders have led to at least 20% of older adults requiring sodium restriction, weight management, drug therapy, and cholesterol control (Schlenker, 1984).

Drugs and Nutrition. Prescription and over-the-counter drugs are commonly used by older adults. Medication can decrease appetite, the sense of taste and smell, and cause gastrointestinal distress. This subject will be treated in more detail in a later chapter. Drugs may also interact with food and lead to serious drug-induced nutritional deficiencies. For example, drugs can increase nutrient excretion, increase nutrient utilization, and compete with the nutrient at the site of action. Food, in turn, can delay, accelerate, or reduce the efficiency of drug absorption. The reader is cautioned that the nutritional and clinical implications of food and drug interaction are not well understood at this time. Multiple drug use, extended drug utilization, and preexisting subclinical malnutrition, however, are vital factors that need to be carefully considered. Figure 5-2 provides a listing of commonly used drugs and their alterations in nutrient metabolism.

Food Habits. Food habits are influenced by tradition, ethnic, religious, and geographic location, all of which may collectively be called culture. The importance of culture as a nutritional influence cannot be overemphasized. An older adult's desire to follow a prescribed nutrition plan for a specific health condition can be sabotaged by the lack of availability of cultural food in supermarkets and restaurants. Although rigidity of food habits increases with advancing age, older people are more likely to change nutrition patterns that are based on their cultural interest and needs.

Fads and Special Diets. Older adults are very vulnerable to quackery and fad diets that promise miracle cures for the diseases, aches, and pains that accompany late life. Special fad diets for arthritis and diabetes are especially noteworthy. Schenkler (1984) estimated that between 18 to 43% of older adults follow a prescribed diet that restricts sodium intake, fat, cholesterol, calories, or carbohydrates. Many of these special diets are expensive, useless, and dangerous. Professional counseling and education is needed to help the elderly sort through the avalanche of fad diets targeted for special health conditions.

Drug	Nutrient	Nature of Action
Cholestyramine (cholesterol-lowering agent)	Fats and fat-soluble vitamins	Inhibit absorption
Aspirin	Iron	Increasing bleeding
	Folic Acid	Compete for transport
Laxatives	Fat-soluble vitamins (A.D.K.)	Inhibit absorption
	Phosphorus	Depletion from bones
Antacids	Phosphorus	Inhibit absorption
Diuretics	Potassium	Increase excretion
	Calcium	Increase excretion
Anticoagulants	Vitamin K	Inhibit utilization
Anticonvulsants	Vitamin D	Inhibit utilization
	Folic acid	
Corticosteroids	Vitamin D	Increase utilization
	Vitamin B^6	Increase requirements
	Zinc	Increase excretion
Alcohol	Folic acid	Decreased absorption
	Thiamine	Increased requirement & decreased absorption
	Vitamin B^6	Impaired conversion to active form
Nicotine (cigarettes)	Zinc & magnesium	Increased excretion
	Vitamin C	Uncertain
	Vitamin B^6	Uncertain
	Vitamin B^{12}	Uncertain

Figure 5-2. Commonly used drugs and their impact on nutrient utilization.
Source: From M. Bogaert-Tullis and S. Samuels, *A Resource Guide for Nutrition Management Programs for Older Persons,* Administration on Aging, Department of Health and Human Services, 1985, pp. 1-7.

Summary: Nutritional Factors and Aging

Physiological changes associated with aging and psychosocial adjustments have a tremendous impact on the nutritional practices of older adults. A number of the changes and adjustments involved affect nutrition practices. A number of these changes involve loss of friends, neighbors, relatives, income, mobility, self-esteem, and independence. One of the most difficult adjustments for the elderly is the loss of a spouse. Women outnumber men in the older age category. Although living alone may preserve independence, isolation can have a dramatic impact on eating habits. Loneliness, lack of motivation, and inadequate cooking or storing may lead to irregular snacking rather than the consumption of regular, balanced meals. People often eat more, more slowly, and with more pleasure in the company of others. Thus, senior centers, congregate meal facilities, and social clubs play a viable role in blending the needs of social interaction and better nutrition practices.

The physical changes associated with aging, as well as social and economic changes, may alter the ability of the elderly to move within their environment. Rigors of driving, lack of transportation, and the replacement of corner grocery stores with large supermarkets have had a dramatic impact on the elderly. Declining income makes it exceptionally difficult to maintain a former standard of living. Reluctant to accept charity, many elderly may sacrifice a former standard of living by choosing foods that are inexpensive rather than foods necessary for good health. For example, the elderly may substitute high carbohydrate foods such as breads, pastries, and cereals for more expensive foods, such as fruit produce, meats, and milk. The lower priced, high carbohydrate foods are usually lacking in vital nutrients, such as essential protein, minerals, and vitamins.

NUTRITIONAL GUIDELINES

Eight of ten older Americans say eating right plays a significant role in preventing illness. But many may not be pursuing the proper nutritional practices for maintaining good health. A five-year project released by the Nutrition Screening Initiative (NSI) reported that 20% skip at least one meal a day, 45% regularly consume multiple prescription drugs that affect appetite or absorption of nutrients, and 36% don't worry at all about proper diets (Bogaret-Tullis & Samuels, 1985). The NSI survey was a survey project involving a coalition of medical, health care, and aging groups. This project initiative focused first on the elderly due to their high nutritional risk. Many of the nutritional needs exposing the elderly to an at risk category are discussed in this section.

K-Calories

A reduced basal metabolic rate, combined with reduced physical activity, results in decreased caloric need. In 1980, the RDA tables for the first time recommended energy intakes for the elderly. These estimates reflect an estimated daily reduction of

5% K-calories per decade in general output. The variation is great and so are the ranges, but average figures for people age 75 and older are 2,050 K-calories per day for males and 1,600 for females.

Although obesity is a common problem in late middle age, increasing susceptibility to chronic diseases (arthritis, diabetes, hypertension) leads to extreme underweight as a prevalent problem among those adults over 70. The lack of sufficient calories needed for biochemical reactions vital to life processes causes a breakdown in cellular metabolism. Protein K-calorie malnutrition is quite common in the elderly and often goes unnoticed. Older people trying to lose weight or eating monotonous or bizarre diets are most likely to be affected (Gambert & Guansing, 1980). Clinical symptoms of K-calorie malnutrition include lack of vigor and interest in the surrounding, increased susceptibility to disease, and appearance of wasted muscles or weaknesses.

In addition to concerns about energy intake, the elderly must also be concerned with energy expenditures. Increase in physical activity should be emphasized for any adult interested in maintaining good health in the later years. Thus, health professionals need to encourage all kinds of physical activity for the elderly and shorter recuperation periods in bed following illness.

Protein

Lean body mass decreases with age. Women experience a greater decrease than men. A decreased rate of protein anabolism (tissue formation) and a reduction in physical exercise are the principal causes of decreased body mass. For most elderly, total essential amino acids are greater. Moreover, the elderly person needs to acquire these essential nutrients from less food; so care must be taken to assure that the protein is of high quality. Protein should also be protected from being used for energy by the inclusion of complex carbohydrates in the diet.

The RDA for protein for the age 50 and older population is 56 gm for men and 44 gm for women. Because the daily K-calorie intake for this age group is reduced, although the protein recommendations are similar to those for other age groups, a greater proportion of the dietary intake should be in the form of protein. The Food and Nutrition Board recommends that 12% or more of the caloric intake be in the form of protein. Yet difficulties in chewing, purchasing and storing have led many of the elderly to omit such vital protein foods as milk and cheese in their diet. Low hemoglobin levels leading to general apathy are a common symptom of omitting these valuable protein foods.

Fats and Cholesterol

High intake of dietary fat has been associated with increased risk for obesity, some types of cancer, and possibly gallbladder disease. High saturated fat intake has been consistently linked to high blood cholesterol and increased risk for coronary heart disease (U.S. Department of Health and Human Services, 1989). Conversely, the reduction of blood cholesterol levels reduces the risk for coronary heart disease; a reduction of 2% in blood cholesterol reduces the risk by 1%. Excessive saturated fat consumption is the major dietary factor contributing to high blood cholesterol levels.

The relative risk from atherosclerosis increases at twice the rate as serum cholesterol level increases. For example, if one's cholesterol level is 10 ml/dl higher than another person's--then one's risk for developing atherosclerosis may be 20% higher. Despite this concern, serum cholesterol levels in the later years are more complicated for the relationship between high serum cholesterol and risk for atherosclerosis is not clear. As Yeagle (1991) observes,

> for people in their 50s or older, total serum cholesterol is not as good a predictor of trouble. In fact, other studies have suggested that one must use LDL cholesterol, not total serum cholesterol, in those past their early 50s. (p. 39)

The reader is reminded that the cholesterol relationship to heart disease has been clearly established. Although serum cholesterol levels may not be as important in later years, the individuals with high levels of HDL (high-density lipoproteins) and low LDLs (low-density lipoproteins) are at a lower risk level. In fact, individuals with high levels of HDL (70 and above) have been found to rarely have coronary heart disease (Yeagle, 1991).

Fat should be limited in the elderly person's diet for other diseases than cholesterol. Cutting fat helps cut K-calories (fat delivers two and a half times as many K-calories as the other energy nutrients) and may help retard the development of cardiovascular disease. High fat intake also interferes with calcium absorption and promotes osteoporosis. On the limited daily K-calorie allowance recommendations for the elderly, it would be difficult to obtain the many vitamins and minerals that come from proteins and complex carbohydrates if too much of the energy intake was supplied by the empty K-calories of fat. Yet fat does provide fat-soluble vitamins and essential fatty acids. Thus the appropriate lower limit for fat is approximately 20% of the K-calories. Of those, approximately half should come from polyunsaturated fat (Whitney & Hamilton, 1984).

Fiber, Sugar, and Salt

Older adults should consume foods with adequate starch and fiber, such as vegetable, fruit, and cereal fibers. A recommended intake of fiber is 15 to 35 grams per day. Dietary fiber is important for maintaining normal bowel activity and is a possible factor in reducing the risk for colon cancer, diverticular disease, and constipation. Fiber has also been shown to lower serum cholesterol levels (Chernoff, 1990).

Sugar is primarily targeted for reduction due to its impact on dental caries. But for the elderly the "empty" calorie contribution of sugar is of more concern. Sugar has no nutritional quality. Limiting intake of foods containing high levels of sugar helps decrease the amount of nutrient-poor (empty), calorie-rich foods. Sodium reduction in the diet may be advisable due to its possible link to hypertension, stroke, and heart disease.

However, the older adult's medical history and medication should be closely monitored before stringent sodium reductions are introduced into the diet.

Complex Carbohydrates and Fiber

Dietary patterns emphasizing complex carbohydrates and fiber facilitate the absorption of water, increase bulk, and improve intestinal motility. This diet also prevents constipation, hemorrhoids, and diverticulosis and reduces calorie intake. Some fibers (except wheat bread) bind cholesterol and execrete it from the body. Moreover, there is an association between diets high in complex carbohydrates and reduced risk for coronary heart disease and diabetes mellitus, however difficult this association has been to interpret (U.S. Department of Health and Human Services, 1989). A recommended intake of fiber is 15 to 35 grams per day (Chernoff, 1990).

Current evidence suggests that all adults should increase their consumption of whole grain foods, cereals, vegetables, and fruits. Unfortunately, older adults often omit fruit and vegetables from their diets. It is not known whether this omission is caused by earlier consumption patterns or is due to cost or storage problems. Any nutrition educational program needs to pay special attention to conveying the importance of complex carbohydrates and fiber. The consumption of foods that are softer but still have high fiber content (e.g., cooked carrots) is especially recommended.

Vitamins

Vitamin deficiency is likely among the elderly unless particular care is given to include food from each of the food groups. Vitamin C (fruits and vegetables), Vitamin B (whole-grain breads and cereals), Vitamin D (milk), and Vitamin E deficiency are of special concern. Elderly who are homebound or who live in smog-filled cities are especially affected by Vitamin D deficiency. Inadequate intake of Vitamin D contributes to the development of osteoporosis and decreased immunocompetence. Older adults may have reduced or eliminated dairy products, the principal source for Vitamin D, because of a perceived or real dietary intolerance.

Deficient intakes of Vitamin B^{12} and B^6 can cause chronic anemia. Hematopoietic reserves may be compromised by inadequate intakes of Vitamin B. Subjects with compromised hematopoietic reserves are at risk for inadequate responses to stress. Insufficient intake of Vitamin C and the mineral zinc deters the healing of wounds. The destruction of Vitamin E by heat processing and oxidation is well known. Processed and commercial foods so often used by the elderly in nursing homes are also thought to contribute to Vitamin E deficiency. Laxatives and drugs have also been shown to cause vitamin deficiency; anticonvulsant drugs, for example, produce a folacin deficiency.

The recommended intakes for most of the vitamins are thought by some nutritionists to be too low for the age 65 and older group. They recommend vitamin supplements, particularly for the water-soluble vitamins. Large amounts of water-soluble vitamins do not pose a toxicity threat. However, other vitamin experts consider vitamin supplements as a "cop out" laying the elderly open to exploitation by health quacks. As a balance between these arguments, Whitney & Hamilton (1985) recommend a vitamin-mineral supplement if the K-calorie intake is below 1,500--not a megavitamin, just a once daily supplement. Differential handling of nutrients by the kidney, liver, and gastrointestinal track puts the elderly at a greater risk of nutritional toxicity from the use of vitamin and mineral supplements. Nutrient imbalance caused by the use of high levels of one substance can interfere with metabolism and absorption of other substances.

Minerals

Iron deficiency anemia is not as common in the elderly as has been believed in the past. But iron deficiency still occurs in some elderly, especially those with low K-calorie intake. Aside from diet, factors in older adults' lives increasing the likelihood of iron deficiency include (1) chronic blood loss from ulcers, hemorrhoids, or other disease conditions; (2) poor iron absorption due to reduced stomach acid secretion; (3) antacid use which interferes with iron absorption; and (4) use of medicines that cause blood loss, including arthritis medicine, anticoagulants, and aspirin (Whitney & Hamilton, 1985). Health professionals counseling the elderly should not forget to ask about these possibilities.

Zinc deficiencies resulting in loss of taste, smell, and slowed wound healing, and calcium deficiency and fluoride deficiency causing bone demineralization are also common mineral concerns for the elderly. But replenishment of proper zinc intake restores appropriate taste, smell, and wound healing (Chernoff, 1990). Salt, which contains the mineral sodium, should be curtailed in all older adults' diets and not just among those suffering from hypertension, congestive heart failure, or cirrhosis of the liver. Salt is conducive to the retention of fluid, which results in raised blood pressure. Convenience foods and processed foods high in sodium content are widely used by elderly living alone, thus making it difficult for them to restrict their salt intake. In sum, to obtain the needed minerals, the elderly should consume food from every good group, milk and milk products, meat and meat alternatives, fruits and vegetables, and grains.

Fluids

As stated earlier in this chapter, the number of functioning nephrons per kidney decreases with age, and therefore the solute load per nephron is greater. To facilitate the excretion of this solute load, adequate fluid intake is essential. In conditions of additional water loss (such as excessive perspiration, vomiting, diarrhea, or the prescribed use of diuretics), the need for ample fluid is even greater (Gasper, 1988). Increased fluid is not only needed to prevent confusion associated with dehydration but is necessary for people taking specific medications (e.g., depression drugs). The elderly need to be reminded of the essential need for fluids because they are likely to be somewhat insensitive to their own thirst signals. The recommendation is the consumption of six to eight glasses of fluid per day. Gasper (1988) identified some key variables that influenced fluid intake of institutionalized elderly: speech, ability to request fluids, visual impairment, opportunity (time) to obtain water, functional ability, and sex. Moreover, Gasper's study suggested that the semi-dependent patient is at greater risk for inadequate fluid intake than independent or dependent patients. Health professionals working in long-term care settings need to work together in building an intervention plan for maintaining adequate patient intake.

Institutionalized older adults are especially vulnerable to dehydration. Acute or long-term care settings operating under scheduled procedures that prohibit eating or drinking by mouth for a set period rarely equalize the need for hydration at the day closure (Ebersole & Hess, 1990). Adams (1988) found that some institutionalized patients go as long as 15 hours without fluid. Older adults unable to acquire fluids on their own should be provided liquids hourly. A scheduled hydration intake may be kept on the patient's door in order to assure adequate fluid intake.

Milk/Lactose Intolerance

Milk and other dairy products are a major and efficient source of protein and calcium for the aged. But many older adults experience lactose intolerance which resembles milk intolerance. Symptoms of lactose intolerance include gas, bloating, cramping, and diarrhea. These symptoms may be displayed when more than eight ounces of milk are consumed. It is theorized that lactose intolerance is a genetic characteristic more common among Blacks, Orientals, American Indians, Eskimos, and other groups who do not consume milk as a traditional food (Rorick & Scrimshaw, 1979). However, White American adults also begin to experience some degree of lactose intolerance at approximately age 45. Older adults prone to lactose intolerance need to be counseled on food substitutes, such as chocolate milk, and calcium derived from greens and dried beans. The older adult's diet may also need to be supplemented with calcium lactate, sodium fluoride, and B complex vitamins in order to maintain skeletal integrity.

Alcohol

Immoderate drinking contributes to malnutrition by replacing nutritional foods in the diet. This causes inflammation of the stomach, intestines, and pancreas (results in malabsorption of many vitamins); rapid excretion of magnesium, zinc, calcium, and potassium; impairment of the body's ability to utilize nutrients properly once they are absorbed; and interference with the activation of vitamins by liver cells, particularly thiamin. In sum, alcohol impairs the body's physiological absorption metabolism of nutrients as well as having toxic effects on the liver. Both of these impaired functions have significant effects on the nutritional status of the elderly (Luks and Barbato, 1989).

Malnutrition

An estimated 30 to 40% of older Americans suffer from malnutrition (Luks & Barbato 1989). Malnutrition refers to a deficiency in essential dietary nutrients and calories and significant deviations in dietary patterns, producing undesirable disease risk factors. For example, protein calorie malnutrition includes such symptoms as weight loss, pallor, dry skin, loss of muscle mass, fatigue, weakness, and dyspnea. Older adults exposed to the psychosocial factors addressed earlier in this chapter are at a high risk for malnutrition.

Sodium

Empirical studies have suggested a relationship between high sodium intake and the occurrence of high blood pressure and stroke. Salt contains almost 40% sodium by weight and is used widely in the preparation, processing, and preservation of food. Sodium is a vital ingredient for normal metabolic function, but is consumed at levels far beyond the recommended 1.1 to 3.3 gram per day intake. Average sodium intake for adults is in the range of 4 to 6 grams per day (Whitney and Hamilton, 1984).

Not all individuals are equally susceptible to the effects of sodium. For example, Blacks and persons with a family history of high blood pressure tend to be more "salt sensitive." But assessment devices are not available for determining whether an individual is salt sensitive or not. Therefore, recommendations for all adults include a reduction in sodium intake by choosing foods low in sodium and limiting the amount of salt added in food preparation and at the table. This is an important recommendation for older adults as high blood pressure is more prevalent in the later ages (Chernoff, 1990).

Caffeine

Caffeine is a stimulant drug that increases the respiration rate, heart rate, blood pressure, and the secretion of "stress" hormones (e.g., adrenalin). It is found in such products as coffee, tea, soft drinks, chocolate, over-the-counter and prescription allergy pills, pain pills, and cold medications. Caffeine is also found in baked goods, desserts, puddings, and many processed foods as a flavoring agent. In moderate amounts, 50 to 200 milligrams a day, caffeine appears to be relatively harmless. But almost 30% of American adults exceed a daily caffeine intake of 500 milligrams. This is a "high" intake level and is a serious cause for concern. Caffeine influences our gastrointestinal, renal, pulmonary, and cardiovascular systems. It has been associated with anxiety, hypertension, malignancy, and fibrocystic breast cancer (Watson, 1988).

Older adults find it more difficult to tolerate caffeine as well as they could in their younger years. The health effect of caffeine depends not only on the amount and frequency but on the amount absorbed, its distribution to targeted organs, and the time it takes for the body to metabolize and excrete the drug. The metabolism, storage, and clearance rate for caffeine declines with age. Moreover, the use of medications that are common in late life may increase or decrease the clearance rate dependent upon the type of medication. Maintenance of caffeine levels below 200 milligrams per day for older adults is, therefore, advisable.

Phosphorous and Calcium

The amount of calcium absorbed by the body is, to some extent, governed by the body's need for calcium and the extent to which calcium is included in the diet. A negative balance in calcium means that we are in a process of losing more calcium than we are absorbing. This progressive loss of calcium contributes to bone demineralization. Reversing this process cannot be attained simply by increasing the amount of calcium in the diet. Effective dietary practices require that the increase in dietary calcium be complemented by a decrease in phospherous and protein intake. The American diet is very high in protein and phosphorous food; thus, attaining this dietary recommendation is difficult. Our typical intake in protein in the form of meats, poultry, fish, and dairy products is twice that recommended by the National Academy of Sciences. The major sources of phosphorous foods, meats and soft drinks, further complicate the calcium and phosphorous dietary recommendation.

Summary: Nutrition Vulnerability

The elderly are vulnerable to nutritional problems for several reasons. First, physical changes that occur as part of the aging process decrease the ability of the body to absorb and use certain nutrients. Second, in the later years foods move slowly through the intestine and thus makes constipation a common problem. In turn, constipation prompts many elderly to avoid certain foods, decrease food intake, or to use too many laxatives. Third, loose or missing teeth and ill-fitting dentures may lead to the omittance of such nutritious foods as meats, fresh fruits, and vegetables. Fourth, some elderly are homebound and find it impossible to shop for nutritious food. Fifth, depression and loneliness may cause disinterest in food. Sixth, chronic illness and medications can alter food tastes and appetites. As a result, the body's ability to use nutrients is impaired and malnutrition and weight loss become critical. And seventh, an increasingly sedentary lifestyle in the later years demands diets consisting of less calories.

NUTRITION INTERVENTION PROGRAMS

The link between diet modification and health outcomes is controversial. But it is clear that well-designed nutrition intervention programs can reduce risk factors associated with many chronic diseases. Adherence to good nutritional principles and practices for many elderly is difficult due to physiologic changes of the aging process and sociocultural conditions (income, transportation, marital status). An advantage of a nutrition intervention program, instituted in a formal organizational setting, is that active support of a health promotion staff and support groups (family, friends) may help overcome nutrition problems.

Nutrition Program Foundation

Recently, protein consumption has come under an aggressive attack by nutritionists. Traditionally, meat, fish, or poultry have been viewed as the main dish for the American diet and vegetables, grains, and breads as a side dish. However, nutritionists now argue that this diet is backward and deadly. Protein has been found to decrease the level of enzymes in the blood that prevent precancerous cells from turning into malignant tumors. Animal studies have also shown that high protein diets lead to increased blood cholesterol levels. This research led the Physicians Committee for Responsible Medicine to recommend that the Department of Agriculture drop meat, fish, poultry, eggs, and milk products from the Basic Four food group guide (Podolsky, 1992).

Despite the research on the dangers of animal protein, most scientists argue that a full scale indictment of protein is premature. The government appears to agree. Yet the Basic Four food group guidelines (meat, fish, and poultry; grains; dairy products; and fruits and vegetables) has been expanded into six food groups. One controversial plan attempting to integrate these six food groups is called the "Eating Right Pyramid." Podolsky (1991) summarizes the Pyramid guidelines as follows:

> The base of the four-tiered triangle is composed of breads, cereals, rice and pasta, as a single food group, suggesting it should constitute the major component (6-11 servings a day) of a healthy nutritious diet. The second level is made up of vegetables (3-5 servings) and fruits (2-4 servings). The narrow third tier is shared by the milk, yogurt and cheese group (2-3 servings), and one composed of meat, poultry, fish, dry beans, eggs and nuts (also 2-3). The tip of the pyramid belongs to fats, oils and sweets and could carry the label "use sparingly." (p. 71)

The Eating Right Pyramid has been criticized by the Center for Science in the Public Interest for not making clear distinctions within the dairy and meat groups for what is healthy and what isn't. The U.S. Department of Agriculture (USDA) unveiled the Mediterranean Pyramid in 1994 and the Asian Pyramid in 1995. In 1992, the initial USDA pyramid was based on four basic food groups with the intent to encourage Americans to eat more fruit, vegetables, and grains (Figure 5-3). Critiques of the 1992 USDA pyramid argued that the guidelines did not differentiate between plant and animal nutrients. Serving sizes were suggested, however, in the 1992 guidelines but not in the 1994 Mediterranean and 1995 Asian pyramids.

Despite this criticism, the new recommendations appear to be better than the old four food group guidelines. These guidelines are based on the simple principle of eat a variety of foods in moderate amounts. Protein, vitamins, minerals, fiber, and starch are needed in sufficient amounts. Older adults, like other aged populations, also need to curb the consumption of fat, sodium, sugar, calories, and alcohol. Health professions can play a vital role by helping older adults (1) to understand the Eating Right Pyramid; (2) to differentiate between healthy and unhealthy dairy and meat products; (3) to know about proper serving sizes; (4) to properly read and understand food labels; (5) to eat right when eating out; (6) to prepare foods with less sodium, sugar, and fat; (7) to assess the older adult's nutritional status. Health professions can also assist in

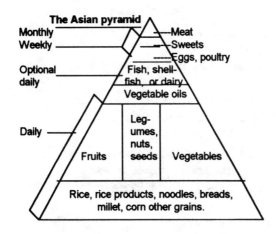

The Asian pyramid

Monthly — Meat
Weekly — Sweets
— Eggs, poultry
Optional daily — Fish, shell-fish, or dairy
Vegetable oils
Daily — Fruits | Leg-umes, nuts, seeds | Vegetables
Rice, rice products, noodles, breads, millet, corn other grains.

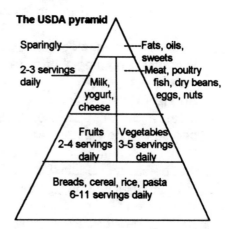

The USDA pyramid

Sparingly — Fats, oils, sweets
2-3 servings daily — Milk, yogurt, cheese — Meat, poultry fish, dry beans, eggs, nuts
Fruits 2-4 servings daily | Vegetables 3-5 servings daily
Breads, cereal, rice, pasta 6-11 servings daily

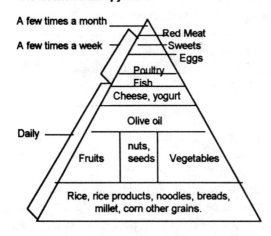

The Mediterranean pyramid

A few times a month — Red Meat
A few times a week — Sweets
Eggs
Poultry
Fish
Cheese, yogurt
Olive oil
Daily — Fruits | nuts, seeds | Vegetables
Rice, rice products, noodles, breads, millet, corn other grains.

USN&WR—*Basic data: Oldways Preservation & Exchange Trust*, Harvard School of Public Health, Cornell University, U.S. Department of Agriculture.

(8) developing programs that use community physicians as a means for nutrition education.

Specific program ideas include the following:

- Provide an ongoing nutrition education class for older adults that offers certificates for participants.
- Establish a library or resource center of books, articles, brochures, and audiovisuals.
- Encourage local libraries to purchase nutrition education materials that you can borrow or recommend to clients.
- Sponsor a nutrition education poster contest, recipe contest, or bake sale. For example, have a contest for converting favorite recipes to low-fat, low-salt versions and offer prizes for the healthiest recipes.

Nothing is as convincing as a taste of a modified recipe that tastes good.

- Publish a cookbook of healthful favorite recipes.
- When serving meals, provide nutrition education information about the meal.
- Sponsor an educational seminar series on nutrition. Classes that offer ideas about shopping, or storing and preparing food for one or two people can be very helpful.
- Contact local food markets and develop an "easy access program" that helps older adults locate low-fat, low-sodium foods; provides easy-to-reach placement of foods on the shelves; and offers large print information about foods.
- Hold a series of demonstrations at the local supermarket on nutritious snacks, shopping for one, shopping "specials" wisely, brand names and generics, and reading ingredient and nutrition labels.
- Prepare a nutrition education column for local publications with large readerships among the older populations.
- Make a video or publish a special bulletin for shut-ins with tips on nutrition; include a shopping list that highlights healthy versions of foods that they can give to a caregiver or aide who shops for them. (Perspectives in Health Promotion and Aging, 1991, p. 3)

A new publication from the Department of Agriculture entitled "USDA's Eating Right Pyramid" (HG249) may be of particular interest for health promotion professionals planning nutrition programs. This publication is a colorful booklet that provides a guide to the relative amounts of different types of food for a healthy diet. Health professionals will find the pyramid a valuable tool for providing more detailed dietary strategies for advising older adults who have elevated blood cholesterol or high blood pressure. Unfortunately, the Department of Agriculture's pyramid for nutrition has resulted in controversy. This controversy has stalled the publication of the aforementioned material. However, the Human Nutrition Information Service (HNIS), an agency of the U.S. Department of Agriculture, sponsors the "Eating Right Campaign." This campaign has developed feature articles, reproducible graphics, and color slides for the new dietary guidelines.

Program Flow

The program flow for a nutrition intervention program is illustrated in Figure 5-4. Nutritional assessment is initially performed to determine the level of nutrition intervention. Two levels of intervention programs are provided. The first level contains nutritional awareness programs that enhance the older adult's knowledge and appreciation of good nutritional principles and practices. Three sublevels of nutritional awareness programs are emphasized: (1) self-help education, (2) group presentations, and (3) experiential opportunities.

Behavior change programs are contained in the second intervention level. Based on an anthropometric and environmental nutritional assessment, the health promotion staff may require a more in-depth nutritional assessment of the elderly participant. This in-depth assessment may include a biochemical assessment, clinical assessment, and dietary assessment. The in-depth assessment is used to help structure a behavior change program for the prevention or treatment of nutrition-related health problems. The key is to focus on the reduction of health risk factors that can be changed or controlled by the parti-cipant. Two behavior change programs are illustrated in Figure 5-4: (1) diet modification and (2) weight control.

Nutrition Awareness Programs

Awareness programs are designed to foster knowledge and appreciation of nutritional needs. Recent research suggests that many of the elderly know what not to eat but do not know what constitutes a well-balanced diet (American Hospital Association, 1985). Programs that incorporate self-help educational materials, group presentations, and experiential opportunities can be used to convey dietary needs. Table 5-3 provides a series of program recommendations for the various awareness program levels. Principle program components using these devices should include:

- Basic concepts of good nutrition--what constitutes a balanced diet-- basic food groups;
- Knowledge about nutrients and benefits, and clarification of confusing facts such as the role of fiber in the diet, saturated fats and cholesterol, vitamins, weight control;
- Food selection and preparation--shopping tips (where to shop, what to buy, how much, cutting costs, etc.), interpretation of labeling and cooking methods to retain nutritional value;
- Choosing substitutes for foods high in fat and carbohydrates and eating good-tasting foods--methods for seasoning and cooking with less salt and fat, substitute foods, importance of proteins, mixing complementary vegetable proteins, food flavor and texture;
- Food problems in later years--under/overweight, diabetes, digestive disorders, lack of appetite, dentures and chewing, cooking for one, small budget, etc. (American Hospital Association, 1985, pp. 34-35)

Many national organizations such as the Food and Drug Administration, U.S. Depart-ment of Agriculture, American Red Cross, American Diabetic Association, American Heart Association, universities, hospitals, and public health departments provide a variety of nutrition education materials and fact sheets. For example, the American Red Cross chapters provide a course entitled "Better Eating for Better Health." Some organizations offer services entitled "Dial-A-Dietician" and nutritional in-home inspec-tions. Appendix D provides some useful nutrition materials for the elderly.

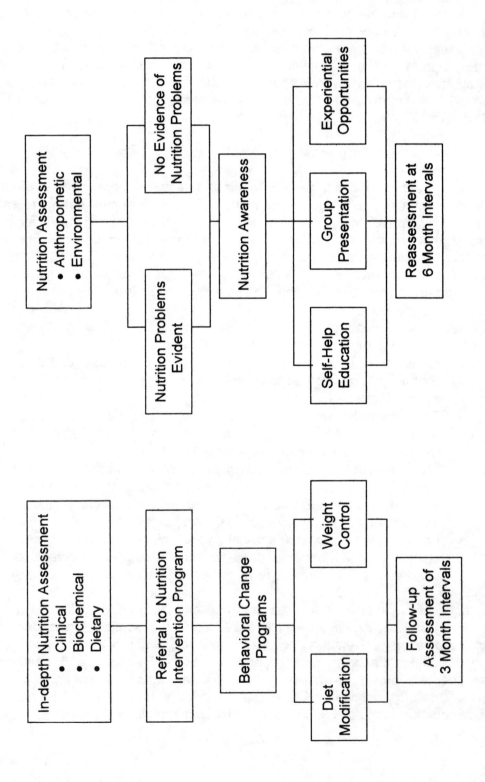

Figure 5-4. Flow of participants through a nutrition intervention program. (Based on the work of M. O'Donnell and T. Ainsworth, *Health promotions in the workplace*. John Wiley & Sons, 1985).

Table 5-3. Types of awareness nutrition program goals and examples of topics.

Type of Nutrition Program	Goals	Examples of Self-Help Programs	Group Presentations	Experiential Opportunities
Nutrition awareness	Knowledge & awareness of good nutritional habits	On-site reference books, publications, tapes, films	Large group	Cooking classes
	Knowledge & awareness of nutrition risk factors	Newsletters, posters, signs, displays	Lectures, workshops, films, panel presentations	Classes for recipe modification, tasting, food preservation, food budgeting, nutritious snacks, planning meals for traveling, vegetarian meals
	Dietary goals of United States	Computers programmed with nutrition assessment and dietary information	Small group discussions using buzz sessions, brainstorming, role playing, case studies	
	Food economy and marketing	Signs, posters, pamphlets		Family potlucks
	Evaluating nutrition information			Health fairs, food cooperatives, community gardens
	Relationships between diet, exercise, and weight control			Games, contests, dramatizations, debates

Based on the work of O'Donnell & Ainsworth, 1984.   From M. L. Teague and R. D. MacNeil, *Aging and Leisure: Vitality in Later Life*. Prentice Hall, 1989.

The implementation of nutrition awareness programs in the community requires very careful planning. To facilitate this planning, the Administration on Aging (AOA) developed a nutrition resource management manual. The AOA manual was authored by Bogaret-Tullis and Samuels (1985). Five basic planning components are presented: (1) setting goals, (2) assessing existing resources, (3) developing new resources, (4) sharing information, and (5) publicizing the program. The manual also provides an excellent presentation on three nutrition awareness programs for older adults: (1) supermarket demonstrations, (2) basic cooking class series, and (3) a cookbook for seniors.

Behavior Change Programs

Many common chronic diseases have been referred to as "diseases of civilization" or "diseases of mechanized society"--a society characterized as sitting, smoking, stuffing, sipping, and stressed. The typical American diet contains copious amounts of calories, cholesterol, fat, sugar, and salt. These dietary factors contribute to the development of high blood pressure, obesity, high blood cholesterol levels, and glucose intolerance. Thus diet modification and behavior change programs focus on the reduction of risk factors by changing behavioral nutritional practices.

The principal emphasis of the diet modification and behavioral change components is to enhance awareness of current diet quality toward adopting new behavior by, for example, incorporating new healthy foods in meal planning and preparation. Because of the interrelationship between eating habits, stress and exercise, fitness programs and stress management programs are also incorporated into behavior change programs. Table 5-4 provides a summary of diet modification and behavioral change programs that may be used to meet the needs and interests of elderly participants.

Intervention Summary

The perception of a negative attitude on the part of the elderly toward nutrition education is generally misstated. This perception is often a reaction to the manner in which nutritional information is presented. Health professionals must identify the unique needs of the elderly and adjust their learning environments to accommodate aging changes that affect learning (e.g., vision and hearing impairment). It is important to remember that the elderly value their independence and fear any illness or disease that may cause them to be disabled, homebound, or institutionalized. An astute health professional can use this concern to advantage by promoting the axiom that proper nutrition is essential. The elderly will be far more receptive to new nutritional ideas if they feel that awareness and behavior change programs can help them maintain their independence.

Table 5-4. Types of behavioral change, nutrition program goals, and topic examples.

Behavioral Change Programs	Examples of Diet Goals	Examples of Weight Modification Programs	Control Programs
	Reducing risk factors that can be changed by the individual	Alternative food choices	Self-monitoring techniques
		Food preparation	
			Setting personal goals
	Nutrition principles	Shopping and reading product labels	
	Methods for estimating nutrient and caloric need	Meal planning	Self-management and behavior modification techniques
		Eating away from home	
	Methods for estimating dietary intake		Reinforcement
	Methods for incorporating low-caloric, high nutrient foods		Support systems
		management	Stress
	Methods for evaluating nutrition, diet, and weight control information		Popular diets, exercise programs for weight control
	Information on modifying recipes		
	Managing dietary needs while traveling, entertaining		

CHAPTER SUMMARY

The elderly are a group prone to more health problems than younger age groups, and these health problems can have a dramatic impact on their nutritional status. Chronic diseases and changing physiologic processes can influence the way the elderly view food, the ways in which they get food, and the ways in which they use food. Because one of the principal effects of aging is gradual loss of functioning cells from organs and body tissues, one may assume that these effects may be prevented or minimized by improving nutrition practices. Many of the nutritional programs cited in this chapter are developed based on that assumption.

Although nutritional deficiency is related to physiological changes, psycho-social factors also play a critical role. Inadequate income and social isolation are especially important dimensions. In fact, adequate dietary intake and nutritional status has been shown to be influenced more by income level than age. Moreover, many gerontology professionals believe that the lack of work, poor use of leisure time, and social isolation are the most prominent factors that lead to inadequate nutritional practices and poor nutritional status.

The intent of this chapter was not to debate the relative importance of physiologic changes and psycho-social dimensions that lead to poor nutritional health. Both of these factors obviously have a dramatic impact. But one of the major problems of the elderly is that they have limited access to a competent nutrition professional. In many cases, access to nutrition information, correct or incorrect, is gained through the local health food store, questionable nutrition publications, and health quacks. Health promotion programs that offer constructive nutrition programs can help offset this nutritional information void and, at the same time, provide a means of social interaction that can play an important role in the lives of the elderly.

The reader may be particularly interested in three nutrition resources provided by the National Council on Aging. First, Eating Well to Stay Well is a 50-page booklet dedicated to older consumers. Topics include dietary guidelines, lifestyle issues, and the link between nutrition and chronic disease. Second, the publication entitled *A Resource Guide for Nutrition Management Programs* is a vital component for any comprehensive health promotion program. This publication includes planning steps for developing and implementing supermarket demonstrations, cooking classes, and a cookbook for older adults. Third, Supermarket Survey is a group of materials directed toward health planners for implementing supermarket tours that teach basic nutrition principles, help participants read and understand labels, and help individuals locate nutritious products in their local grocery store. The training kit includes a manual, two audio cassettes that address marketing and program planning, reproducible handouts, a 52-minute video of an actual supermarket tour, and an extensive list of brand foods.

CHAPTER 6

DRUG MANAGEMENT AND OLDER ADULTS

The use of medication by older adults has become an important topic of discussion in the health care industry. This accelerated interest is due to the prevalence of chronic diseases in later life, the increasing number of medications used to treat chronic diseases, and the growing awareness that adverse drug reactions among older adults have become a critical problem. This chapter reviews medication use among older adults, adverse drug reactions, and drug management intervention strategies.

PREVALENCE OF MEDICATION USE
BY OLDER ADULTS

The elderly account for a highly disproportionate amount of prescription drugs, psychoactive drugs, and over-the-counter (OTC) drugs. Approximately 25 to 30% of all prescription drugs are consumed by the elderly population. By the year 2020, this consumption will increase to almost 50%. Moreover, the elderly consume 70% of the OTC drugs as compared to 30% by the general population. This over-reliance on prescription and OTC drugs has created some very special health concerns for the elderly.

Categories of Drugs Prescribed

Drugs can be wonderful health tools for the care of patients. We can certainly attribute part of our increased life expectancy to the success of medicines and the availability of vaccines. Used appropriately, drug therapy can increase both the length and quality of life. However, the use of drugs in geriatric medicine is complex as many classical signs and symptoms of aging may be absent or exacerbated. Virtually all medications have the potential to produce side-effects. Wolfe, Fugate, Halstrand, and associates (1988), in their book *Worst Pills, Best Pills*, note that of 287 prescribed drugs, 104 should not be used by older adults. Unfortunately, the 104 drugs recommended for non-use account for one out of every four prescriptions filled by older adults.

According to numerous pharmaceutical specialists, older adults are receiving far too many prescription drugs. A wrong initial diagnosis and reluctance to try nondrug therapy are but two reasons why the prevalence of medications in late life has led to significant health concerns. Dr. George Carruthers, a British geriatric drug expert, acknowledges this problem:

> Unfortunately, for a variety of reasons, medications are often used to
> treat the physical, psychological, social and economic problems

associated with aging, even when there is scientific evidence that drugs are the least appropriate way of managing some of these problems. Rather than having the quality of life improved, the elderly patient may actually suffer adverse effects of drug intervention which was initiated, presumably, with the best intentions. Overuse of medications in the elderly may result. (Wolfe et al. 1988, p. 2)

Three categories of drugs often overprescribed and misprescribed are: mind affecting drugs, cardiovascular drugs, and gastrointestinal drugs.

Mind-Affecting Drugs. The common mind-affecting drugs prescribed include tranquilizers and sleeping pills, antidepressants, and antipsychotic drugs. Although comprising only one-sixth of the population, older adults are prescribed one-third of the minor tranquilizers (Valium, Librium, Xanax, Tranxene), one-third of the major tranquilizers (Thorazine, Mellaril), one-half of the sleeping pills (Dalnane, Halcion, Restoril), and one-third of the antidepressants (Elavil, Butisol, Triavil). Many of these drugs are prescribed for one month or longer even though there is no evidence that their usage is effective for that period of time (Wolfe et al., 1988). Table 6-1 provides a summary of the more common mind-affecting drugs and their potential side-effects.

Table 6-1. Mind affecting drugs.

Antipsychotic Drug	Sedative (sleepiness, disturbed sleep)	Anticholinergic (dry mouth, urine retention, confusion)	Hypertensive (lowering of blood pressure to levels that are too low)
Chorpromazine/ Thorazine	strong, adverse effects	strong, adverse effects	strong, adverse effects
Thioridazine/Mellaril	strong, adverse effects	strong, adverse effects	moderate, adverse effects
Antidepressant			
Doxepin/Adapin, Sinequan	strong	moderate	moderate
Amitriptyline, Elavil, Triavil	strong	strong	moderate

Source: Data from S. M. Wolfe, et al., *Worst Pills, Best Pills,* 1988, Public Citizen Health Group, Washington, D. C.

Cardiovascular Drugs. The 287 drugs cited in Wolfe et al.'s (1988) book involve almost 558 million prescriptions each year for older adults. Forty-six percent of these prescriptions are for 58 cardiovascular drugs. Twenty-three of the 58 cardiovascular drugs are considered unsafe due to their adverse health effects. Moreover, a study by Hansen, Jensen, Langesen, and Peterson (1982) suggests that 41% of patients age 50 and older, taken carefully off their prescribed high blood pressure medications, returned to normal blood pressure 11 months after the drug was stopped. Wolfe et al. (1988) conclude, "This suggests that a large proportion of older adults are being put on or kept on antihypertensive drugs who would do very well off them, gladly foregoing the adverse effects and the unnecessary expense" (p. 9).

Some of the "Do Not Use" medications cited in the *Worst Pills, Best Pills* book include high blood pressure drugs containing reserpine. Reserpine is a chemical that has been linked to drug-induced depression, sometimes resulting in suicide. Ser-ap-es, Diupres, and Hydropro are common prescribed medications that include reserpine. Wolfe et al. (1988) noted that 69% of high blood pressure drugs containing reserpine are used by older adults.

Dilating drugs (e.g., Digoxin, Parabid, Vasodilen, and Cyclospagmal) are commonly used by older adults to offset the narrowing and hardening of the arteries in the legs or head. Older adults actually consume 84% of the blood vessel dilating drugs used in the United States. Lee, Johnson, Bingham, and associates (1982) found that 40% of persons using Digoxin were receiving absolutely no benefit from this dilating drug. Moreover, Digoxin has dangerous side-effects thus raising serious ethical questions concerning its usage for older adults. The findings by Lee et al. (1982) were later substantiated by Fleg and Lakatta (1984).

Gastrointestinal Drugs. Forty-three percent of all gastrointestinal drugs used in the United States are by people age 60 and older. Wolfe et al. (1988) list 27 gastrointestinal drugs, 12 of which are included in the "Do Not Use" category. Drugs used for treating nausea and heartburn--Reglan, Tigan, Phedergan, Compazine, and Antivert-- are among the most dangerous prescribed gastrointestinal drugs; Drug-induced Parkinsonism (tremors), similar to antipsychotic medications, has been a potentially dangerous side-effect. Together, these five drugs account for 48% of gastrointestinal prescriptions. Antispasmodic drugs (Bentyl, Lomotil, Librax, and Donnatal) are also gastrointestinal medications producing serious side-effects.

Many of the gastrointestinal complaints experienced by older adults may be suited to nonmedication treatment. In fact, most gastrointestinal problems may be caused by the use of other medications. Wolfe et al. (1988) write:

> A knowledge of the patient's life situation and health concerns often allows the therapist [doctor] to use frequent visits, prescribed physical or social activities, detailed diet instructions, and the use of innocuous

medications (vitamins, antiflatulents [we disagree about the antiflatulents, see p. 255, Mylicon]) to overcome boredom and preoccupation with an unoptimistic future. Often patients are treated with substantial amounts of cathartics (laxatives), antispasmodics, when a more appropriate course would be to address diet, preoccupation with a daily bowel movement, and a monotonous daily existence.

Modern treatment of gastrointestinal conditions usually favors four or six small meals daily, increases [in] the fiber content of the diet for all conditions. Most gaseous conditions are controlled more effectively by deliberately chewing food (to lessen air swallowing). (p. 10)

High Cost of Drugs

Older adults are a lucrative market for the pharmaceutical industry because their collective income exceeds $600 billion per year. By the year 2000, older adults will control almost 20% of all discretionary spending in the United States. The availability of discretionary income and the heavy utilization of prescribed drugs by older adults make them a primary target of pharmaceutical advertisement. In fact, the pharmaceutical industry spent approximately $3.6 billion in 1989 developing new drug therapies for the 28 major diseases that afflict older adults (Walsh, 1990). This $3.6 billion represented almost 50% of the pharmaceutical industry's research and development budget.

Although the pharmaceutical industry may be flourishing, the same cannot be said for adults facing the problem of drug affordability. The escalating cost of drugs today has seriously dampened the ability of many older adults to afford necessary prescriptions. For example, the Medicare Catastrophic Coverage Act of 1988 was repealed, but the price of drugs was one component that did not die with this legislation. The debate as to whether the federal government should become more active in controlling drug costs has become very vivid in the early 1990s. As Pryor (1990) notes,

Access to health care in the United States is increasingly imperiled by the combined effect of surging medical costs and the clearly expressed will of taxpayers who do not trust public officials to spend their tax dollars wisely. As this climate of political and economic stalemate settled in on our state and national legislatures during the 1980s, it became more and more unlikely that major new public health insurance programs would be enacted. Incremental improvements in health coverage, such as those established in the Medicare Catastrophic Coverage Act of 1988 (P.L. 100-360) or those proposed by the U.S. Bipartisan Commission on Comprehensive Health Care (the Pepper Commission), either perished or have been largely drowned out by disputes over taxation. Statutory commitments to existing publicly financed benefits, too, have been steadily eroded as medical costs exceeded government's fiscal resources.   Nowhere has this crisis of affordability been more apparent than in the joint federal/ state Medicaid program's $3.5 billion outpatient prescription drug bene- fit for the nation's poor.

In recent years, as medical costs have risen, state Medicaid budgets have become a source of major concern. Medicaid overall has been growing faster than every other state budget category except correc- tions. But even within this context, the growth of prescription drug costs has been conspicuous: Medicaid prescription drug outlays for states with drug benefits rose 224 percent between 1980 and 1988. Between 1984 and 1988, drug benefit expenditures in the average Medicaid plan rose by 75 percent, and spending more than doubled in ten states. (p. 101)

The failure of states to hold down drug costs is due to the inability of health cost containment measures to address drug price inflation. Thus, efforts to control rising prescriptive medication costs are likely to fall under a national plan rather than state initiatives. Development of such a national plan cannot help but have a tremendous impact on the health of older adults. The need by older adults to receive financial assistance for prescriptive drugs must not be lost in the cost containment shuffle. This financial assistance is critical to both the elderly and society in general.

To control soaring drug outlays, states resorted to the previously well-tested measures that attempt to hold health budget lines. The most common state cutting lines include reducing pharmacy reimbursements, raising the coinsurance paid by the poorest poor who qualify for Medicaid, limiting the number of reimbursable prescriptions, and constructing limited lists of approved drugs that fall under reimbursement provisions. As a result of these state measures, many poor older Americans (the Medicaid-qualified) are finding it more difficult to find necessary prescriptive medications. Yet, despite these cost containment efforts, Medicaid prescription drug costs continued to rise more rapidly in the latter half of the 1980s as compared to all other Medicaid expenditures except home health care and nursing home care for the mentally retarded (Pryor, 1990).

ADVERSE DRUG REACTIONS

Adverse drug reactions are difficult to measure because of an unclear definition and difficulty of identification. There is tremendous difficulty in differentiating drug-age effect, drug-drug interaction, drug-food interactions, and symptomology of chronic diseases. Moreover, as is well documented, many older adults manifest their medical problems in vague and nonspecific symptoms that are difficult to interpret by attending physicians (Ostrow, 1984). In discussing these concerns, we will use the U.S. Food and Drug Administration's definition for an adverse drug reaction as follows:

Any adverse event associated with the use of a drug in humans, whether or not considered drug related, including the following: an adverse event occurring in the course of the use of a drug product in professional practice; an adverse event occurring from drug overdose, whether accidental or intentional; an adverse event occurring from drug abuse; an adverse event occurring from drug withdrawal; and any significant failure or expected pharmacological action. (German & Burton, 1989, p. 12)

Some adverse drug reactions are not very serious, but others can lead to serious illness health consequences that could have and should have been avoided. Although adverse drug reactions occur at all ages, they are much more likely in the later years. Above age 50, the amount of prescription drugs and the odds for adverse reactions increase sharply. The risk for adverse reaction is about 33% higher for people age 50 to 59 than it is for people age 40 to 49. Moreover, after age 60 the risk may increase two to three times higher (Bogaret-Tullis, 1985). In this section, we will entertain two questions: How significant is the problem of adverse drug reactions for older adults? and . . . Why do adverse drug reactions occur?

How Extensive Is the Adverse Drug Reaction Problem?

Larry, an otherwise healthy 58-year-old man with diarrhea believed to be due to "irritable bowel syndrome," was given Stelazine, a powerful antipsychotic tranquilizer, to "calm down" his intestinal tract. Stelazine is not even approved for treating such medical problems. Six months after starting Stelazine, Larry developed severe Parkinsonism and was started on L-Dopa, a drug for treating Parkinson's disease. The Stelazine was continued because the doctor presumably did not realize the Parkinsonism was drug-induced. For seven years, Larry took both drugs. Then a neurologist specializing in Parkinson's disease saw Larry, recognized the real cause of his problem, stopped the Stelazine and slowly withdrew the L-Dopa over a six-month period. Larry's severe, disabling Parkinsonism cleared completely (Wolfe et al., 1988, p. 15).

The adverse drug reactions such as Larry's are not uncommon. Over 61,000 older adults develop drug-induced Parkinsonism each year. At least 80% of them should never have been prescribed drugs that cause Parkinsonism in the first place. But drug-induced Parkinsonism is not the only startling adverse drug reaction experienced by older adults. Wolfe et al. (1988) detail the extent of the problem:

- In 1985, an estimated 243,000 older American adults were hospitalized because of adverse reactions to drugs they were taking before their hospitalization.
- Each year in hospitals alone, there are 29,000 cases of life threatening heart toxicity from adverse reactions of Digoxin, the most commonly used form of digitalis in older adults.

- 32,000 older adults a year suffer from hip fractures attributable to drug-induced falling.
- 163,000 older Americans suffer from serious mental impairment either caused or worsened by drugs.
- 2 million older Americans are addicted or at risk of addiction to minor tranquilizers or sleeping pills because of using them daily for at least one year.
- 73,000 older adults have developed drug-induced tardive dyskinesia, the most serious, common, and often irreversible adverse reaction to antipsychotic drugs. (pp. 14-15)

Measuring the actual extent of adverse drug reactions is confounded by the problem of definition. Many of the past epidemiological studies focused on the incidence of events presumed to be drug adverse reactions. But these studies tended to have serious methodological limitations (Klein, German, Levine, 1981). For that reason, several governmental and institution-based attempts have been initiated to monitor the occurrence of adverse drug reactions in special populations. Post-marketing surveillance which depends on spontaneous reports of adverse reactions from clinicians is one of the primary initiatives. Medicaid data bases have also been used to determine adverse drug effects. Despite these efforts, German and Burton (1989) conclude that more rigorous methods are needed to determine the true impact of adverse drug reactions.

Why Do Adverse Drug Reactions Occur

In Chapter 1, we discussed the three medical revolutions entitled the Engineering Era, the Medical Era, and the Post-Medical Era. The Medical Era (1920-1960) may as well be called the Chemical Era, for it saw the first vast production and distribution of magical pharmaceutical drugs. During the early stages of the Medical or Chemical Era, both prescription and OTC drugs were fewer and were tailored to children and young adults. Thus substance abuse problems for the elderly were largely limited to alcohol abuse. But as life-sustaining technologies advanced, the potential problems of improper use of medications by older adults came to the forefront. Seven principal factors lie behind the adverse drug reactions that have brought drug abuse into the limelight as a major substance abuse issue: (1) multiple pathology, (2) polypharmacy, (3) drug mismanagement, (4) medical quackery, (5) OTC drugs, (6) physician education about pharmaceuticals and the elderly, and (7) pharmacodynamic and pharmacokinetic changes.

Multiple Pathology

As presented earlier in this book, 75% of older adults are afflicted with at least one chronic disease and of those, almost 40% may be affected by two or more chronic diseases. Anemia, cardiac failure, degenerative vascular disease, diabetes, hypertension, arthritis, and liver and kidney damage are likely to alter the older adults' response to drug therapy. Little is known about the influence of multiple chronic diseases on drug effects in older adults. However, it is known that uncontrolled cardiac failure and cirrhosis of the liver can have dramatic effects on drug absorption. The progressive loss of organ reserve in the cardiovascular and central nervous system combined with increased pathology are certain to increase adverse drug reaction susceptibility. For example, when the heart is not able to pump as much blood as it used to, which occurs following heart failure, blood flow is also decreased to the kidneys. This decreased blood flow will impair the drug excretion ability of the kidneys.

Polypharmacy

Multiple pathology, a common phenomenon among the elderly, fosters a practice called polypharmacy, which attempts to treat several disorders simultaneously. An estimated 77% of the elderly take at least one prescription drug daily, 65% two to three prescription drugs, and 20% more than five prescription drugs daily. Adverse drug reactions accelerate with increased drug exposure (Frisk, 1986). For example, hospital patients who were given one to five drugs had an adverse drug reaction incidence of 18.8%, whereas patients ingesting six or more drugs experienced an incidence of 81.4% (Weg, 1978).

Multiple drug use among the elderly has serious implications because of pharmaco-kinetic (differences in metabolism, distribution, absorption, excretion) and pharmacody-namic (alterations of actions of receptor sites) considerations (Ruben, 1990). Pharmacokinetic and pharmacodynamic changes will be discussed later in this chapter. Potentially harmful are such commonly prescribed drugs as antidepressants, antirheu-matics, cardiac glycosides, diuretics, barbiturates, and tranquilizers. The point is that drug therapy among the elderly should proceed with caution. Multiple pathology of the elderly leads to polypharmacy, which in turn may cause a greater number of iatrogenic reactions, frequently treated with an even greater number of drugs. This cycle needs to be broken by greater awareness of polypharmacy by health professionals, policy-makers, and the elderly themselves.

Drug Mismanagement

It is estimated that more than 50% of older adults mismanage the administration of their drugs (Michocki, Pharm, & Lamy, 1988). The National Association of Retail Druggists estimates that 25% of hospital admissions for older adults are the result of drug errors (Perspectives on Health Promotion and Aging, 1990). Drug-induced delirium, confu-sional states, and vision and hearing impairment can lead to many of the drug mismanagement problems. However, the principal mismanagement causes are threefold: drug interactions with food, drug misuse, and noncompliance.

Interactions of Drugs with Food. The elderly are at special risk from the effects of drugs on nutritional status. Drugs commonly used in the treatment of chronic or long-term health conditions particularly alter a person's nutritional status. For example, Digoxis (a heart stimulant) can suppress appetite; antirheumatic drugs (e.g., aspirin) can cause stomach irritation and lead to nausea and vomiting; mineral oil laxatives can block absorption of Vitamin D; and antidepressant drugs can increase the appetite and lead to obesity. Thus drugs that have an impact on nutritional status need to be closely monitored by a physician (Nelson, Roberts, Simmons, et al., 1986).

Drug Misuse. Forms of drug misuse include overuse, underuse, erratic use, and contraindicated use. Most misuse is caused by the inadequate geriatric training of the prescribing physician (Ebersole & Hess, 1990), and underuse (Ruben, 1990). Yet drug misuse may, at times, be deliberate. Personality responses under stress may lead to both overuse and underuse of drugs (prescribed or over-the-counter). Actual misuse may be the elderly individual's means of asking for help--a response to isolation, alienation, or low social status. Drug misuse can also be a manifestation of certain pscyhophysiological states. However, in most instances, drug misuse by the elderly is unintentional, as in forgetting to take drugs, misplacing the drugs, or using outdated drugs.

Noncompliance. Noncompliance is often considered a deliberate misuse of medication. But most elderly clients make a deliberate choice to limit drug consumption (National Institute on Drug Abuse, 1982). Health professionals tend to forget or ignore that individuals will not comply with a prescription or treatment plan that is incompatible with the practicalities of life, such as disabilities, or finances. Moreover, the individual may distrust the information source (Bower, 1985). Ebersole and Hess (1990) provide excellent examples of such incompatibilities:

> The aged individual cannot take medication three times a day with meals if he only eats two meals daily; the aged person may not continue to take a medication if it makes him lethargic and unable to participate in his social activities. This is no different than the aged person who is told to soak in the bathtub twice a day for 20 minutes when he only has a shower and that must be shared. (p. 275)

The elderly person may also not comply with medication prescriptions because of unclear directions presented in a rapid-fire fashion or in medical jargon. Health professionals must remember that it takes longer for the elderly to process information. Visual and hearing impairments and cultural or language barriers can also interfere with adequate communication of important instructions. Economic difficulty is also a critical noncompliance factor. The elderly have been known to omit expensive drugs by not purchasing them or to alter the drug dosage in an effort to stretch the medicine over a longer period. When the elderly person feels better, he or she will sometimes stop taking the medication. Persons with little educational background and in economic difficulty are the most likely not to comply with drug prescriptions or treatments.

In summary, noncompliance to a medication regimen can occur in two ways, either intentional or unintentional. When an older adult knowingly deviates from his or her prescribed regimen (e.g., taking too little or too much of a drug, not filling a prescription), they are intentionally noncompliant. Unintentional noncompliance may involve forgetting occasional dosages, misinterpreting directions, or inappropriately selecting nonprescription drugs. According to Ostrom (1985), noncompliance with drug therapy occurs almost 75% of the time. Intentional noncompliance is assumed to account for more than 70% of noncompliant behavior (Wolfe et al., 1988), underuse being the most common noncompliant behavior.

Medical Quackery

Be it a medical elixir made from the horn of a unicorn, or merely the familiar snake-oil sales pitch, medical quackery remains a gullibility problem for the elderly. The promise of a "quick fix" for vitality or of a longer life through magical brews and special potions creates a sense of false hope. Today's magical products include vitamins, bee pollen, ginseng, and many more. Not only can these products lead to economic waste for the elderly, but such special cures can actually be quite harmful to health.

Estimates for money wasted on bogus medical remedies are $4 to $5 billion on cancer cures, $2 billion on arthritis, $10 billion on diet gimmicks, and $3 billion on odds and ends such as products to prevent baldness (Barrett, 1980). Although some of these medical remedies may be harmless and inexpensive, they may also lead the elderly to delay seeking medical attention. Complicating this situation are the tendency of the elderly to diagnose their own ailments and their susceptibility to advertisements of nonprescription drugs, assorted vitamins, health foods, and over-the-counter remedies that purportedly provide relief for a great variety of ailments. The net results are experimentation and total preoccupation with medications, both leading to an irrational regimen of drug ingestion.

Over-the-Counter (OTC) Drugs

The actual number of OTC drugs taken by older adults is difficult to determine. However, it is estimated that over 40% of persons age 60 and older use OTC drugs for such conditions as arthritis, insomnia, and gastrointestinal disorders.   Six factors contribute to self-medication with OTC drugs: (1) retrenchment of Medicare coverage for prescriptive drugs, (2) lessening affordability of prescription drugs, (3) increase in the number of OTC products, (4) increased cost for medical care and professional consultation, (5) increased self-advocacy activities of older adults, and (6) greater exposure of older adults to drugs in their youth (Wolfe et al., 1988).

A significant problem in OTC drug utilization is the simplistic assumption that if a drug is readily available and a nonprescription, then it must be safe and harmless. Many people do not realize that the Food and Drug Administration (FDA) cannot possibly review the safety of all OTC drugs. Proper labeling often escapes the FDA for OTC drugs. Additionally, many powerful prescription drugs are now being reclassified under a nonprescription status. Thus, the potential for OTC drug interaction and subsequent adverse effects has become a critical issue.

Physician Education About Pharmaceuticals and the Elderly

Ferry, Lamy, and Becker (1985) have assessed the level of knowledge among physicians practicing as general practitioners, family practitioners, and internists. The authors conclude that the mean score on a 23-item drug questionnaire was significantly lower than the score judged satisfactory by a panel of six experts. Lower scores were associated with greater number of years since date of licensure and with physicians' reliance on drug advertisements. Physicians relying solely on advertisements rather than on continuing education outlets appeared to have a less clear understanding of prescribing drugs for older adults. Moreover, Williamson, Gorman, Skinner, and associates (1988) found that the lack of information about new pharmaceuticals was the most frequently identified problem for continuing medical education.

The ability of physicians to remain informed of new drug information and potential adverse drug effects has been questioned. Most states require continuing education for licensure renewal. Drug therapy information is usually considered a viable part of such continuing education efforts; however, little evidence suggests that these efforts include clinical pharmacology information for the geriatric patient (German & Burton, 1989).

Pharmacodynamic and Pharmacokinetic Changes

The physiological scatter in response to drugs is much wider in the later than the younger years. This wider response decreases the ability of physicians to predict typical drug action. These physiological changes are partially explained by both the pharmacodynamic and pharmacokinetic hypotheses. The pharmacodynamic hypothesis attributes altered drug reaction with age to changes in the brain, central nervous system, cardiovascular system, receptors, and endocrine system (Michocki et al., 1988). The pharmacokinetic hypothesis attributes altered drug reaction with age to pronounced changes in the rate with which a drug moves through the body. Our discussion will focus on the pharmacokinetic changes.

The rate with which a drug moves through the body involves absorption, distribution, metabolism, and excretion. Absorption is the time required for a drug introduced into the body to enter general circulation. Distribution is the drugs transport to different body sites. Metabolism is the breaking down of the drug into a form that permits its elimination. And excretion is the removal or elimination of the drug through the kidneys. Figure 6-1 details the changes with age for these four vital functions.

The age changes in pharmacokinetic functions are largely due to a normal alteration of the body systems over-time. Nearly all medications are metabolized and excreted by the liver and kidneys, rendering the medications harmless once they have produced their desired effect. However, the function of these vital organs declines steadily with age, even in the absence of a major illness or disease. Thus the elderly possess a diminished ability to absorb, distribute, metabolize, and excrete any chemical they ingest, making the possibility of drug overdose and underdose much higher (Frisk, 1986).

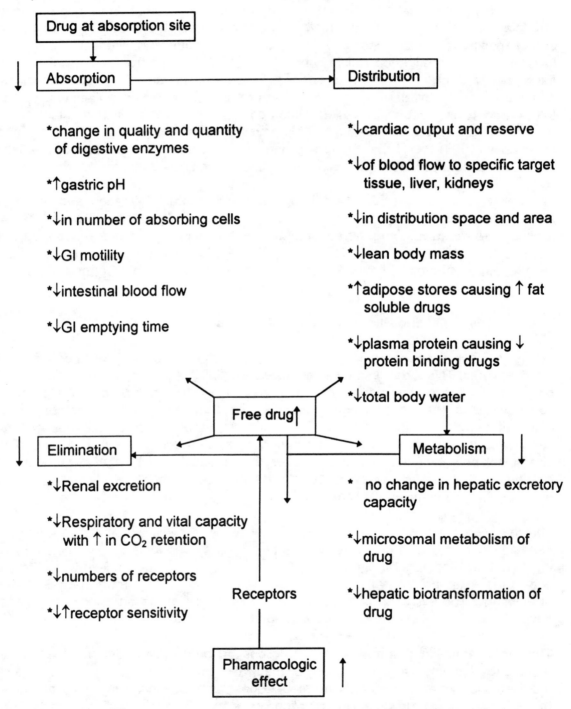

Figure 6-1. Physiologic age changes influencing pharmacokinetics in the elderly.

DRUG MANAGEMENT FOR OLDER ADULTS

Approximately 70 to 80% of drug-related problems experienced by the elderly are predictable and preventable through medication management programs. Regardless of the setting, the elderly can be educated and assisted in proper medication management through multifaceted programs. These programs should minimally include the following components: (1) drug use assessment and intervention, (2) patient education, (3) protective dispensing procedures, (4) improved communication between the physician and the older adult client, and (5) over-the-counter (OTC) drug education.

Drug Use Assessment and Intervention

Knowledge of the factors that lead to adverse drug reactions for older adults has not substantially reduced the drug mismanagement problem. An approach that focuses more specifically on adequate medication history may be a more viable strategy. An individualized and comprehensive drug history would potentially maintain a therapeutic medication regimen and eliminate unnecessary and dangerous medications. Either the pharmacist or a nurse is usually charged with constructing the medication history.

Questions pertaining to the medication history should include motivations and beliefs about taking certain medications; current prescriptions; over-the-counter prescriptions; current administration schedule; client's knowledge about his or her medications; medication side-effects; medication noncompliance; number of prescription drugs taken; frequency of visits to the physician; level of sensory, physical or mental disability; ability to afford medications; and the use of social drugs such as alcohol, tobacco, and caffeine. Typical foods and vitamins consumed and the use of "street" drugs (i.e., opiates, marijuana, cocaine) should also be discussed. Once this information is acquired, the physician should question whether the drug is necessary, as well as investigate the drug's potential for causing side-effects and consider the possibility of polypharmacy and malnutrition (Ebersole & Hess, 1990).

"Medication Brown-Bag Check" has been a popular program used to reassess medications on a periodic basis. The elderly clean out medicine cabinets and bring in all prescribed and over-the-counter medications. Health professionals review shelf-life, appropriateness of drug treatment, potential drug interactions, and answer questions about drug usage and storage. In conjunction with this program, many pharmacists offer assistance through educational programs and computerized profiles to help the elderly better understand and monitor medications for possible interactions and side-effects. The reader may find the publication "Brown Bag Prescription Evaluation Manual" (no date) published by the Department of Pharmacy Practice at the University of Rhode Island very helpful.

Patient Education

Drug education includes both formal and informal classes designed to educate older adults on medication practices and compliance behavior. These classes can prove helpful to older adults and their relatives because the classes help them to better understand the purpose and management of medications (prescription and OTC), and what to expect. Ascione and Shimp (1988) suggest a two-prong strategy for such drug education programs: (1) medication information dissemination and (2) proper management of medications.

The objectives of medication information dissemination are to provide appropriate knowledge for proper taking of medication, for understanding the reasons behind the medication, for minimizing potential drug side-effects, and for avoiding allergic drug reactions that may be caused by potential interactions (with food or vitamins). Both written and oral information should be used; however, one should take particular care not to deluge the older adult with too much information.

Proper medication management is concerned with reducing the complexity of the medication regimen and improving self-medication, especially for OTC drugs. Guidelines for OTC drugs should cover proper reading of labels, potential adverse reactions of OTC drugs, OTC expiration dates, and the importance of informing one's physician and pharmacist of OTC utilization. The reader is encouraged to consult Graedon and Graedon (1988) for an excellent article on understanding the self-medication behaviors of older adults and on counseling older adults based upon this understanding. This article is particularly worthwhile as it includes the pharmacist as a key figure in the drug management education program. Additionally, the reader may find the "Elder-Health Program" at the University of Maryland's School of Pharmacy quite worthwhile. This organization provides a series of brochures developed specifically for pharmacy-based medication education programs.

Protective Dispensing Procedures

Containers and container labels are a concern that should be included in drug management programs. Most child-proof containers are also "geriatric-proof." Older adults with arthritic hands are likely to face difficult and frustrating situations opening medications that are child-proof. It is now possible for older adults to request that their medication be placed in a screw or flip-top container. Individuals in health care settings responsible for ordering medications from the pharmacy should intercede and make this request for the older adult.

Table 6-2 provides a listing of problems older adults experience in taking medications. Older adults experience special problems with medication labels. Labels should be in large print, color coded, and contain international signs and symbols. The use of Braille labels may be advisable. Medication boxes, pill wallets, and medication charts are now used as protective dispenser-type devices to offset many of the medication problems cited in Table 6-2. Technological interventions such as simple, inexpensive bottle cap devices that sound an alarm when it is time to take a medication have also been employed.

Table 6-2. Problems with taking medications.

Trouble taking at nighttime	8.0%
Trouble remembering	22.9%
Trouble opening bottle	36.5%
Trouble separating or breaking tabs	4.6%
Trouble mixing or preparing medication	1.1%
Trouble keeping adequate supply	6.2%
Trouble reading label	9.0%
Taking more or less than label says	4.3%
Medications look alike	1.1%
Other	2.3%

Source: Data from The National Institute on Drug Abuse, "Drug Taking Among the Elderly," 1982, The Institute, Washington, D. C.

Medication charts can help assure that the elderly adult takes each medicine as directed by a physician. Information on the chart should include, (1) name of drug, place purchased, and prescription number, (2) reason for taking drug, (3) date started taking drug, (4) date stopped taking drug, (5) dosage and schedule, (6) results or side-effects, and (7) cost of drug. A daily calendar for checking off medicine may also be beneficial.

Communication Between Physicians and Older Adults

Common drug prescription misjudgments between the physician and the older adult include lack of time in the health care industry to adequately collect necessary information, failure to try nonprescription drug treatment in the early stages of treatment, lack of general communication between the physician and the patient, not constructing a complete medical history of the patient, complexity of the physical problems that can be inherent in an older patient, and administering too strong a medication dosage because of failure to consider pharmacokinetic and pharmacodynamic changes associated with aging. An important step in offsetting these problems is to focus directly on the dialogue between the physician and the older adult.

Specifically, drug management programs can aid the older adult by focusing program components on (1) the importance of telling the physician about all medications being taken, (2) how to ask doctors and physicians questions about safe medication management, (3) side-effects to be aware of with certain medicines, (4) purposes of medications, (5) potential drug interactions, (6) how to follow prescribed medication regimens, (7) generic drug information, (8) medical quackery, and (9) health insurance coverage. The American Institute for Preventive Medicine provides an excellent program for building a health promotion program focusing on these components.

In many instances, the elderly person's drug problems are not corrected by family members, friends, or health professionals. Judgments and decisions related to drug usage are usually left with the elderly. Brady (1978) notes that "friends and family are mostly lay persons who are not expected to know much about drugs, so if they defer to the judgment of the patient who is using the drugs, the inference is that they may also defer any responsibility" (p. 3). However, one would hope that family, friends, and health professionals would become more actively concerned about medication management. Informed vigilance by health professionals in detecting signs and symptoms of adverse drug reactions and aggressive educational awareness programs can serve as prevention devices. The point is that most adverse drug interactions and reactions can be prevented, but prevention begins with a respect for drugs. Appendix F provides useful materials about medication management for the elderly.

OTC Drug Education

OTC drugs treat symptoms not conditions. They are powerful medications that can potentially produce serious side-effects. The Food and Drug Administration (FDA) has established a safety review process for OTC drugs that requires extensive labeling information for consumers. The labeling information required includes the following:

- The name and address of the manufacturer, packer or distributor, and the lot and batch number. This allows the consumer to identify a particular drug should there be any problems with quality or tampering.
- The name of the product and the type of drug it is, such as antacid or decongestant.
- The active ingredients--essential for identifying ingredients to check for potential allergy or sensitivity.
- Yellow Dye #5 will be listed if included in the product. People who are allergic to aspirin are also allergic to this dye.
- Inactive ingredients such as colors, alcohol, binders, flavors, and preservatives are listed by most companies voluntarily, but are not required to be listed by the FDA. The consumer needs to look at these substances for possible allergy or sensitivity.
- Amount--number of tablets, ounces of liquid or ointment.
- Indications for use--conditions or symptoms the product should be used for.
- Directions for use--how much to take, how long to wait between doses, and the maximum number of doses. How to take the drug: chewed, taken with water, etc. These instructions should be followed carefully to get the best results and to avoid potential problems.
- Warnings and cautions--who should not take the drug, when the drug should not be taken, possible adverse reactions, reactions that indicate the need for professional help.

- Drug interaction precautions--an interaction can simply negate the effect of the drug or cause a harmful reaction.
- Expiration date--a drug that is expired can be useless or harmful. (Perspectives in Health Promotion and Aging, Volume 5, No. 1, 1990, p. 5)

The OTC drug label information is certainly needed by consumers. But this information does not replace the importance of maintaining an active dialogue between the older adult and his or her pharmacist and physician. Many OTC drugs, unfortunately, are purchased in grocery stores where there may be no one to answer questions. Drugs such as vitamins, laxatives, cold remedies, and alcohol can all lead to serious problems if used too often or in combination with other medication. A valuable resource for teaching older adults about OTC drugs is a slide/tape show called "Treating Yourself with Care." This show is available by loan through the AARP Pharmacy Service, One Prince Street, Alexandria, VA 22314.

CHAPTER SUMMARY

The use of medications has become an important issue in the health and the health care of older adults. Demographic changes resulting in the aging of American society, coupled with the higher prevalence of chronic disease, focus critical attention on prescriptive and nonprescriptive drug use and the inherent problems associated with such use. This chapter detailed the prevalence of adverse drug reactions among older adults and why such adverse reactions occur. Additionally, we focused on drug management programs as a critical element in the field of health promotion. The need for strong and substantial information concerning drug management in health care for older adults is readily apparent.

The reader interested in drug management for older adults may find the publication by the U.S. Department of Health and Human Services entitled Health Promotion: A Resource Guide for Drug Management for Older Persons (Borgaret-Tullis, 1985) especially helpful. This resource guide was prepared to assist local health and service agencies in developing drug management programs. The guide consists of five sections. The first section provides an introduction to drugs and the older adult. The second section focuses on community organizations and strategies for developing and utilizing community resources. The final three sections describe program models that may be developed at the community level. A listing of resource material is provided at the end of each section.

The reader may also consult Managing Medications published by the National Council on Aging. This publication is a series of six brochures for caregivers and includes information on the purposes of and precautions concerning particular medications. The book by Wolfe et al. (1988) entitled *Worst Pills, Best Pills* provides a more exhaustive treatment of this subject. Finally, the reader may consult the publication *Using Your Medications Wisely: A Guide for the Elderly.* It is published in large print and includes practical suggestions for improving communication between physicians and older adults. The book is published by the National Clearinghouse for Alcohol and Drug Abuse Information, P.O. Box 23245, Rockville, MD 20852.

CHAPTER 7

SUBSTANCE DEPENDENCY AND THE ELDERLY

Some drug and alcohol abusers "mature out" as they age, but many maintain their substance dependency and become elderly addicts. Moreover, a number of previously nonaddicted individuals turn to drugs and alcohol as they age and become elderly addicts. In recent years there has been increasing attention paid to the population of elderly who are drug and alcohol dependent. Yet the field of addiction and aging is very young. Thus, it is not a surprise that there is sparse empirical literature on the complex interacting problems of adults who are both aged and addicted.

The term addiction has inappropriately conjured visions of derelicts, back alleys, and wasted lives. The reality of the situation is that millions of people who are addicts do not fit the wasted-life scenario that has been assigned to the alcoholic or the junkie. Addictions are actually habits gone awry as is evident in the elderly's use of substance abuse to cope with problems, symptoms, and conditions that could be more effectively dealt with by other means. We discuss these "awry" habits by focusing on the semantics of substance dependency and on three substance dependency programs relevant to the elderly--alcohol dependency, tobacco dependency, and food dependency. Drug dependency, due to its critical importance, will be discussed in Chapter 8.

THE SEMANTICS OF SUBSTANCE DEPENDENCY

In order to understand substance dependency, it is essential to differentiate the terms substance abuse and substance addiction. For example, not everyone who drinks alcohol regularly or heavily is an alcohol abuser or alcoholic. To understand the semantics of substance dependency and to apply its principles to intervention programs, one must address the defining characteristics of substance dependency. These characteristics may then be applied under a continuum view of drug dependency.[1] This continuum allows one to separate the terms substance use, substance abuse, and substance addiction.

Defining Characteristic of Drug (Substance) Addiction

A drug is viewed as abusive when it threatens or impairs a person's health or impairs social or economic functioning. For example, cigarette smokers with lung disease are obviously abusing tobacco; alcoholics unable to hold down steady employment are abusers of alcohol. Yet there are many people who consume tobacco, alcohol,

---

[1]Drug is defined here as any substance that in small amounts produces significant changes in the body, mind, or both.

marijuana, and even cocaine without abusing their health or social and economic status. Thus, drug abuse is not simply a matter of what drug an individual chooses to use; rather, it depends on the relationship of the individual to the drug in question.

Recently, addiction problems (i.e., harmful drug relationships) have been labeled as overmedication, dependency, abuse, problem usage, and habituation. These terms are often used as euphemisms for addictive involvement. But each term may mean different things to different people. Because addiction can take so many forms, there is a tendency for researchers and professionals to view the behavior of substance abusers as being unique to a particular substance. O'Donnell and Ainsworth (1985) suggest, however, that the state of being addictively dependent has five common defining characteristics.

Tolerance. Tolerance is defined as the necessity to increase the dosage of a drug in order to obtain the initial psychotrophic effect. Although an essential ingredient in addiction experience, tolerance can occur without addiction. The mechanism of tolerance is not entirely understood. However, it is theorized that tolerance is related to biochemical alterations produced by the drug in the organism, mainly in the liver and the brain. When decreased tolerance accompanies other characteristics of addictive behavior, attempts to reduce consumption are usually not successful. Thus, addicts become unable, despite acts of will, to control dosage.

Abstinence Distress. Abstinence distress is the distressing and painful symptoms caused by sudden deprivation of the habitual use of a drug. These withdrawal symptoms are dependent upon the nature of the drug used, but the psychological manifestations of withdrawal are far more pertinent to management and prevention of relapse than are physiological reactions to discontinuation. The aroused state, a feeling of intense need, can be abated if an addict believes the drug gratification will not occur.

Cognition. As the addiction process develops, an addict recognizes that continued redosing is essential for maintaining a sense of normalcy and for avoiding withdrawal symptoms. The hook of addiction may not be the pleasurable euphoric effect, but rather a need to avoid the unpleasant symptoms of withdrawal. Abstinence distress acts as a precursor to the "normalcy feeling" required by continued drug maintenance. It is during repeated failures of trying to reduce frequency of dosage that the addict becomes cognitively aware that he or she is "hooked."

Craving. The addictive syndrome is actually an endless cycle of craving and satiation. Degree of craving is dependent not only on the length of time an addict has been without a drug, but on the possibility of redosing (availability). Maintenance of the addicted state is dependent on craving and abstinence discomfort, not on the gratification of redosing. Yet craving can reappear unexpectedly years later and thus presents a continuous threat of relapse to the ex-addict. "Extinction of craving is dependent on the permanent loss of any anticipation of the drug use experience" (O'Donnell & Ainsworth, 1985, p. 451).

Relapse. Once the state of addiction is cognitively and effectively realized, a preoccupation with becoming unaddicted commences. However, an individual who has become hooked on a substance has permanently altered his or her relationship with that substance, making resumption of nonaddictive use virtually impossible. This altered relationship is characterized by irrational feelings or rationalizations: "Everybody else is doing it," "I felt bored," "I can stop any time I want to." Relapse begins with a vague thought that, under certain circumstances, the drug may be appropriate or possible to use again. In turn, this rationalization leads to drug-use anticipation and eventually craving. Relapse becomes unavoidable once intense craving has been promoted. Thus short-term abstinence will not end the individual's relationship to a drug addiction.

Drug Dependency: A Continuum Process

The state of dependence as a behavioral syndrome is characterized by the inability of a person to live without the drug he or she is on. This inability takes form and grades dependent upon the type of drug; a person can abstain from alcohol addiction, for example, then heroin addiction. Regardless of the type of drug addiction, a state of inner tension leading to feelings of craving will eventually occur after abstinence distress.

It is useful not to view dependence, including addiction, as a separate entity only, but to regard dependency as the final state of a process. Van Dijk (1985) illustrates this process in Figure 7-1.

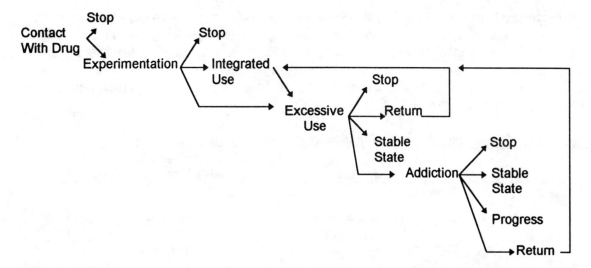

Figure 7-1. Stages in process of drug use. Developed by W. K. Van Dijk. "Complexity of the Dependence Problem." In *Addictive Behavior*. Englewood, Colorado: Morton Publishing Company, 1985, p. 31.

Contact with the drug is represented by the first stage. After one or more drug contacts, the process may cease or enter into a second stage of experimentation. The experimentation stage assumes different forms dependent on several factors to be discussed later in this chapter. After a period of time has elapsed, the second stage may cease or lead into a socially tolerated use stage (integrated mode of use) or may lead to an excessive use stage.

The stage of excessive use is marked by several risks and damages that may be of a physical, social, economic, or moral nature. It is very important to note that what is regarded as a risk or a damage depends primarily on the prevailing social habits and customs. The stage of excessive use is distinguished from incidental excessive use and from periodic excessive use caused by psychiatric factors, such as epilepsy, or depression. In other words, excessive use is more or less a continuous state. For a percentage of cases, excessive use may develop into an addiction syndrome. The addiction syndrome is a terminal state. Yet the addiction syndrome may be avoided by stopping the excessive use or by returning to integrated use.

Van Dijk's (1985) stage process of dependency characterizes addiction as an extreme form of dependence. Considered an illness, the addiction syndrome displays three main features: (1) damaging to the individual, (2) relatively autonomous, and (3) self-perpetuation. Damage to the individual is self-explanatory. Relative autonomy means that for most cases merely removing the initiating addiction factors is not sufficient; special measures must be aimed directly at the overall syndrome. Self-perpetuation suggests that if no help is provided, there is a tendency for the addiction syndrome to spiral into further deterioration.

Dependency Etiology. The actual course the dependency process may take in individual cases, successive stages, and the final stage is very heterogeneous due to the drug nature, personality structure of the user, and the social context. As the dependency process develops, there are several dramatic changes in characteristics associated with the earlier and later phases of drug use. These characteristics are described in Table 7-1.

Table 7-1. Some shifts in characteristics of stages of drug use.

Earlier Phases (Contact, Experimentation)	Later Phases (Excessive Use, Addiction)
More Freedom	Lack of Freedom
Less Risks and Damage	More Damage
Abuse Possible	Abuse Present
No Illness	State of Illness
Operating Factors Linear	Vicious Circles

Reprinted from *Addictive Behavior,* W. K. Van Dijk, "Complexity of the Dependency Problem," page 32, Copyright 1985, with kind permission from Elsevier Science Ltd., The Boulevard, Langford Lane, Kidlington OX5 1GB, UK.

A critical question of interest to health promotion programs is why dependence continues despite its unfavorable impact on the individual. There are no widely accepted answers to this question. However, Van Dijk (1985) suggests the underlying answer is a vicious circle in which a cause generates a result which maintains or reinforces the initial cause. Four vicious circles are distinguished: (1) pharmacological, (2) cerebro-ego-weakening, (3) psychic, and (4) social.

Pharmacological. Repeated use of drugs may cause a change in the phenomenon of tolerance; an increased dose becomes necessary to attain the same effect and the same withdrawal syndrome. A persistent need for a drug and the inclination to increase dosage leads to further metabolic changes and, in turn, the need to repeat drug use again. Thus, cause and effect influence each other by means of pharmacological mechanisms.

Cerebro-Ego-Weakening. In some types of dependency, the quantitative and qualitative excessive use of a drug may directly damage cerebral functions. Cerebro functions form the basis for regulation and integration of behavior. The outcome of excessive use is a weakening of cerebro-ego strength; personal psychical powers to regulate and control use are reduced. In turn, reduced control implies that motives influencing the use of a drug have the opportunity to assert themselves more fully and readily.

Psychic Vicious Circle. Dysfunctional use is marked by feelings of guilt and shame, unpleasant notions that abstaining or decreasing use would be better, and a disagreeable future perspective. The most effective and simplest way to rid oneself of these feelings is to escape through drugs. Moreover, an infantile effect may occur with drug use. Levy describes this effect as a regression to a more infantile behavioral form with an increase in affective and instinctive behavior aspects, and a decrease in the controlling and synthetic fractions of the ego (cited in Van Dijk, 1985).

Social Vicious Cycle. The social circle may be described as a dysfunction, and finally, a disintegration within an addict's social network (spouse, friends). Quarreling, disdain, and withdrawal are examples of social repercussions of drug abuse that foster feelings of isolation and rejection. These negative feelings eventually lead an addict toward feelings of helplessness.

Summary: Dependency and Addiction

Shaffer and Kauffman (1985) view addiction as "an extreme of a continuum of involvement with drug use and refers quantitatively rather than qualitatively to the extent that drug use pervades the total life-activity of the user" (p. 250). Anyone currently addicted would be viewed as drug-dependent, but those who are physiologically or psychologically dependent may not be addicted. Shaffer and Kauffman (1985) provide an illustration of this point:

> The use of alcohol is not considered abuse unless it is used in a
> socially unacceptable manner. For example, drinking a quantity of

alcohol with dinner and becoming loud, threatening, and abusive can no longer be considered simple drug use; it is now likely to be defined as drug abuse. Substance or drug abuse is not necessarily determined by the amount of the substance used, but rather by its effect on individuals within their social context. In addition, what might be drug use for one may be drug abuse for another. That is, people react to alcohol, for example, in a variety of ways (e.g., becoming playful, destructive, sleepy). Playfulness at a party may be a desirable effect of alcohol (use) but at an important business luncheon an inappropriate consequence (abuse).

If a person feels it necessary to drink in order to tolerate a social affair, feel confident at a luncheon meeting, or relax at night, then such use of alcohol might be considered indicative of psychological dependence. Conversely, when one must have a drink before a family function, or a business meeting, in order to prevent shakiness, anxiety, nausea, sweating, weakness, etc., then the person is manifesting signs of physical dependence. Both of these dependent states are considered drug abuse. Finally, when one becomes so overwhelmingly involved with alcohol that its use is compulsively carved into one's daily routine (e.g., hiding a flask at work or slipping alcohol into one's morning orange juice), then the pattern of substance use becomes addiction. (pp. 250-251)

Thus, the language of addiction theory tends to be rich with connotative, confusing, and associative meanings. For example, is being "high" the opposite of being "low," or is "stoned" the opposite of "straight"? The decision to call some substances drugs and others not is often arbitrary. Most people think of chocolate as a food or flavor, but it contains a chemical related to caffeine, is a stimulant, and can be addictive. The point is not that drugs themselves are good or bad but rather whether these substances are put to good or bad use.

SUBSTANCE DEPENDENCY INTERVENTION PROGRAMS

During most of the 20th century, Western society has attempted to deal with its drug problems through negative actions--repressive laws and outrageous propaganda. These negative actions have had a minimal impact. In fact, today more people abuse drugs than ever before. To be successful, intervention strategies must include treatment not only after drug abuse has occurred but as a strategy to prevent abuse from developing. This premise is a consistent theme in substance dependency intervention programs that have been directed toward (1) alcohol dependency, (2) tobacco dependency, and (3) food dependency.

Alcohol Dependency

Simon (1980) defines an alcoholic as a person whose dependence upon alcohol has reached such a degree as to interfere with his or her health, interpersonal relationships, social adjustment, or economic functioning. Most empirical literature on nonadaptive correlates of alcohol abuse has been devoted to the individual's functioning in the first half of life. Relatively few investigations have explored alcohol abuse in mid- and later-life. Despite this void in research, common sense and common experience suggest that the elderly are a highly susceptible group for having alcoholic problems. This section reviews the general findings on alcohol problems in late life, types of elderly alcoholics, differences between late onset and early onset alcoholism, physical effects of alcohol, and treatment strategies.

General Findings. The topic of alcohol and aging has received attention only in the past decade. Perhaps, in the past, we assumed that alcohol was not a major problem in later life. Recently, however, we have realized that alcohol is a problem in late life that can have a devastating impact. Approximately 10 to 15% of adults age 65 and older have alcohol-related problems. Recent research suggests that this percentage of alcohol abuse may be over-stated (Omenn, 1990). Regardless of this discrepancy between alcohol abuse statistics, we can surmise that as the younger and middle-aged adults graduate to their retirement years, the statistics for alcohol abuse will rise dramatically. What we do know about the alcohol problems of today's older adults has been summarized by Maddox and Blazer (1984):

- Approximately one-third of the adult population abstains from alcohol consumption. Older adults are more likely to abstain than younger adults. Women are more likely to abstain than men. Among adults 70 years of age or older, 40% of males and 60% of females abstain from alcohol.
- Longitudinal research has not convincingly established the age when alcohol consumption declines. It is believed, however, that a decrease in alcohol consumption occurs around age 60.
- About 5% of the adult population exhibits alcohol-related problems that may be defined as severe abuse or alcohol dependency. Younger men (age 30 or younger) are four times as likely as older men (age 60 or older) to exhibit severe alcohol problems. Men are also four times more likely to exhibit severe alcohol problems than women. If alcohol problems are defined to include intoxication-related matters (e.g., driving under the influence), alcohol problems are five times lower for the age 60 and older population than younger populations.
- Older clients and patients seen by welfare agencies or in clinics do constitute special subgroups exhibiting relatively high rates of problems with drinking. It is common, for example, to find that in all admissions to general and to psychiatric hospitals, alcohol problems among older persons admitted range from a low of 15% to a

high of 49%. In selected studies of nursing homes, estimates of alcohol-related problems among residents range from 25% to 60%.

- Alcohol-related problems exhibited early in adult life (early-onset alcoholism) tend to persist late in life. Only 1% of the population age 65 and older are thought to develop late-onset alcoholism.

A study by the National Institute of Mental Health on alcohol problems in late life has received particular attention. This study was noteworthy because it used a uniform definition for alcohol abuse and dependence and included a large sample size (4,600 people) from three different sites. Poor education, low income, and a history of depression were the principal factors tied to alcohol-related problems (Maddox & Blazer, 1984). Men (1.9 to 4.6%) were found to exhibit more alcohol problems than women (0.1 to 0.7%). Clark and Midanik's 1982 study also reported higher alcohol problems for men than women. Cohen (1985) found that social drinking was related to income, health, living arrangements, and social networks.

The number of older Americans with alcohol problems is expected to increase as America's population ages. A significant increase is particularly projected for older women. The current group of older women are not heavy drinkers. According to the National Center for Health Statistics, approximately 2% of women age 65 and older consume five or more drinks per day at least five times during the past year (AARP, no date). Women age 45 to 64, however, had substantially higher alcohol consumption rates. Approximately 8% consumed five or more drinks at least five times during the past year.

Types of Elderly Alcoholics. There are two distinct groups of elderly misusers of alcohol. The first group consists of elderly who use alcohol socially and always in moderation. Individuals in this group may compromise their personal safety by mixing drinking with driving, drugs, or walking. The second group of misusers is subdivided into elderly alcoholics who began drinking in later life (late onset alcoholics), and alcoholics who have been drinking for many years and have managed to survive into old age (early onset alcoholics).

Epidemiological studies indicate that well over 10% of individuals age 60 and over are heavy drinkers (Nowak, 1985). Two-thirds of these heavy drinkers are represented in the late onset alcoholic category. Mortality rates are very high for mid- and late-life alcoholics; the greatest incidence in death ranges between 50 to 59 and 60 to 69 respectively.

Differences Between Late Onset and Early Onset Alcoholism. Etiological investigations have reported distinct differences between early and late onset problem drinkers. Late onset drinkers are viewed as stress-reactive rather than process alcoholics. For example, Bland (1985) reports the following factors that lead to late onset drinking:

- The elderly appear to be a high-risk group for problem drinking and alcoholism. Changes in metabolism and in central nervous system functioning may increase the intoxicating effect of alcohol, and the presence of chronic illness may tend to exacerbate the body's response to the ingestion of alcohol.

- Social and psychological aspects of aging can become predisposing conditions causing older people to drink with harmful effect. These include the necessity of living on a limited and fixed income, reduced income, reduced mobility, changes in role and social status, and the feelings of loneliness and isolation associated with the death of friends and family members.

- Problems stemming from the combined use of alcohol and other drugs occur more frequently among the elderly than in younger age groups. Prescription and over-the-counter drugs are both heavily used by older Americans, thus increasing the incidence of interactions between alcohol and drugs that may have toxic or lethal effects.

- Late-onset drinking problems usually occur as a result of situational problems, exacerbated by failing physical and mental health, and emotional and environmental stresses. Early-onset drinkers are those who began to have drinking problems prior to old age, usually during their thirties and forties.

- Diagnostic problems constitute a substantial barrier to treatment of older alcoholics. Medical personnel often mistake signs of frailty, senility, or brain disorder conditions which may in fact be signs of alcohol abuse and alcoholism.

- Evidence suggests that older people may be more responsive to treatment and prevention strategies than younger populations. (pp. 275, 276)

Thus late-life onset alcoholism is principally caused by related environmental stresses such as empty nest, bereavement, retirement, loneliness, and interpersonal conflict. Nowak (1985) writes,

Where investigations have even tangentially explored the characteristics of late-life onset alcoholics, they have found them to be more inundated with stress; more depressed; more likely to have developed inappropriate or unchallenged reserves of strength to cope with stress in their adult years; more involved in situationally anchored rather than psychologically elusive incidents of stress; more likely to have better prognosis for recovery; and more responsive to and active in their plans for treatment and rehabilitation. (pp. 21-23)

Physical Effects of Alcohol. It is not our intent to summarize the many related problems associated with alcohol consumption. In terms of the Healthy People 2000 report, however, moderate alcohol consumption and heavy alcohol consumption have been related to coronary heart disease, diabetes, certain forms of cancer, emphysema, pneumonia, and some other common chronic diseases in late life. Moderate drinking is generally assumed to be more than two ounces of alcohol per day for males and one ounce for females. Alcohol-related medical problems are usually associated with 21 drinks or more per week for men and 14 or more for women (Geller, 1996).

Problem drinking is not a major problem among the elderly. Yet the problem does exist, and it certainly troubles the people who comprise the social network of the elderly person. Although controversial whether the elderly adapt better or worse than younger people to life events, it is tragic when the coping response used is alcohol. Parenthetically, there is no apparent reason why the elderly cannot drink moderately unless there are illnesses or medications which contraindicate alcoholic consumption. There is, however, accumulating evidence that alcohol has unusual effects on the elderly.

The elderly appear to be less tolerant of lower doses of alcohol. Moreover, alcohol may affect the body in unusual ways, making certain medical problems very difficult to diagnose. For example, the effects of alcohol on the cardiovascular system can mask pain that may otherwise have served as a symptom of an oncoming heart attack. Alcoholism can also produce symptoms that mimic dementia, such as forgetfulness, confusion, and lethargy. Over time, alcohol may alter blood sugar metabolism, cause liver disease, create gastrointestinal aggravation, lead to nutritional deficiencies, and damage the brain.

Alcohol, itself a drug, mixes unfavorably with many prescription drugs and over-the-counter drugs frequently used by the elderly. This unfavorable interaction may intensify the older adult's reaction to alcohol, leading to more rapid intoxication. Alcohol can also dangerously slow down performance skills (driving, walking), impair judgment, and reduce alertness when taken with "minor" tranquilizers (e.g., Valium, Librium, Miltown, Mellaril), "major" tranquilizers (e.g., Thorazine), barbiturates, pain killers, antihistamines, and diuretics. Knowledge of drug and alcohol interactions is limited. The possibility that reaction may be idiosyncratic and dangerous, even in small doses, is disquieting. The biggest problem associated with alcohol in late life, however, is the increased number of accidents due to intoxication.

Treatment Strategies. Alcohol abuse among older adults is a more serious problem than people generally realize. Past neglect occurred for several reasons: our elderly population was small, and few were identified as alcoholics; chronic problem drinkers (early onset alcoholics) often died before old age; and because they are often retired or have fewer social contacts, the elderly have often been able to hide drinking problems. Yet older problem drinkers and alcoholics have an unusually good chance for recovery because they tend to remain with treatment programs for the duration. Signs of alcohol abuse include facial puffiness (especially in the morning), rhinophyma, dilated capillaries, sweating, facial flush, tremulousness, easy bruising, nail infections and spider angiomas.

Treatment of alcoholism in old age may be divided into the classic typology of primary, secondary, and tertiary prevention. Table 7-2 illustrates the principal program characteristics for these three typologies. Primary prevention, efforts to reduce incidence of alcoholism, involves society at large or specific target groups. Interventions focus on life-event causes of alcoholism (e.g., bereavement, forced retirement) and include such strategies as improved housing quality, pre-retirement planning, outreach to isolated elderly, and aid to families with dependent older adults. More radical and controversial prevention efforts include substituting less harmful psychotrophic medications for the readily available alcohol--marijuana as a chemical substitute for miseries (Mishara, 1985).

Secondary prevention concerns late onset problem drinkers and focuses on a lasting cure. Unfortunately, candidates in secondary prevention categories are seen well after the alcoholism problem has started. Clients need to be convinced to seek help.

Table 7-2. Models of prevention and treatment of alcoholism in old age.

	PROGRAM CHARACTERISTICS			
	CASE FINDING	PROGRAM IDENTIFICATION WITH ALCOHOL ABUSE	ACTIVITIES	FOCUS
PRIMARY PREVENTION	Society wide programs Identify high risk groups Identify critical life events (crises?) or developmental stages	Not necessary	Education Consultation Advocacy Social change	Society High risk groups
SECONDARY PREVENTION	If has family/support system: family initiates contact client is con-vinced or pressured to obtain help. If limited social supports: client is convinced to seek help (e.g., by physician) crisis event leads to treatment (e.g., acci-dent/hospitalization	Debatable	Outreach Family support Crisis intervention Direct treatment Follow-up and follow-through Medical care	Families Clients
TERTIARY PREVENTION	Habitual referral methods: self, police, interested parties, social service, agencies, hospital/medical	Necessary	Sheltered environment Direct treatment Medical care Creating non-institutional alternatives	Clients

From B. L. Mishara in *Alcoholism, Drug Addiction and Aging,* edited by E. Gottheil et al., 1986. Courtesy of Charles C. Thomas Publishers, Ltd., Springfield, Illinois.

Families, physicians, friends, or any interested party may serve the role of convincing late onset drinkers to seek help. Often, a medical crisis may lead to the realization that alcoholism is a problem. But the principal barrier to secondary prevention remains the stigma associated with a socially unacceptable disease. Mishara (1985) notes this controversy:

> For many families and clients, the idea of going into a general hospital for some "physical care" seems more socially acceptable than telling friends that you are going to the "addiction treatment program." Others feel that unless the problem is openly identified as "alcoholism," avoidance or denial of the nature of the problem inhibits treatment. (p. 251)

Tertiary prevention efforts are not meant to cure alcoholics but to reduce the impact of alcoholism on the life of the alcoholic and society. Chronic alcoholics may enter tertiary programs after their social support network has failed, they are picked up by the police, or they enter the hospital due to a medical crisis. Organic impairment is always present, and thus only skilled neuropsychologists can satisfactorily differentiate between organic impairment due to alcoholism, concurrent organic impairment unrelated to alcoholism, and reversible brain syndromes which are readily treatable (Mishara, 1985, p. 249). Activities in tertiary prevention constitute the majority of available services for the elderly alcoholic.

Summary: A Balanced View. It is very important to maintain a balanced view about alcohol and old age. Alcohol beverages consumed in moderate amounts do not appear to be unhealthy. In fact, there is some research suggesting that restrained alcohol use should be encouraged (Mishara, 1985). However, it is also easy to brush aside problem drinking in old age as a device that offers solace for an individual; it is much harder to create social alternatives to the life events that lie behind alcoholism.

Secondary prevention efforts have not been fruitful. Families and individuals tend to avoid seeking help for alcoholism until it is almost too late--termed the "tardive referral syndrome." This delay in referral results in a higher proportion of physical illness related to alcohol abuse and increases difficulties in attaining successful treatment. Tertiary prevention experiences the major difficulty of attempting to cure the client of his or her illness only to face the client's goal of surviving to drink again. Both secondary prevention and tertiary prevention face the added problem of returning clients to the same psycho-social environments which led to their alcoholism in the first place.

Primary prevention programs must attempt to overcome strong cultural characteristics and patterns. For example, the alcohol industry is firmly entrenched in our society. Alcohol is thus readily available and marketed. Despite cultural patterns, primary prevention efforts seem to offer the most promise of the three prevention intervention categories. "If alcoholism can be prevented before it begins, the costs of alcoholism in resources and social ramifications would be greatly reduced" (Mishara, 1985, p. 251).

The most helpful primary prevention programs are self-help programs, stress management programs, educational programs about alcohol dangers, and link-ups to community support agencies. Unfortunately, very little of society's resources are directed toward primary prevention efforts. The reader may wish to consult Appendix E for a description of types of community programs relevant to alcoholism and illegal drug treatment.

Tobacco Dependency

Smoking is the nation's number one health problem. It is also considered the most preventable cause of mortality and premature morbidity. For example, Scholl (1980) estimated that one-third of all deaths occurring in men age 50 to 60 could have been avoided if all smokers had quit at age 50. Schuman (1981) presented evidence that suggested a decrease in mortality for men who quit smoking for one to four years between the ages of 50 to 69. Although the benefits of smoking cessation should not be extrapolated for the elderly based on studies of middle-aged men, the general evidence still suggests essential health benefits for individuals who cease smoking in older age. This is a very important point when one considers that today's older smoker tends to be more addicted to chewing and heavy tobacco use than do younger smokers.

Health Risks of Smoking. On April 30, 1884, the modern cigarette was born in the North Carolina factory of W. Duke and Sons. The new Bonsack-rolling machine marked the end of the inefficient hand-rolling era and allowed cigarette output and the number of smokers to increase substantially. Approximately 80 years later, January 11, 1964, to be precise, the cigarette's golden age fueled by the Bonsack cigarette-rolling machine came to an end. On this date, the U.S. Surgeon General's Report on Smoking and Health presented scientific evidence on the hazards of cigarette smoking. Today, over 20 years after the Surgeon General's report, we know that smoking is even more dangerous than was believed in 1964. Figure 7-2 summarizes these concerns by addressing the risks and benefits of smoking cessation.

In sum, cigarette smoking is addictive and increases the risk of developing and dying from cancer, heart disease, and chronic lung disease. People who smoke one pack per day have a 50% higher hospitalization rate and a 50% higher general illness, and have a 70% higher over-all death rate than nonsmokers. Despite the tremendous amount of warnings about the dangers of smoking, many elderly people believe that smoking cessation is effective only for younger age groups. This unfortunate myth is also shared by some health professionals. Approximately 65% of smokers age 50 and older wanted to quit smoking. But fewer than 40% of older smokers were ever counseled by health providers about smoking cessation (AARP, no date).

Why you should quit smoking

Risks of Smoking	Benefits of quitting	Low-tar, low-nicotine
Shortened Life Expectancy Risk proportional to amount smoked. A 25-year-old person who smokes two packs a day can expect to live 8.3 years less than a non-smoking contemporary.	After 10 to 15 years ex-smoker's risk approaches that of those who never smoked.	Reduced risk of death from certain diseases suggested increased life expectancy.
Lung Cancer Cigarettes are major cause in both men and women. Overall, smokers' risk is 10 times greater than non-smokers'.	After 10 to 15 years risk approaches that of those who never smoked.	Filter tips reduce risk, but the risk is still 5 times that of non-smokers. Low T/N brands reduce risk to men by 20%, to women by 40%.
Larynx Cancer Smoking increases risk by 2.9 to 17.7 times that of non-smokers.	Gradual reduction in risk, reaching normal after 10 years.	No identified benefit.
Mouth Cancer Smokers have 3 to 10 times as many oral cancers as non-smokers. Alcohol may act as synergist, intensifying effect.	Reducing or eliminating smoking/drinking lowers risk in first few years. Risk drops to level of non-smokers in 10 to 15 years.	No identified benefit.
Cancer of Esophagus Smoking increases risk of fatal cancer 2 to 9 times. Alcohol acts as a synergist.	Since risk is proportional to dose, reducing or eliminating smoking/drinking should lower risk.	No identified benefit.
Cancer of Bladder Smokers' risk is 7 to 10 times greater. Synergistic with certain occupational exposure.	Risk decreases gradually to that of non-smokers.	No identified benefit.
Cancer of Pancreas Risk of fatal cancer is 2 to 5 times higher than for non-smokers.	Since risk seems related to dose, stopping smoking lowers risk.	No identified benefit.
Coronary Heart Disease Smoking a major factor, causing 120,000 heart deaths each year.	Risk decreases sharply after one year. After 10 years risk is the same as for those who never smoked.	With low T/N brands, men have 12% lower risk, women 19% than smokers of high T/N brands.

Why you should quit smoking *(cont'd.)*

Risks of Smoking	Benefits of quitting	Low-tar, low-nicotine
Bronchitis and Emphysema Smokers face 4 to 25 times greater risk of death; lung damage even in young smokers.	Within weeks, cough sputum disappears. Lung function may improve; slower deterioration.	No identified benefit.
Stillbirth, Low Birth Weight Smokers have more stillbirths, more low birth weight babies, and more vulnerability to disease and death.	If smoking is stopped before fourth month of pregnancy, risk to fetus is eliminated.	No identified benefit.
Peptic Ulcer Smokers get more ulcers and are more likely to die from them; cure more difficult in smokers.	Ex-smokers get ulcers, too, but they heal faster and more completely than smokers.	No identified benefit.
Drug and Test Effects Smoking changes pharmacological effects of many medicines. It changes results of diagnostic tests and increases the risk of blood clots from oral contraceptives.	Most blood factors raised by smoking return to normal. Non-smokers on birth control pill have much lower risk of hazardous clots and heart attacks.	

Figure 7-2. What are the real benefits of nonsmoking? (Adapted from "Dangers of Smoking, Benefits of Quitting," prepared by the American Cancer Society. Used by permission.)

Elderly and Smoking Cessation. Data from the American Cancer Society's Cancer Prevention Study (CPS-II) clearly supports the benefits of smoking cessation in later life. CPS-II data was used to estimate the impact of smoking cessation at various age intervals (Table 7-3). For example, a healthy man aged 60 to 64 years smoking a pack of cigarettes or more per day (21 or more) is projected to have a 56% chance of dying in the next 16.5 years. If this individual quits smoking, his chance for premature death decreases to 51%. Although this drop of 5% in death chance may appear to be trivial, investigators from the Framingham studies estimate that smoking cessation between the ages of 65 to 69 increased life expectancy for men by 1.3 years and 1.0 years for females (U.S. Department of Health and Human Services, 1990).

Three important facts may be drawn from our discussion of health benefits associated with smoking cessation in later life: (1) 7 million smokers are age 60 or older; (2) smoking is a major risk factor for 6 of the 14 leading causes of death among the population age 60 and older and is a complicating factor in three others; and (3) life-expectancy gains from smoking cessation in later life are not trivial. Immediate benefits of smoking cessation include: (1) lower blood pressure, reducing risk of stroke; (2) improved respiratory function, especially when exercise programs are combined with smoking

Table 7-3. Estimated probability of dying in the next 16.5 year interval for quitting at various ages compared with never smoking and continuing to smoke, by amount smoked and sex.

Age quitting or at start of interval	Never smokers	Males			
		1-20 cig/day		>21 cig/day	
		Continuing smokers	Former smokers	Continuing smokers	Former smokers
40-44	0.05	0.11	0.05	0.14	0.07
45-49	0.07	0.18	0.10	0.22	0.11
50-54	0.11	0.27	0.17	0.31	0.21
55-59	0.18	0.39	0.28	0.46	0.33
60-64	0.30	0.54	0.46	0.46	0.33
65-69	0.46	0.68	0.59	0.67	0.64
70-74	0.40	0.61	0.55	0.58	0.52

Age quitting or at start of interval	Never smokers	Females			
		1-20 cig/day		>21 cig/day	
		Continuing smokers	Former smokers	Continuing smokers	Former smokers
40-44	0.03	0.06	0.03	0.08	0.04
45-49	0.04	0.09	0.06	0.13	0.05
50-54	0.07	0.14	0.07	0.19	0.09
55-59	0.11	0.21	0.12	0.27	0.15
60-64	0.18	0.30	0.19	0.38	0.32
65-69	0.30	0.46	0.39	0.52	0.32
70-74	0.26	0.41	0.27	0.45	0.31

Source: Data from the Surgeon General, *The Health Benefits of Smoking Cessation,* 1990, page 83. U. S. Department of Health and Human Services, Public Health Service, Rockville, MD.

cessation; and (3) improved taste which contributes to better nutrition (American Hospital Association, 1985).

In addition to the functional benefits of smoking cessation, it is important to note that smoking is a major risk factor in 8 of the top 15 causes of death for older Americans (AARP, no date). Coronary heart disease (CHD), atherosclerotic peripheral vascular disease, lung and laryngeal cancer in women, oral cancer, esophageal cancer, and chronic obstructive lung disease have been found to have a direct causal relationship with smoking. Diabetes, osteoporosis, and ulcers have also been found to be related to smoking. The American Medical Association (1984) summarizes the impact on smoking on the lives of older adults as follows:

> You can have a similar impact on lessening your chances of developing lung cancer. Let us assume that you are a fifty-year-old man who decides to quit smoking. You toss out the pack, wash the ashtrays and never take another puff on a cigarette. You have no guarantee of avoiding the number-one cancer killer for men in the country--lung cancer--but by approximately age fifty-seven you will have reduced by one-half your changes of getting the disease. By the time you are sixty-five years old, you will have brought the odds down to less than 1 percent, the same as those for a man who has never smoked. There's even an added bonus, according to researchers at the Gerontology Research Center. As a fifty-year-old smoker, you had the lung function of a man ten to fifteen years older. But within one or two years of quitting smoking, your lung capacity will equal that of the average nonsmoker your age. (It should be noted, however, that in some case damage to the alveoli--the air cells of the lungs--is irreversible.) (pp. 10-11)

Does Smoking Affect Older Adults Differently. A longitudinal study by Jajich, Ostfeld, and Freedman (1984) focused on smoking and CHD for 2,674 adults ages 65 to 74 years. The authors reported CHD death rates as 52% higher for nonsmokers and ex-smokers. This excess risk due to smoking declined within one to five years after smoking cessation. A cross-sectional study by Rogers, Meyer, Judd et al. (1985) investigated the effects of cerebral blood flow after smoking cessation. Substantial benefits by increased cerebral blood flow were found within a relatively short period after smoking cessation.

Smoking has been found to complicate the healing process and to encourage bone demineralization. The rate of medication metabolism is also impaired by smoking. Moran (1990) states that,

> Of the many compounds in cigarettes, some are microsomal liver enzyme stimulators that influence the metabolization of drugs. Heavy smokers may need higher doses of certain medications to maintain the same serum levels as nonsmokers. For instance, propoxyphene hydrochloride (Darron), a minor analgesic, has been found to be ineffective in about 20 percent of smokers, double the rate for the general population. Smoking aggravates peripheral ischemia that can occur with B-blockers. Cigarettes shorten the half-life of heparin, which may be given to dissolve blood clots. Heavy smokers may need doses up to 50 percent higher than nonsmokers of theophylline of aminophylline to maintain serum levels. (p. 48)

In spite of the benefits of smoking cessation for older adults, the Office of Legislation of the U.S. Department of Health and Human Services had not introduced legislation, as of 1989, related to smoking and older adults. The Office of Legislation had, however, been directed toward preventing the young from beginning to smoke and the creation of smoke-free environments. Yet as argued in this section, the normal effects of aging make older adults especially vulnerable to the adverse health effects of smoking.

Year 2000 Health Objectives and Smoking. Smoking was a critical component in the year 1990 health objectives for the nation released by the Public Health Service (1986) in the 1980s. Four of the five smoking objectives were concerned with awareness issues, such as increasing the awareness of health risks associated with smoking. None of these objectives, however, were targeted to a special population group such as older adults. This situation has been remedied with the release of the Healthy People 2000 report.

One of the primary smoking objectives in the Healthy People 2000 PHS report is to "increase to at least 50 percent of the population of current smokers age 20 and older who made a serious attempt to quite smoking" (U.S. Department of Health and Human Services, 1989, p. 3-3). This national focus on smoking cessation for young adults will also benefit older adults. A specific objective directed toward older adults states, "Increase to at least 50 percent the proportion of older smokers ages 65 through 74 who know that quitting smoking even late in life is one of the most important actions a person can take to preserve his or her health" (p. 7-4). The introduction of health promotion programs directed specifically to smoking and older adults will be needed to attain this objective. Bridging awareness and behavioral change, however, will require health professionals to focus directly on barriers to quitting that are peculiar to older adults.

Barriers to Smoking Cessation. Psychosocial factors such as the need to control or make choices in life significantly affect smoking behavior. Smoking may actually be a display of autonomy for older adults who have lost control of many life aspects due to age decrements (Fisher, Bishop, Goldmuntz et al., 1988). Smokers may also use smoking to regulate emotional states. Nicotine and other cigarette substances may condition emotional states during feelings of anxiety (Leventhal & Cleary, 1980). Self-image for body weight control may be especially important for women (Sorensen & Pechacek, 1987).

Common sense tells us that it is difficult to stop a behavior like smoking that can be viewed as both beneficial and enjoyable. For example, the Clear Horizons Survey (Ferguson, 1989) reported that the nicotine in cigarettes is seen as a substance that can regulate moods, improve attention and concentration, help learning and memory, stimulate creativity, dull the sensation of pain, produce mild euphoria, shed pounds without dieting, and help control stress. To be successful, smoking cessation programs will need to address barriers that may be seen by smokers as beneficial.

Smoking Cessation Programs. For years, smoking was thought of as a habit--a nasty habit, Mark Twain called it. Smokers can break themselves of smoking, and every year hundreds of thousands do, but such cessation efforts can be very difficult. One-third of the people who try to stop smoking, start smoking again one week later and only one-fourth remain abstinent for longer than six months (O'Donnell & Ainsworth, 1985). To assist individuals interested in smoking cessation, a variety of programs has been developed. Although these programs are principally directed toward younger age groups, program options can be expanded or tailored to include the elderly.

In-House Programs. In-house programs are directed and staffed by health promotion employees and involve distribution of "how to quit" materials, presentations by the staff, and individual or group counseling. Particular program components include facts about smoking, identification of smoking patterns and cessation obstacles, motivation to stop, how to change behavior, cessation strategies, and maintenance techniques to prevent backsliding. The advantage of an in-house approach is the use of existing resources and the provision of on-going support to elderly participants as the need occurs. Variables that influence the success of in-house programs include staff expertise, department commitment, and the seriousness with which the cessation program is addressed.

Community Service Programs. Organizations such as the American Cancer Society, American Lung Association, and Seventh Day Adventists offer smoking cessation programs at little or no cost. The American Cancer Society has the best known and most widely available program. The programs provided are relatively short (5 to 8 group meetings) and may be conducted over a one to four week period. Development, staffing, and program delivery are allocated by the community service agency. Space and dissemination of material is usually the responsibility of the user organization. Community service programs use a health education approach laced with bits and pieces of behavioral techniques. The simplicity of this approach has led to a low smoking-cessation rate (O'Donnell & Ainsworth, 1985).

Commercial Programs. There are several large commercial smoking cessation programs that are offered on a nation-wide or regional basis. The largest commercial programs contain a series of lectures conducted over an 8-week period. The strategy employed principally consists of categorizing cigarettes on a one to four importance scale, followed by progressive elimination of the least important category. Delaying tactics (postponement of taking a cigarette), behavioral modification techniques, aversive conditioning, and pep-talks are also used. Problems with commercial programs center around the qualifications and expertise of program providers and program appropriateness. Outside evaluations of the supposedly high success rate of commercial programs are rarely initiated. Thus, it is advisable for the user organization to evaluate commercial services according to their staff training and expertise, evaluation documentation, materials provided, and level of satisfaction expressed by past clients.

Packaged Programs. Packaged smoking-cessation programs are presented in written form, audio-cassette, videotape, or on film. The simplicity of these programs is appealing due to minimized personnel requirements and access to large numbers. Despite this attractiveness, packaged programs are probably most helpful to individuals who are least in need of smoking cessation help and least helpful for those who most need help. The content of packaged programs tends to neglect the hardships, difficulties, and negative aspects associated with a substance dependency. Superficial treatment is not likely to be successful for an addictive problem (O'Donnell & Ainsworth, 1985).

Treatment of Withdrawal: Nicotine Replacement Techniques. Nicotine products produce both tolerance and dependence. The actual intensity of withdrawal symptoms will vary according to the abrupt cessation of continuous use. Gelder 1996 writes:

> . . . 80% of smokers who quit experience some withdrawal, which starts within hours, peaks at 48 hours, and may continue with diminishing intensity for 2 to 5 weeks. Increased appetite and weight gain may continue for 10 weeks. Craving for cigarettes may persist for months and is probably more related to the powerful and pervasive association than to physiological drug withdrawal itself. Most relapses occur during the first 2 weeks after cessation, when physiologic withdrawal is at its height. (p. 28)

Frequent withdrawal symptoms include irritability, impatience, anxiety and dysphasia. To ease the process of withdrawal, nicotine replacement techniques have been used. Nicotine gum, for example, is a common initial step. This gum is available in doses of 2 mg or 4 mg. The 4 mg dose is typically used in highly dependent clients. Nicotine gum is kept in the mouth for 30 minutes between the gum and cheek. The gum is slowly turned in the mouth and not chewed. Clients are advised to use one piece of gum per hour during the day since it is important to maintain a steady level of nicotine in the blood.

Transdermal nicotine patches are also used as a nicotine replacement technique. These patches are available in different mg strengths and are delivered in a steady dose over a 24-hour period. The Fagerstrom test for nicotine dependence is used to determine the mg dose. This dose is administered in a stepwise fashion. Detoxification patterns will vary between clients (Gelder, 1996). The average detoxification period is between 6 to 10 weeks.

Other nicotine replacement techniques are also being developed. Nicotine nasal spray and vapor-inhalation methods are under development. Nicotine replacement techniques are only effective, however, if they are used in conjunction with other intervention strategies. Cognitive-behavioral therapy with pharmacotherapy is more successful then when pharmacotherapy is applied alone. Nicotine replacement techniques are approved for detoxification but not for maintenance. Cognitive behavioral therapy is employed to assist the client in the process of learning, unlearning, and extinction. This process is used to help smokers decrease the reinforcing value of smoking. Both external and internal triggers to smoking are identified and alternative ways to offset these triggers are taught. Stress reduction techniques and exercise programs tend to be used as adjunct treatment programs.

Summary: Two Critical Issues. The benefits of smoking cessation programs are valuable for the continued health of the elderly. Several organizations offer programs that use behavioral modification and group interventions or support groups. Some groups sponsor smoking cessation at age 50 or older clubs and combine smoking-cessation efforts with nutrition, weight control, stress management, and drug and alcohol use programs. Successful programs include a combination of these program strategies. Generally, programs with success rates of 15 to 20% are considered excellent.

The key is to recognize that tobacco is an addictive product. Frequency of use, method of administration, psychosocial and pharmacological rewards, craving syndrome, abstinence distress, and relapse all point toward the compulsive nature of smoking behavior. Thus, health professionals designing smoking cessation programs for the elderly face two critical issues: (1) convincing the elderly that smoking cessation has immediate benefits for their health; and (2) designing programs that are based on the addictive nature of tobacco dependency.

Food Dependency

The reader may be surprised by the inclusion of food as a substance dependency category. However, food dependency contains the same defining characteristics of substance addiction discussed earlier in this chapter. For example, individuals who have become accustomed to large quantities of sugar or caffeine will experience withdrawal symptoms when they abstain from these products. In fact, O'Donnell and Ainsworth (1985) convincingly argue that the principal reason behind the high failure rate of traditional diet plans is due to their failure to recognize the addictive qualities of food. To illustrate the addictive quality of food, we will explore the schools of thought behind obesity and traditional versus addictive intervention strategies.

Two Schools of Thought. Obesity has seldom been viewed as a substance dependency problem. However, it is common knowledge that compulsive eaters do engage in addictive behaviors with food. Whitney and Hamilton (1984) provide an excellent illustration of this intense relationship:

> *Scene*: Your place. *Time of day*: Afternoon or evening. You are doing nothing in particular, when suddenly you feel like eating something sweet. You resist, but the feeling gnaws at you. With guilt fluttering in your conscience you head for the cookie jar, telling yourself, "Just one. Maybe two. Not more than three. Or four." But you already have calculated about how many cookies are in the jar. A few minutes later, the jar is empty.

176

Not all people see themselves in this description, but many more do than you might think--probably the majority of people in our society. We all have a complex and intense relationship with our food that no one completely understands. Many factors are involved, from the body's purely chemical interaction with food to the emotional involvement of the self with food and the consciousness of its social meaning. One factor is the tiny entity, the sugar molecule itself, which provides the sweet taste we all find so attractive. (p. 263)

Obesity is a process whereby excess body fat accumulates when K-calories are eaten beyond those needed for the day's metabolic, muscular, and digestive activities. Two schools of thought govern why obesity is a problem. One attributes obesity to inside-the-body causes, the other to environmental factors. The set-point theory, appestat theory, and the glucostatic theory are represented by the inside-the-body school of thought. Proponents of the environmental school argue that we overeat because we are pushed to do so by factors in our surroundings, such as advertisements and food availability. The two views are not mutually exclusive, and research suggests that both schools are possible.

A discussion of the inside-the-body and environmental theories are beyond the scope of this chapter. The reader is encouraged to consult Whitney and Hamilton (1984) for such a review. However, the salient point is that there are valid reasons to view an overeater's difficulty in overcoming an excessive need for food as parallel to a person's addictive response to other substances. Addiction may be too strong a word here; the behavior may be more adequately described as a habit or abuse.

Traditional Versus Addictive Intervention. Group support interaction and behavioral modification strategies are commonly employed to assist overeaters in reducing their K-calorie consumption. Yet many weight reduction plans give the mistaken impression that a diet is an abnormal, temporary regimen to be adhered to until the desired weight loss is attained, at which point "normal" eating may be resumed. The problem with weight loss, however, is not a lack of knowledge. Most people who have addictive eating disorders resulting in obesity are knowledgeable about caloric contents of food, the energy balance equation concept, what represents a normal food portion, and the need for a well-balanced regimen of three meals per day. O'Donnell and Ainsworth (1985) clearly convey the problem as follows:

Weight reduction diets interfere with an addictive treatment approach when they lack a sense of permanent normalcy, fail to eliminate those foods that the overeater consumes only to obtain addictive gratification, and maximize the number of food choices and taste experiences to put emphasis on the joys of eating. Many diet programs acknowledge "out of control" eating behaviors but then reinforce food involvement by endlessly enumerating all the pleasures that can be derived from foods on the free list (allowable in unlimited quantities) and by providing recipes intended to enhance the experience of consuming such low-calorie foods. (p. 457)

O'Donnell and Ainsworth (1985) are suggesting that perpetual involvement with food and eating helps maintain addictive involvement rather than discouraging it. In other words, diet plans are not addressing the most pertinent issues of craving or the compulsive nature of the eating experience--the influence of availability and acceptability. The point is not that diet plans and behavioral modification strategies are not important. They are! However, some aspects of a drug abuser rehabilitation plan might be used effectively in weight control programs. Such an approach would elevate overeating from the status of a bad habit to the level of importance encouraged by a substance addiction. Viewed as a food dependence (addiction), individuals would be encouraged to act in their own behalf and realize the degree of seriousness needed for effective intervention programs.

The focus of a food dependency approach is to provide long-term support to prevent relapse rather than achieve short-term weight loss. Extinction of the addictive eating behavior would be a main program goal for directing a compulsive overeater's attention away from any involvement with food not motivated by nutritional need.   Active lifestyles, coping systems, and alternative reward systems would play an integral program role.   O'Donnell and Ainsworth (1985) suggest the following principles for integrating addictive behavior principles for integrating addictive behavior principles into weight control programs:

- The program's focus should shift away from issues of food intake, such as menu planning, food allowances, calorie counting, and graphic descriptions of food binges. Any behavior that encourages the anticipation of food availability is discouraged.
- Concepts of normal eating behavior based on good nutritional practices should be established. In other words, food should be consumed based on nutritional need and not to alleviate hunger sensations.
- Although difficult to achieve, participants should be encouraged to minimize food involvement, as in food shopping and meal preparation.
- The concept of addiction is incorporated to allow participants to identify specific eating behaviors, experiences, and attitudes about food that must be relinquished if a non-addictive food relationship is to be attained. Concepts about craving states and false attribution caused by emotional needs are emphasized.
- Quality of life and lifestyle changes are developed. The key is to develop the need for active rather than passive participation in life's activities.
- On-going, long-term support is available for all participants.

Summary: Food Can Be Addictive. As you can see, some of the principles used in an addiction approach to food dependency are very different from most weight control plans. The point is that food can be addictive, and its treatment requires a serious and long-term approach. Overeaters need to identify their problem as an addictive involvement with food rather than as excessive body weight. Availability (craving) and acceptability (social eating) are addictive stages that require principal program attention. Thus, when food addicts are not made aware of their misuse of the eating function as the basic problem, are not helped to eliminate addictive eating behaviors, and are treated for obesity only on the basis of weight loss, they will almost certainly fail in their attempts to control food dependency.

CHAPTER SUMMARY

The salient theme in this chapter is that substance abuse is not the use of a disapproved substance; rather, abuse is the use of any substance in ways that impair physical or mental health, or social functioning and productivity. Bad drug relationships commence with ignorance or loss of awareness of the nature of a substance and its effects and overuse. These bad relationships were categorized under three substance dependency programs: (1) alcohol, (2) tobacco, and (3) food. Prescription and nonprescription drugs were covered in Chapter 6.

Elderly adults need to learn to look at and analyze their own relationships with drugs. Because it is difficult to view one's own behavior, health professionals can play a viable role in helping the elderly to make an effective drug appraisal. However, recognizing drug abuse is not a simple process such as merely looking for dilated eyes or certain styles of dress or types of behavior. Learning to recognize drug abuse is imperative because drug treatment is not easy. Prevention of drug abuse is always much easier than treatment.

CHAPTER 8

THE ELDERLY AND THEIR MENTAL HEALTH: CHOICES AND CHALLENGES

Consider Ruth: Ruth is 91 years of age. She was widowed when she was in her late 70s. After her husband's retirement, the couple continued to live in the home he had built nearly 50 years before. They traveled occasionally to visit friends and family in other communities, but were content to remain close to home. After retiring, Ruth continued to cook and garden. Her husband kept very busy doing jobs around the home and for others. They had frequent contact with other family members who lived in and near their community. Always an important component of their lives, they remained active members of a local church. They attended services regularly and also participated in many social activities that were organized for church members. Retirement afforded the couple opportunities to do more of the things they had always liked to do.

Ruth's husband suffered his first heart attack at the age of 67. Two others followed over the next seven years, the last of which was fatal. Other losses were experienced as well. Within months of her husband's death, several elderly friends also died. Following an understandable period of extreme sadness, Ruth decided to get on with her life. She returned to many of the activities that had been enjoyable to her in the past. Regular contacts were reinitiated with family and friends. Ruth also decided that she needed to replace the friends that she had lost. Although she had been "too busy" to do so before, she decided to participate in activities at a senior center. She regularly attends movies with several of her 'new friends.'

Except for a slightly elevated blood pressure (that is controlled with medication), Ruth is quite healthy. She sees her doctor regularly and follows his recommendations. Ruth takes pride in the fact that her doctor says she doesn't look a day over 80! She exercises regularly at the senior center. Last year Ruth took a nutrition class; she now makes healthier food choices. With very little prompting, Ruth says that she is 'happy' and that she has 'a good life.' Although she has slowed down considerably in recent years, she still lives on her own and continues to enjoy (and be enjoyed by) her family and friends.

Consider Sally: Sally and her husband had moved to a rural community shortly after his retirement. Retirement proved to be very difficult for the couple. Years later, Sally admitted that she thought that their move had been a mistake. Precipitated in part by lingering tensions within their extended family, Sally and her husband used retirement as an excuse to get away. Although the move provided a buffer between the couple and other members of the family, it also separated them from a number of close friends. Sally and her husband had difficulty meeting people. They both spent little time doing things that they hoped would fill their retirement--travel, fishing, gardening, woodworking--and more time being inactive. They watched a lot of TV. On those rare occasions when other family members came to visit, they often were alarmed by what they saw. Both physically and emotionally, Sally and her husband seemed to be deteriorating rapidly. Despite the fact that they now had lived in the community for almost five years, they remained disconnected from those around them. Sally, a diabetic, saw their physician far too infrequently. As she put it, "He only tells me what I don't want to hear." She also suffered from glaucoma. Her vision had become very compromised over the past few years. Sally's husband complained that she couldn't remember things anymore. Efforts to convince the couple to move back home were vehemently opposed. Sally's husband's health declined very rapidly. Five years before her move to the nursing home, he died of a previously undetected cancer. His death intensified her isolation and seemed to accelerate her own physical and emotional decline.

During a visit to her mother, Sally's daughter became convinced that her mother's vision difficulties were significantly compromising her health and safety. Although groceries were delivered to her home, her nutritional status was in question. Sally consumed a lot of canned food. She joked that since she couldn't really see the labels, every meal was a "surprise." Sally's daughter was also concerned that a fire might result from her mother's efforts at food preparation. She was also concerned that her mother seemed very depressed. Sally angrily refused to consider moving to an apartment community for elders, even one that would be close to her daughter. A compromise was reached: instead of going to the retirement community, Sally would be visited ("spied on" was the phrase Sally used) several times each week by a woman from a local social service agency. The compromise failed, however, when following her daughter's return home, Sally simply refused to answer her door when the woman visited.

Following the visiting nurse's unsuccessful efforts to check on Sally, the daughter was contacted. Arrangements were soon made that resulted in a nursing home placement. Sally was angry and reported feeling betrayed by her daughter. Upon admission, a number of health issues required immediate attention. The admitting physician was very concerned about how confused she seemed, and about her obvious depression.

Although the names have been changed, these are glimpses at the lives of two real people. Although they grew up at approximately the same time in our culture, Ruth and Sally have distinctly different histories. In combination, the stories of these women anchor two ends of a continuum: Ruth's end of the continuum can be described with terms like "connection," "activity," "prevention," and "continuity." Sally's end of the continuum is characterized by terms such as "denial," "resignation," and "decline." Their stories provide a suitable opening for a discussion of the topics pertaining to geriatric mental health.

PREVALENCE OF MENTAL ILLNESS

George (1992) reports that approximately 7% to 12% of community-dwelling older adults have one or more diagnosable psychiatric disorders. This figure is lower than the prevalence estimates for adults under age 65, which range from 14% to 19%. The estimated prevalence range for the elderly is also lower than a number of earlier estimates that were in the vicinity of 25% to 35%. This rate reduction can be accounted for in part by progressive improvements in case identification in more recent epidemiologic studies (George, 1992). Marie Haug and her associates (Haug, Belgrave, & Gratton, 1984) have suggested that the higher prevalence rates in early studies typically resulted from failures to distinguish different types of psychiatric disorders. Quite frequently, depression (a treatable condition) was not differentiated from dementia (an untreatable, often chronic organic brain syndrome). Since the rate of organic psychiatric disorders was (and still is) more common in older people (George et al. 1988), the comparative rates of mental disorder tended to be severely skewed in the direction of the elderly. These data, in combination with the fact that the elderly often underutilize potentially helpful mental health services (Waxman, Carner, & Klein, 1984), strengthened at least two unfortunate impressions regarding geriatric mental health: first, that mental disturbances must be the inevitable accompaniments of advancing age, and second, that such difficulties in the elderly are often unchangeable. Although the elderly are clearly not immune from what Anthony and Aboraya (1992) referred to as "disturbances of mind and behavior" (p. 92), in contrast to the gloomy view that characterized earlier epidemiologic investigations, others have stressed more recently that the majority of elderly persons experience happiness and satisfaction throughout the later years of their lives (Row & Kahn, 1987).

ETIOLOGY

Epidemiologic investigations in recent years have clarified some of the general characteristics of the mental illnesses experienced by the elderly (George, 1992). It is estimated, for example, that 40% of late-life mental illnesses are organic in nature, as in the case of the various dementias. Many of the disturbances in the remaining 60%, however, including the so-called reactive or situational disturbances, are *not* the result of organic factors. And although genetic influences are likely with reference to the etiology of a number of major mental disturbances (e.g., schizophrenia, biopolar conditions, major depression, etc.), it has been argued that genetic influence may be a less crucial factor in mental illnesses that first appear in old age (Zung, 1980). Affective disorders and anxiety are very common among the elderly (George); they are also very treatable (Gallagher-Thompson, Hanley-Peterson, & Thompson, 1990; George, 1992; Woods, 1993). A number of researchers have speculated that many of the nonorganic disturbances experienced by the elderly (e.g., adjustment difficulties, dysthymia, non-major depression, anxiety, etc.) are possibly the result of increases in social stress and accompanying decreases in social support (Green, Copeland, Dewey, et al. 1994; Rubinstein, Lubben, & Mintzer, 1994; Woods, 1993; Zung, 1980).

In advance of a discussion of some of the psychotherapies that are used to treat nonorganic mental disturbances, attention will be devoted to: (1) a survey of some of the predictable (often stressful) issues that must be addressed in old age; and (2) some of the factors that appear have a protective influence on the mental health of many elderly persons.

PREDICTABLE ISSUES

The elderly experience a number of stressors that typically are not experienced by persons in other age groups. These stresses and their resulting outcomes (e.g., adjustment difficulties, affective difficulties, anxiety, etc.) can often be viewed as artifacts the stage of life that the elderly have reached. Although the following list certainly does not exhaust the universe of possibilities, some of the predictable issues that commonly must be addressed by the elderly are summarized below.

Retirement

Transitions from one stage of the family life cycle to the next are often more difficult than might be expected (Haley, 1973). It is not uncommon for difficulties to arise as retirement approaches, or shortly after it has occurred. Although there certainly are variations across cases (Vinick & Ekerdt, 1995), many couples need assistance recalibrating their relationship at this time. Previous family routines that may have been organized around the work schedule of one or both spouses may no longer be necessary or desirable. Many couples must come to terms with spending considerable amounts of time with one another; in many instances, more extended time than at any other point in their relationship. A person's (or couple's) adjustment can be influenced by a number of factors including, for example: whether work before retirement was viewed as a source of stress or reward; the degree of planning that was done in advance of retirement; and views that retirees hold of their retirement (e.g., retirement as a time to enjoy new things, versus retirement as a time to dwell on unattained goals, etc.) (Woods & Britton, 1985). It could be predicted, for example, that people who miss their work, planned poorly for retirement, and blame themselves for not having accomplished more, might have more stressful retirements than their more planful, optimistic counterparts.

The Loss of Friends and Family Members

With increasing age many elderly persons are confronted with deaths in their family and friend networks. These losses can significantly alter the elderly person's interpersonal environment (Woods & Britton, 1985). A wide range of grief reactions are possible, however. Comparatively mild periods of bereavement have been reported in some studies involving the elderly (Averill & Wisocki, 1981; Woods & Britton, 1985), although other investigations have documented more intense reactions, including significant increases in physical symptoms (Doherty & Campbell, 1988), and prolonged periods of psychological distress (Woods & Britton, 1985).

Health professionals can be very helpful to elderly persons (and other family members) who are struggling with such losses. Ultimately, a number of specific objectives may need to be accomplished to facilitate their long-range adjustment. These may include helping them to: (1) transform shared experiences into memories; (2) deal with important issues pertaining to daily living (e.g., task demands, loneliness, etc.); and (3) develop new interests and activities (Walsh, 1980).

Illness and Physical Decline

As people age, the chances increase that they will experience at least one chronic illness or some other disabling condition (McGinnis, 1988). Problems sometimes arise regarding the adjustment (or lack thereof) to the diagnosis of a new medical condition in an elderly member, or significant changes in the status of a previously diagnosed condition. Health professionals can help families organize appropriately around the illnesses that are experienced. In instances where the illness is chronic but has a relapsing or progressive course, time should be spent trying to enhance the adaptability of the family system (via education, planning, etc.) to adequately prepare the family for anticipated changes (Rolland, 1988).

The Frequent Interrelatedness of Physical and Mental Illness. Health professionals who work with the elderly should be aware that physical and mental illnesses can occur separately or in combination. Salzman and Nevis-Olesen (1992) stressed that psychiatric symptoms can be the first signs of an underlying physical illness. For example, hypothyroid and hypoadrenal states, and chronic viral infections can significantly alter affective functioning. Similarly, psychiatric symptoms often accompany serious medical conditions. In the case of stroke, for example, depression may result because of complications that are specific to brain damage, or because of the reaction of the patient to the resulting changes in his or her life. Summarizing the results of a number of investigations, Zung (1980) similarly noted a strong correlation between impaired mental health and medical difficulties. It was speculated that this association was due, in part, to the inability of many physically impaired elderly persons to engage in adequate self care.

Cohen (1985, 1992) outlined a typology that summarizes a number of possibilities (and examples) regarding the interrelatedness of medical and mental illnesses among the elderly. Specifically, he proposed that: (1) psychogenic stress can lead physical compromise (e.g., the chronic anxiety of an elderly person could lead to gastrointestinal symptoms); (2) the effects of physical disorders can result in psychiatric disturbances (e.g., a patient's hearing loss could result in the onset of delusional thinking); (3) physical and mental disorders can be recursively linked (e.g., an elderly person's congestive heart failure may lead to depression, which in turn could lead to further cardiac complications); and (4) social factors can influence the clinical course of physical problems (e.g., an elderly diabetic with an infected foot could be at increased risk for loosing his or her foot due to an absence of people to help with medical management and follow-up care).

Health professionals should remain attuned to the impact that medical problems can have on mental health, and the accompanying impact of psychological factors on health. With specific reference to psychological influences on health, the reader should note that there is an expansive literature that addresses the impact that mental health interventions can have on illness outcomes (Cohen, 1992).

Generational Problems

Health professionals should be knowledgeable of some of the potential stresses that can accompany specific family-focused difficulties involving the elderly. Generational conflicts are not unusual (Florsheim & Herr, 1990; Qualls, 1993). In a study of the referral patterns of elderly clients to a community mental health center, Mosher-Ashley (1993) reported that although comparatively few elderly referred themselves for mental health services, when they did so, it often was in an effort to resolve particular family conflicts.

During his or her dealings with elderly persons and their families, the health professional should pay particular attention to interactions in which there is evidence of any of the following: (1) scapegoating of the elderly member by other family members; (2) excessive demands (real or perceived) by the elderly on others in the family; (3) perpetuated family alliances that stand in the way of adaptive problem solving regarding the elderly; (4) symbiotic relationships between the elderly and middle-aged children; (5) incongruence between elderly persons and family members (e.g., major differences regarding expectations, values, plans, acceptable behaviors, etc.); (6) family immobilization--often the result of incongruent expectations--at times when important decisions about care for the elderly family member must be made (Herr & Weakland, 1979). Such interactions can have a powerfully constraining influence on the overall functioning of the family. When such difficulties are identified, the family should assisted by the health professional, or referred elsewhere for appropriate services.

Anticipatory Loss

Another common source of stress arises when families are coming to grips with the eventual loss of an elderly member of the family. Either by virtue of direct service or referral, the health professional can be of assistance to the family in helping them confront: (1) the family's reactions and fears regarding the anticipated loss of the elderly person; (2) the elderly member's anticipated loss of his or her family; and (3) the elderly person's expectations regarding disability and/or death (Rolland, 1991). One particularly noteworthy situation that needs to be counteracted occurs when the family prematurely interacts with a sick elderly member as if he or she is already absent from the family. Often an effort to distance themselves from the intense emotionality of the situation, this occurrence can prevent meaningful family interactions at this crucial time in the life of the elderly person.

Caregiver Stress

The burden that accompanies the care of some elderly persons can be a major problem in some families. The possibility of caregiver stress must be evaluated by health professionals who are working with families who provide extensive care for elderly members, including of course, elderly spouses who care for their partners. The degree of burden--from nonexistent to extreme--can be powerfully influenced by a number of interrelated factors, including: (1) the kind of relationship the caregiver currently has (and had) with the elderly person receiving care; (2) the nature and characteristics of the elderly patient's illness (e.g., its onset, course, and likely outcome, in addition to whether the condition is exclusively physical in nature or has accompanying cognitive components as well--see Rolland, 1984); (3) the emotional capacities of the people providing care; and (4) the kinds of family and community resources that are available both short- and long-term (Houlihan, 1987; McDaniel, Campbell, & Seaburn, 1990).

A substantial research literature has developed in recent years that details a variety of physical and psychological outcomes that can sometimes accompany prolonged caregiving (Fuller-Jonap, 1995; Houlihan, 1987; Jutras & Lavoie, 1995; Monahan & Hooker, 1995). Health professionals should intervene whenever necessary to minimize the potentially devastating effects of caregiver stress.

RESILIENCE

In the section above, some of the stressful changes and challenges that can accompany old age were summarized. However, as the contrasting stories of Ruth and Sally (see start of chapter) clearly suggest, people differ considerably in terms of their overall experience of aging. Given the evidence provided, it can be argued that although Ruth is older, she appears to be much more resilient than Sally.

Garmezy (1991) defined resilience as "the capacity for recovery and maintained adaptive behavior that may follow initial retreat or incapacity upon initiating a stressful event" (p. 459). Similarly, Rutter (1987) described resilience as "the positive role of individual differences in people's response to stress and adversity" (p. 316). Resilient elders are those who for one reason or another experience aging differently (often more positively and in better overall health) than those who are less resilient.

An expansive literature (both conceptual and empirical) has emerged in recent years that focuses on a delineation of processes (physical, cognitive, and social) that appear to distinguish more resilient elders--those who age successfully--from those who do so less successfully. It is beyond the scope of this text to summarize this literature in its entirety. However, in the section immediately below, several factors will be summarized that appear to have a protective influence on the mental health of the elderly.

Remaining Active

Although the cross-sectional nature of the data makes it impossible to determine the direction of causality (i.e., does better overall functioning lead to more activity, or does more activity lead to better overall functioning?) an association between activity and better functioning has been reported in the research literature. In a study of community-dwelling older men and women, Berkman, Seeman, Albert, et al. (1993) reported for example that people in the "high functioning" group were more likely to report continued involvement in productive activities and to engage in strenuous exercise. Although such participation undoubtedly explained some of the differential physiological findings of the study (i.e., in contrast to the other group participants, those in the high functioning group had better pulmonary functioning, higher self-assessed ratings of health, etc.) increased activity was associated with particular social and mental health findings as well. Members of the high functioning group were less likely to report feelings of anxiety or depression, and to report "greater feelings of self-efficacy, mastery, and life satisfaction" (p. 1138). These findings suggest that continued activity (including exercise) with advancing age may have a positive impact on at least selected aspects of mental health. The capacity of elderly persons for continued activity of course varies from person to person. To the extent that it is possible, however, efforts to promote both the physical and mental health of the elderly should include recommendations for continued activity and exercise.

Making and Maintaining Social Connections

There is growing evidence that a person's ability to remain connected with others throughout their old age can have a powerful impact on a number of outcomes (Thompson & Heller, 1990; Thomas & Chambers, 1989). Summarizing the findings of three epidemiological studies, Rowe and Kahn (1987) reported that continued participation in a network of family members and friends was associated with lower risks of mortality. Heidrich and Ryff (1993) also documented the positive effects of continued social participation. In a study of 243 community-dwelling elderly women, they discovered that continued participation mediated the effects of physical health status on a number of mental health outcomes. "For elderly women, having meaningful and valuable roles, reference groups, and normative behaviors is strongly related to multiple aspects of psychological well-being in terms of decreased psychological distress as well as increased perceptions of life-satisfaction, affect balance, personal growth, positive relationships, and autonomy" (p. 333).

It is through ongoing social participation that the elderly person continues to feel connected. These relationships provide another valuable function as well. If the elderly person remains an active part of a social group, ongoing comparisons of the self to others are possible. Assuming that the comparison groups are appropriate, the resulting comparisons can serve an important protective function as the elderly person manages the changes that accompany advancing age (Staudinger, Marsiske, & Baltes, 1993). Heidrich and Ryff (1993) reported, for example, that elderly women who had continued access to others, and who continued to compare themselves to others as a way of generating self-specific information, reported higher levels of psychological well-being and lower levels of distress. Continued social participation and social comparison appear to be processes that allow the elderly to remain mentally healthy "in the face of age-related losses or threats" (p. 328, Heidrich & Ryff, 1993). People who are interested in promoting the physical and mental health of the elderly should encourage their continued involvement with others. This includes encouraging new relationships with the deaths or departures of others from their established social networks.

Striving for Autonomy and Control

There is also evidence that older persons who continue to make autonomous decisions regarding activities, how and with whom they will participate, etc., do better than people who have others making decisions for them. In contrast to those who are less autonomous, those who remain in control tend to have better emotional, performance, and physiological outcomes (Rowe & Kahn, 1987). This literature is important too in that a crucial distinction is made concerning the kinds of interactions with others that can either foster or hinder control. Rowe and Kahn (1987), noted for example, "Teaching, encouraging, enabling are autonomy-increasing modes of support. Constraining, "doing for," warning, and the like beyond the requirements of the situation may convey caring but they teach helplessness" (p. 147). Although this of course will vary on an individual basis, where appropriate, the elderly should be encouraged to remain in control of important aspects of their lives as long as possible.

Remaining Adaptive

People differ considerably in terms of their ability to adapt and respond to change. A number of writers in recent years have drawn a connection between adaptation and successful aging (Baltes, 1991; Brandtstädter & Greve, 1994; Herzog & House, 1991; Schaie, Dutta, & Willis, 1991). Brimm (1988) stated that the normative physical changes that accompany aging require the elderly to make accompanying shifts in both behaviors and aspirations. Examples include: modifying the behaviors that may be needed to accomplish particular goals; increasing the amount of time that may be needed to meet objectives; altering expectations related to particular desired outcomes; and, if the changes noted above are not sufficient, possibly modifying a particular goal or objective entirely. Those who are less skilled at making these progressive modifications tend to be at greater risk for increased disappointment in the face of additional functional changes. In contrast, those who age successfully appear more able, with evidence of an inability to do previously mastered tasks, to narrow their focus. They devote "their energies to a reduced set of life domains and [compensate] for certain losses by alternative behaviors or devices, thereby preserving their mastery in a few elected domains" (p. 52).

Creating Multiple Roles

There also appears to be a relationship between the extent to which an elderly person fills multiple roles in his or life, and general physiological well-being. Adelmann (1994) found, for example, that elderly persons who defined themselves as currently filling multiple roles (from a list of options that included: employee, spouse, parent, volunteer, homemaker, grandparent, caregiver, or student) were more likely to report higher levels of life satisfaction and self-efficacy, and lower levels of depression. Similar results have been reported by other researchers as well (see discussion of "possible selves" in Staudinger, Marsiske, & Baltes, 1993). These results are also meaningful with reference to the information presented above concerning the positive impact that continued activity can have on late-life mental health.

Reviewing Life

A number of theorists and researchers have argued that the life review process, a periodic reviewing and reminiscing about one's life, can positively impact the mental health of the elderly. It has been proposed, for example, that thinking and talking about past events can help the elderly cope with the losses that accompany aging. Several researchers have documented specific positive mental health outcomes (i.e., higher levels of reported life satisfaction and less depression) for those who actively engage in life review (Coleman, 1974; Staudinger, Marsiske, & Baltes, 1993; Wong and Watt, 1991).

The changes and challenges that accompany aging can significantly impact the mental health of the elderly. Immediately above, a number of activities and processes were outlined that appear to enhance the reserves and resilience of many elderly persons. Two facts are obvious, however: (1) all elderly people are not equally resilient; and (2) even resilient elders can experience mental illnesses. Although certain organic difficulties (e.g., dementias) are more common among the elderly than other age groups (George, 1992), older persons can and do experience the same reactive difficulties (e.g., adjustment difficulties, depression, anxiety, etc.) that are experienced by others in the general population (APA, 1994; Rabins, 1992).

SELECTED PSYCHOTHERAPIES

The intent of this section is to provide an overview of some of the therapeutic methods that are used to treat the nonorganic mental health difficulties of the elderly. In the early 1990s, Engler and Goleman (1992) published a text entitled The Consumer's Guide to Psychotherapy. This guide provided descriptions of common therapeutic procedures and underscored the fact that the field of psychotherapy is characterized by tremendous theoretical and clinical diversity. At present, persons who are interested in psychotherapy can choose from more than 250 distinct forms of treatment (Strain, 1993). Things become less complex, however, when it is realized that these various forms of treatment can in fact be condensed into five general approaches to psychotherapy (Engler & Goleman, 1992). These approaches--and their accompanying use with the elderly--are summarized below.

Psychodynamic Therapy

Psychodynamic therapy is one of the oldest established forms of psychotherapy (Rieff, 1979, 1987). In this therapy, the relationship that links the therapist and patient is of central importance (Koenig & Blazer, 1992). Depending on the circumstance of the patient, psychodynamic therapy can be either insight-oriented or more supportive in nature. Particularly well suited for patients experiencing less severe difficulties, insight-oriented approaches are intended to broaden the understanding that patients have of the difficulties they are experiencing in their lives. The goal of therapy, for example, might be to help a patient resolve conflicts that are rooted in early relationships, but which nonetheless have been repeated in other significant relationships in the person's life (Engler & Goleman, 1992).

In contrast to this rather broad objective, insight-oriented therapy can also be used to address more specific behavioral difficulties. Writing of the use of psychodynamic approaches with less seriously depressed elderly patients, Moberg and Lazarus (1990) spoke of therapeutic strategies that might include: "communicating empathically how the patient experiences losses and their meaning; working through grief over losses and gently encouraging the patient to rediscover old, and to find new, relationships and activities that provide gratification and enhance self-esteem; clarifying negative transference reactions; and using new insight and understanding to find meaning in life and to improve interpersonal relationships" (p. 93).

A support-focused psychotherapy is often particularly appropriate for more seriously compromised patients. Speaking again of the treatment of elderly patients, Moberg and Lazarus (1990) described some of the immediate objectives of supportive psychotherapy with more severely depressed elderly patients. These include: "providing advice, supporting healthier defense measures, arranging a supportive, nurturing environment, and helping families and health professionals in their caretaking role" (p. 93). Turner (1992) has also discussed the use of psychodynamic procedures when working with the elderly.

There is recent empirical support for the use of psychodynamic psychotherapy in the treatment of elderly depressed patients. In an investigation of the comparative effectiveness of behavior, cognitive, and psychodynamic psychotherapies, in contrast to the results seen in a delayed-treatment control group, all treatment modalities were equally effective in reducing depression. Overall, 52% of the patients in the treatment sample attained remission by the end of treatment while another 18% showed significant improvement (Thompson, Gallagher, Breckenridge, 1987).

Behavior Therapy

In general, this kind of therapy tends to be briefer and more problem-focused than the psychodynamic approach summarized above. Heavily influenced by research on learning and conditioning, this treatment focuses on present behavior rather than on things that happened in the past. Common techniques include the positive reinforcement of adaptive behaviors (e.g., rewards for the weight gain of nutritionally compromised patients, or the increased social or occupational activity of depressed patients, etc.), and the negative reinforcement of problematic behaviors (e.g., alcohol consumption or smoking, or the social withdrawal of depressed patients, etc.) (Brink, 1979; Koenig & Blazer, 1992).

Specialized techniques such as deep muscle relaxation, biofeedback training, assertiveness instruction, and problem-inhibiting procedures such as thought stopping, reciprocal inhibition, and systematic desensitization--each of which may be used to address specific problem behaviors--are also part of the behavior therapy tradition (Brink, 1979). Given their specific focus on the problem, behavioral techniques tend to be less time consuming than some other approaches (e.g., insight-oriented psychodynamic therapy). Besides their efficiency, these approaches are appealing because by virtue of learning specific self-management techniques (e.g., relaxation to reduce anxiety, assertiveness training to reduce shyness, etc.), the patient realizes that he or she has some element of control over the problem situation. This tends to engender hope rather than helplessness (Moberg & Lazarus, 1990).

Behavior therapy has received considerable attention as a method of treatment for elderly individuals (O'Donohue, Fisher, & Krasner, 1986). A number of authors have highlighted the utility of behavioral approaches when treating elderly patients experiencing depression (Thompson et al. 1987), and, in combination with techniques like biofeedback and/or cognitive therapy, physical complaints such as headache (Nicholson & Blanchard, 1993) and other chronic pains (Widner & Zeichner, 1993). Similarly, behavioral methods were used to treat the obsessive-compulsive behavior (i.e., obsessions that harm would come family members, checking rituals, etc.) of an 80-year-old man. The treatment included exposure to the anxiety provoking situations and response prevention. Despite some methodological limitations, a marked improvement (i.e., substantial reductions in reported obsessive thoughts and ritualistic behaviors) was reported at conclusion of treatment. The reported gains had been maintained at the time of an eight-month follow-up (Calamari, Faber, Hitsman, & Poppe, 1994).

Cognitive Therapy

This is a form of therapy that works particularly well with problems like depression, low self-esteem, and anxiety. Cognitive therapy focuses less on the feelings or affect of patients, and more on their thinking: the cognitions that either set the occasion for, exacerbate, or maintain problems. These cognitions often include persistently negative and faulty views of previous experiences, the self, or what is likely to happen in the future (Beck and Emery, 1985; Engler & Goleman, 1992; Koenig & Blazer, 1992;

Moberg & Lazarus, 1990; Whitton, 1994). Examples of faulty thinking include, for example, exaggeration, catastrophizing, overgeneralization, and tendencies to ignore positive evidence (Beck & Emery, 1985). The task of the cognitive therapist is to assist patients in correcting faulty ideas and logic, which if uncorrected, can maintain difficulties such as depression, anxiety, etc.

In terms of specific examples of cognitive therapy with the elderly, Fishback and Lovett (1992) employed a single-case methodology to investigate the impact of 20 sessions of cognitive-behavior therapy on the chronic depression of a 79-year-old woman. Marked changes (reductions) in documented depression were noted between the beginning and end of treatment. These changes had been maintained at four- and five-month post-treatment follow-ups.

Additional support for the use of cognitive therapy when treating depressed elderly patients can be found in the results of a comparative investigation conducted by Thompson et al. (1987). Similarly, Gallagher-Thompson & Steffen (1994) conducted an investigation of the comparative effectiveness of cognitive-behavioral and psychodynamic psychotherapies in the treatment of depressed family caregivers. Although both therapies proved to be effective, they were differentially effective relative to the amount of time caregivers had been providing care to the elderly patient. Psychodynamic psychotherapy proved to be most effective when the time spent giving care had been comparatively short. When subjects had been providing care for at least 44 months, however, cognitive-behavioral therapy tended to be the most effective.

A combination of behavioral, cognitive, and educational procedures were used to successfully treat a group of elderly patients who experienced a number of sleep disturbances (i.e., sleep latency, waking after sleep onset, early morning awakening, and general sleep inefficiency). In the cognitive therapy component of the intervention efforts were made to alter "dysfunctional beliefs and attitudes about sleep and the impact of sleep loss on daytime functioning" (p. 140, Morin, Kowatch, Barry, & Walton, 1993). The substantial improvements that were noted at the conclusion of the 8-week treatment were maintained at 3- and 12-month follow-ups.

Supportive Therapy

In supportive therapy, the therapist tends to either reinforce appropriate actions that a patient may already have taken in his or her effort to address a particular difficult situation, or suggest and encourage solutions that may not have been tried as yet. Empathy (i.e., being able to view the situation from the vantage point of the patient), encouragement, and listening are key ingredients of this form of psychotherapy (Moberg & Lazarus, 1990; Semenchuk, 1994). Supportive therapy can be especially useful when working with elderly persons who are experiencing minor adjustment difficulties that are the likely results of predictable age-related losses and stressors (Koenig & Blazer, 1992). It should be recognized that although supportive therapy is being described as a therapy in its own right, elements of support are evident in many of the different psychotherapies.

Group Therapy

Group therapy has long been recognized as a valuable treatment modality when working with the elderly (Klein, Le Shan, & Furman, 1966). In a very general sense, this type of therapy is often helpful because by virtue of its social nature, it may be possible to counter some of the potentially devastating effects of social isolation: a common problem for many elderly persons (Zung, 1980). Semenchuk (1994) has proposed that group therapy with the elderly can be used to accomplish a number of more specific objectives as well, including: "information sharing, resocialization and remotivation, enhancement of self-esteem, expression of feelings, learning of problem-solving techniques, and dealing with losses and death" (p. 7). A number of special-purpose groups are commonplace in clinical work with the elderly (Capuzzi et al. 1990), including:

Reality-Orientation Groups. These groups are common in structured living facilities for the elderly. They are designed to provide structure, support, and assistance to elderly patients who have shown evidence of organic impairment. Reality-orientation groups meet frequently and often begin with information concerning the day, time, and place. The focus of these groups is sometimes expanded to include discussions of topics such as self-care, grooming, and social interaction once there is an overall improvement in reality orientation. In addition to their more immediate educational focus, it is theorized that these groups may be beneficial in terms of slowing additional mental deterioration (Capuzzi et al., 1990).

Remotivation Groups. An extension of the reality-orientation groups noted above, the members of these groups are generally oriented to time and place. Since these individuals function at a higher level, the objective of the group is to foster communication, stimulate mental capabilities, and motivate members to become more participatory in current and future activities (Capuzzi et al., 1990).

Reminiscence Groups. Members of reminiscence groups come together to share life experiences and memories (see previous section entitled "Reviewing Life"). It has been theorized that these groups may have a beneficial effect in terms of raising the self-worth and esteem of the participants, and in providing general recreation and enjoyment (Capuzzi et al., 1990). There is research-based evidence that supports the idea that reminiscence can facilitate the overall affective functioning of group members. In an investigation of the comparative effectiveness of the reminiscence group therapy and general supportive group therapy, the greatest improvements in the self-reported depression came with participation in the reminiscence group. The authors reported that the benefit gained, however, was quite short-term. Based on this finding, it was recommended that the most enduring benefits of reminiscent group therapy may come when this treatment option is part of an ongoing rather than a short-term treatment program (Goldwasser, Auerbach, & Harkins, 1987).

Psychotherapy and Support Groups. In these groups, members come together in a supportive atmosphere to discuss problems and possible solutions for the difficulties they are experiencing (Capuzzi et al., 1990). Some groups are topic- or problem-specific. Examples include groups of people who are experiencing similar emotional crises (e.g., grief following the death of a family member or friend, etc.), or possibly dealing with stresses that can accompany particular diagnostic conditions (e.g., support groups for arthritis patients, those experiencing cardiac problems, breast cancer, etc.). The primary intent of these groups is to help people deal with the stresses that accompany a variety of potentially overwhelming situations (Capuzzi et al., 1990; Engler & Goleman, 1992). Examples include group therapy programs for depressed and anxious elderly inpatients (Moffatt, Mohr, & Ames, 1995), and for those experiencing functional psychiatric illnesses (Procter & Alwar, 1995).

Systems Therapies

Systems therapies represent a more recent development in the field of psychotherapy. These therapies focus less on individual-level phenomena (i.e., thoughts, feelings, individual behaviors), and more on the relationship patterns and dynamics that are operative, for example, in marital or family systems. Depending on the particular model of family therapy that is being used, treatment goals may include, for example: helping a family change unhelpful, problem-maintaining patterns of interaction (a common goal in strategic family therapy); restructuring the lines of authority and participation in a family (a common goal in structural family therapy); or identifying and addressing problematic intergenerational issues (an objective that is addressed in idiosyncratic ways in a number of family therapy models--structural, strategic, Bowenian, and contextual) (Nichols & Schwartz, 1991).

Based on their extensive clinical work with the elderly, Florsheim and Herr (1990) have described several problem situations in which systems-focused interventions are very important. These may include, for example, situations where there is evidence of marital discord. The reported marital difficulties may be of either short or long duration. More acute marital difficulties are often the result of situational changes that the couple may be experiencing (e.g., retirement, relocation, health-related relationship changes, etc.). Systems therapies are also of use when devising solutions to problems that have arisen between the elderly and their adult children (e.g., negotiating appropriate levels of caregiving by adult children, addressing unsuccessful--possibly inappropriate--efforts on the part of the elderly parent to assist adult children with their own difficulties, etc.) (Florsheim & Herr, 1990; Genevay, 1990; Qualls, 1993; Richardson, Gilleard, Lieberman, & Peeler, 1994).

Clearly informed by a systems tradition, an important literature has developed that specifically addresses the impact that caring for the elderly can have on other family members (Cohen-Mansfield, 1995; Genevay, 1990; Fuller-Jonap & Haley, 1995; Jutras & Lavoie, 1995; Mellins, Blum, Boyd-Davis, & Gatz, 1993; Monahan & Hooker, 1995). Very importantly, this literature also contains a number of recombinations for minimizing the stresses that can result from caring for frail and demented family members (e.g., devising family education programs, support networks, etc.) (Houlihan, 1987). Herr and Weakland (1979) have also written a text that includes a number of valuable recommendations for clinical work with the elderly and their families.

Pharmacologic Treatment

The techniques summarized above are used to treat at least some of the difficulties experienced by the elderly. It should be recognized, however, that a number of medications are available that are of potential use in minimizing the symptoms that sometimes accompany these difficulties (e.g., depression, anxiety, etc.). However, normative physiological changes that accompany the aging process (e.g., increased nervous system sensitivity to psychotropic drugs, and alterations in the body's ability to bind, distribute, and dispose of drugs) can influence the pharmacology of many recommended medications (Salzman & Nevis-Olesen, 1992; Zung, 1980). The medication issue is complicated even further by the fact that since many elderly persons have multiple diseases, it is not uncommon for them to already be taking a number of medications (Conlin, 1980; Salzman & Nevis-Olsen, 1992). Many elderly persons are therefore at risk for adverse drug side-effects (Semenchuk, 1994). A number of references are available for readers who are interested either in the pharmacologic treatment of the elderly (Pirozzolo & Maletta, 1981; Salzman, 1992; Salzman & Nevis-Olesen, 1992; Semenchuk, 1994), or the combined use of medication and psychotherapy to address mental health difficulties (Klerman, 1986; Klerman, Weissman, Markowitz, et al., 1994).

THE ROLE OF HEALTH PROFESSIONALS

Given their frequent contact with the elderly, health professionals are in an important position in terms of assessing and treating the difficulties experienced by the elderly. The importance of their role is underscored by the fact that many elderly people underutilize mental health services (Waxman et al., 1984), choosing instead to visit their doctors, often for relief from a variety of stress-induced somatic complaints (McDaniel et al., 1990; Zung, 1980). Given these realities, it is imperative that health professionals know how to assess the mental health circumstances of their elderly patients, how to initiate at least basic forms of treatment, and how to make successful referrals if additional mental health services are needed.

If the decision is made to refer, a range of professionals are available who can assist in the treatment of mental and/or behavioral difficulties (e.g., psychiatrists, psychologists, marriage and family therapists, clinical social workers, etc.). Although many professionals work in private practice settings, with increasing regularity, treatment is being provided in community mental health centers (Kent, 1990) and in settings that address the combined mental and physical health needs of the elderly (Lustbader, 1990). Mental health services are increasingly being offered in settings that tend to be routinely frequented (or inhabited) by the elderly: retirement communities, senior centers, nursing homes, etc. Peer counseling programs have been developed in a number of communities. Typically, these programs pair a trained peer counselor with one or more persons who are in need of assistance. The peer counselor is trained to offer support and to assist with a number of problems (e.g., depression, adjustment problems, etc.). These programs are appealing for a number of reasons: many older people may be more comfortable discussing their problems with someone their own age; the service is often comparatively inexpensive; and the relationship that is developed is often mutually beneficial to both the "patient" and the peer counselor (Bratter & Freeman, 1990). These programs represent an important addition to an expanding range of services that are available to meet the mental health needs of the elderly and their families.

CHAPTER SUMMARY

Elderly persons and their families often must confront a number of stressful circumstances (e.g., retirement, illness, loss, etc.), many of which are clearly informed by the aging process. Professionals who attend to the physical and mental health needs of the elderly can often be of assistance in reducing the stresses that accompany these events. A number of resilience-enhancing behaviors have been identified that appear to set the occasion for better mental health. In the spirit of prevention, whenever possible, these very learnable behaviors should be brought to the attention of the elderly. Like other age groups in the general population, it is clear, however, that the elderly can also experience a number of diagnosable mental illnesses, some of which are caused by organic or biological factors, while others are more situational in nature. A number of effective psychotherapeutic procedures are available that can be used to treat many of the situational difficulties that are experienced by the elderly. When mental health difficulties do arise, they should not be ignored. Health professionals should either address the situation personally, or refer the patient (and possibly his or her family) to a professional who will work to resolve the difficulty as quickly as possible.

CHAPTER 9

STRESS AND HEALTH PROMOTION

Nick and Kay had been married for 45 years and were both doing well until Kay got diagnosed with cancer. She tolerated treatment and Nick took responsibility for her care, the care of their home and all other life tasks. After one year of struggling with illness Kay died leaving Nick to cope with her death. Up until that point Nick had seemed in good health. Now however, Nick seems to be overwhelmed, forgetful and disinterested.

Charles worked until his 70th birthday. While he felt forced into retirement he believed he was ready for the next stage in his life. His health appeared to be fine following retirement but lately he has appeared tired and old. An active man for most of his life he now appears to have few interests. Following his retirement he also wanted to live in a warm climate but his spouse was unwilling to move away from her community. Now, in winter, he simply stays in his house since he has a hard time coping with the cold weather.

Sarah is 74, lives in a large city and is uncomfortable leaving her home. A number of her old friends have been robbed and she seems genuinely concerned about her own safety. She has a great deal of support from family who often come and visit but she still feels lonely and sad.

David has had arthritis since he was 40 years old yet continued to be active despite the pain. At 65 he has dramatically reduced his physical activity and withdrawn from most social contacts. He often describes himself as feeling tense and irritable, struggling to get a good nights sleep. When he is asked "what's wrong?" he simply says "nothing" and tries to change the subject. He would not describe the quality of his life in a positive manner, feels stuck and seems without options.

All of the above individuals are struggling with stress and the impact it has on their lives. There appears to be a growing recognition that stress can either be a cause of/or make worse any number of illnesses. This evidence seems to suggest that emotional turmoil, our place in society, and the way we perceive life's events can have an effect on almost every body system. For example, "stress-triggered changes in the lungs contribute to asthma, bronchitis and other respiratory conditions. Stress suspends tissue repair and remodeling which in turn causes decalcification of the bones, osteoporosis, and susceptibility to fractures" (Davis, Eshelman, & McKay, 1994, p. 3).

Figure 9-1. Stress response impairment.

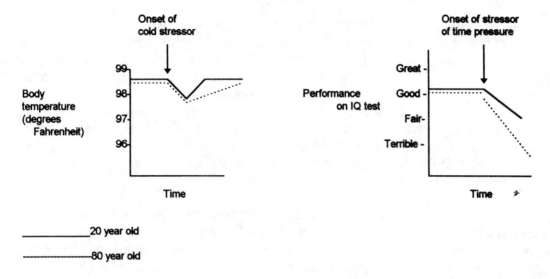

_____20 year old

----------------80 year old

Two ways in which the stress-response may be impaired in an older individual. (Left) Young and old individuals may have the same function under nonstressed conditions (in this case, the same body temperature). However, in the face of a stressor that knocks that measure out of homeostatic balance (chilling the person one degree), it takes the older person longer to reestablish homeostasis. (Right) Young and old individuals may have the same function under nonstressed conditions (performance on an IQ test). However, as the stressor of time pressure is added to the test, performance declines in both individuals--but to a greater extent in the older person.

(Reprinted with Permission) Stress Response Impairment. Sapolsky, R. M. *Why Zebras Don't Get Ulcers: A Guide to Stress, Stress-Related Diseases, and Coping*. W. H. Freeman and Company, 1994.

In elderly populations there appears to be increased difficulty in dealing with stress as the older body seems to respond more slowly to a number of environmental changes (Sapolsky, 1994, Figure 9-1). Older individuals do not easily turn off the stress response and continue to secrete hormones which over time wear on the body. For example glucocorticoid excess brings about fatigue, thinning muscles, adult–onset diabetes, hypertension, and immune suppression (Saplosky, 1994).

Overall, a number of life events contribute to the elderly individuals level of stress. In addition, the persons perception of any particular event also seems to have a large impact on their ability to cope with that particular stressor. Finally, there are a number of learned skills that can help individuals cope with even the most difficult predicaments. Thus a situation exists where the event combined with the perception of that event and individual coping skills determines the impact any given stressor has on an individual.

STRESS DEFINED

Stress has been defined as a "constraining force or influence: as b: physical, chemical or emotional factor that causes bodily or mental tension and may be a factor in disease causation" (Websters, 1963, 868). This relationship between psychological events and physiological responses was first examined by Cannon in 1911 when he demonstrated that psychological stimuli could trigger stressful responses. By noticing that barking dogs had an effect on a cat's adrenal medulla he was able to describe a series of biochemical reactions which occurred in reaction to a threat. Three years later Cannon presented the first paper focused on the stress concept. While he did not use the word stress to describe the fight or flight response he did describe the body's secretion of catecholamines as a response to an external menace.

As Hans Selye, a pioneer in research focused on stress, demonstrated 22 years later, the body reacts to modern psychological stresses as though it were still facing a physical threat. Selye (1936) wrote his first paper, a letter in *Nature,* describing his research on rats. Although he did not use the world stress in that initial paper he later defined stress as "the non specific response of the body to any demand made upon it." This demand can be any perceived threat or challenge and the response is automatic and immediate. The pattern of biobehavioral responses caused by stress Selye called the general adaptation syndrome (GAS) (Internet--Posen, 1995).

The GAS has three stages according to Selye. During the alarm or first stage the individual senses a stressor and a metaphorical alarm suggesting danger sounds. The body responds during this acute stress with a release of adrenocorticotropin and corti-coids. This stage is also marked by faster breathing, a tensing of muscles, increased mental alertness, increased blood flow to the brain, heart and muscles, and less blood to the skin, digestive tract, kidneys and liver. Basically the body is mobilizing resources in order to survive the challenge.

The second or resistance/adaptation stage represents the body's attempt to reach a chemical balance and calm down. Basically as coping mechanisms are utilized the individuals response should, if successful, return to a pre-stressed state. The inability to cope results in the development of the third or chronic stage of stress. It is during this third stage called exhaustion that stress-related diseases emerge.

Under conditions of chronic or long-term stress the individual remains in a constant state of readiness. The immune system tends to be suppressed, blood-cholesterol rises and calcium is lost from bones. "When protracted over time, the normal short-term increases in blood pressure can become hypertension, increased muscle tension can lead to headaches or aggravate pain, unusual changes in the activity of the intestinal tract can lead to diarrhea or spasms, increases in heart rate can raise the risk of arrhythmia. In addition depressed immunity may make an individual susceptible to colds and the flu or more serious diseases" (Pelletier, 1993, 23).

STRESSORS AS MOTIVATORS, CHALLENGERS OR KILLERS

It is impossible to live a life without stress. While individuals could certainly try to minimize the amount of stress they face there are situations that may result in a physiological reaction. For example, someone choosing to be alone may have a stress response triggered by coming into contact with others.

People seem to respond to stress in a number of ways. For example, a student waiting to write a paper for class may simply be waiting for their level of stress to increase enough for them to be motivated enough to meet their deadline. This might be an example of stress as a motivator. A couple deciding to move may struggle with the decision and develop panic attacks as they weigh their options. Following the death of a spouse a person faced with a decision about building new relationships stays home and is simply immobilized. All of the above situations describe individuals dealing with normal life transitions or activities of living. It is not the stressor that will determine one's response since it is no longer believed that individuals react the same way to disruptions. Stress is not the event or what happens to the person--these are called stressors--stress is how a person reacts (Pelletier, 1993).

Therefore, all situations can be considered as motivators, challenges, or potential killers. Basically it is what the individual brings to the situation that will most often determine its overall impact. Psychological factors such as mood, personality characteristics, suppressed anger, coping style, and defensiveness can all effect how a person deals with stress (Pelleitier, 1993).

There also appear to be a variety of coping styles and skills that may buffer a person from stress (Kobasa, Maddi, & Kahn, 1982, 1993; Kobasa, 1979). This style of coping is called hardiness and behaving in a hardy fashion should reduce the likelihood of acquiring stress-related illnesses. The behaviors suggested by Kobasa include:

- perceiving life's demand as a challenge
- having a commitment to something you believe is meaningful
- having a sense of being in control

Handling stress in a constructive manner also means having support from family, friends, and community. Social contacts may also serve as buffers that help individuals modify the way they perceive certain stressors. For example, Sapolsky (1994) describes one study focused on people who were undergoing cardiac-catheterization. Those who talked to their doctors during the procedure seemed to have smaller stress responses when compared to those who were stoic and distant. Pelletier (1993) mentions that people with supportive social networks had shorter hospital stays. Others (Kiecolt-Glaser & Glaser, 1993) support the relationship found between social support and health. They argue that lonely individuals appear to have poorer immune functions and research seems to suggest a relationship exists between stronger immune functioning and support.

In summary, it appears that there are a number of factors which facilitate resiliency and hardiness. Strong support systems, good problem-solving skills, and an ability to feel in control are all factors which allow us to view most stressful situations as challenges to be overcome.

COMMON CAUSES AND SYMPTOMS OF STRESS

The major life stressors for the elderly include: retirement from a job, coping with illness, providing care for an ill spouse, coping with the death of a spouse, coping with the death of peers. Other stressors which seem to effect the elderly include noise, light, temperature, and a number of daily hassles like getting to the supermarket. One additional stressor for many elderly individuals includes frustration due to memory problems.

While there are many other stressors which the elderly face on a daily basis it appears that general reactions to stress manifest themselves in a number of ways. In general the symptoms of stress seem to appear in five major areas.

The first general category includes symptoms that relate to an individual's cognitive functioning. Individuals developing symptoms that indicate cognitive difficulties usually manifest those symptoms by having anxious thoughts, difficulties in concentration and memory problems. Some people struggling in this area also seem to have a fearful anticipation about the future which when taken to a pathological limit can immobilize them.

The second category includes emotional symptoms. Individuals handling stress in an emotional manner usually demonstrate feelings of tension, irritability, restlessness, and an inability to relax. Clinical depression may also be a potential response for individuals struggling with stress over time or who are reacting to what for them might be a particularly difficult situation.

There are also a number of behavioral symptoms that are indicators of a reaction to stress. Avoidance of tasks, sleep problems, difficulty in completing work assignments, crying, and having an overall strained posture or look all appear to be behavioral markers of too much stress. In addition, exaggerating our typical methods for handling stress are also behavioral responses for some individuals. This might include increases in drinking, eating or smoking behaviors.

Social symptoms that are indications of difficulties with stress include responses as different as seeking people out or possibly increased isolation. Relationships seem to change when people are responding to stress but the literature indicates that responses are idiosyncratic.

The last group of symptomatic responses to stress are those that manifest themselves in a physiological manner. Responses to stress that are physiological include stiff muscles, grinding teeth, tension headaches, difficulty swallowing, nausea, vomiting, constipation, reduced libido, general tiredness, weight loss or gain, and shakiness or tremors. These are only a few of the possible physiological responses to stress and they may increase in intensity as the stress becomes either chronic or intensifies.

There are a number of stressors that seem to appear most often in elderly populations. For example, elderly individuals under stress react physiologically with cold hands and feet, sweaty palms, diarrhea, and headaches. Psychological reactions to stress in the elderly also include increased anxiety, panic, memory loss and poor self-esteem. Overall, however, elderly individuals may manifest symptoms of stress in all or just one of the categories mentioned. It is important to remember that stress can effect a number of systems and should not be overlooked as a factor when developing treatment in prevention approaches to health.

STRATEGIES FOR STRESS REDUCTION

In order to master stress or at least reduce its impact on one's life individuals must make lifestyle changes. Using any number of techniques, the individual is first responsible for becoming aware of situations that trigger stress reactions and developing methods for reducing the impact of those reactions. Strategies that appear to be most effective focus on changes in behavior, lifestyle choices, and/or thinking. A recent review authored by the National Institutes of Health Technology Assessment Panel on Integration of Behavioral and Relaxation Approaches into the Treatment of Clinic Pain and Insomnia (1996) also found strong evidence for the use of relaxation and behavioral strategies to treat people with specific disorders.

A review of Table 9-1 describes a number of relaxation techniques and their physiological impact (Benson,1993). It appears that a number of strategies are useful methods for achieving the relaxation response (Benson, 1975) or having some positive benefits for the individual (Lehrer, Carr, Sargunaraj, & Woolfolk, 1994).

The remainder of this chapter will describe a few of those techniques which have been found useful for reducing stress and helping individuals gain control of their lives.

Relaxation Training

One of the most basic methods for achieving a relaxed state is progressive muscle relaxation. This technique was described by Edmund Jacobson in his book *Progressive Relaxation* (1929). He described deep muscle relaxation as a method for reducing physiological tension by helping individuals focus on relaxing their muscles rather than on anxiety-provoking thoughts. The instructions for this relaxation method are rather simple and involve methodically sweeping through your body, tensing and then

Table 9-1. Relaxation Techniques

Technique	Oxygen consumption	Respiratory rate	Heart rate	Alpha waves	Blood pressure	Muscle tension
Transcendental meditation	Decreases	Decreases	Decreases	Increase	Decreases*	(Not measured)
Zen and yoga	Decreases	Decreases	Decreases	Increase	Decreases*	(Not measured)
Autogenic training	(Not measured)	Decreases	Decreases	Increase	Inconclusive results	Decreases
Progressive relaxation	(Not measured)	(Not measured)	(Not measured)	(Not measured)	Inconclusive results	Decreases
Hypnosis with suggested deep relaxation	Decreases	Decreases	Decreases	(Not measured)	Inconclusive results	(Not measured)

*In patients with elevated blood pressure.

PHYSIOLOGICAL CHANGES WITH DIFFERENT TECHNIQUES

Several techniques have now been shown to elicit a constellation of related changes, all part of what we have called the relaxation response. While not every change has been measured with every technique, the overall results suggest that these methods trigger the same natural physiological pattern.

From H. Benson, "The Relaxation Response" in "Mind Body Medicine - How to Use Your Mind for Better Health" in *Consumer Report Books,* S. Goleman and J. Gurin, Eds., 1993. Reprinted by permission of H. Benson.

relaxing each major muscle group (see Appendix G). By continuing to tense muscles and then relax them individuals are able to identify the difference between tension and relaxation.

The research examining progressive relaxation training suggests progressive relaxation may be superior to meditation for relieving anxiety and many believe that learning relaxation skills may enhance coping (Emmelkamp, 1994). In addition, according to Hollon & Beck (1994) interventions such as progressive muscle relaxation appear to be well established for the treatment of chronic pain. Scogin, Rickard, Keith, Wilson, and McElreath (1992) suggested that progressive muscle relaxation is the gold standard against which others must be compared. More recent reviews of the outcome literature examining the use of progressive muscle relaxation for chronic pain and hypertension, however, appear to be mixed and suggest continued examination of the overall effectiveness of PMR. In cases of insomnia it also appears that progressive muscle relaxation yields the poorest outcome when compared to other behavioral procedures (Blanchard, 1994). Most recently (National Technology Assessment Panel, 1996) it was again suggested that "cognitive forms of relaxation were slightly better than soma-tic forms of relaxation such as PMR" for individuals struggling with insomnia.

In a study examining 30 elderly volunteers (Rankin, Gilner, Gfeller, & Katz, 1993), anxious elderly individuals seemed to reduce their levels of state anxiety following one session of progressive muscle relaxation. Participants, however, did not perform better on memory tests and as opposed to previous studies (Yesavage, 1984), a one-session relaxation program was not found to be sufficient for modifying memory outcomes.

Others have found that relaxation training may be an effective method for reducing subjective anxiety. Scogin, Rickard, Keith, Wilson, and McElreath (1992) reported an increase in relaxation, less anxiety, and fewer psychological symptoms in a group of elderly participants when compared to a delayed treatment control group. A one-year follow-up (Rickard, Scogin, & Keith, 1994) also found significant positive changes on relaxation level, psychological symptoms, state anxiety, and trait anxiety.

The use of progressive muscle relaxation with elderly individuals must be done cautiously. While it appears that its use has some clinical utility it may not be well suited for many older adults who are unable to do muscle tension and joint tightening exercises. In particular these activities may be impossible for arthritic individuals (Zeiss & Lewinsohn, 1986).

Biofeedback

Biofeedback is a treatment technique in which people are trained to improve their health by using signals from their own bodies. It is often aimed at changing habitual reactions to stress that can cause pain or disease. Emerging in the 1970's biofeedback methods use sensitive instruments to increase the individuals awareness of bodily changes. The person uses the information about skin temperature or muscle tension as a guide as they learn how to increase control over physical tension. The five most frequently measured bodily processes monitored by biofeedback have been described by (Schwartz & Schwartz, 1993) and a brief description of each approach follows:

- Electromyographic (EMG) Biofeedback. During this procedure muscle tension is measured using sensors attached to the skin in the particular muscle area being treated. The goal is to learn to relax those areas that seem to be related to the particular problem. Tension headaches, muscle pain, incontinence all appear to be treated through EMG.
- Thermal Biofeedback. This from of biofeedback uses skin temperature as a method for assessing blood flow. The feedback from biofeedback instruments usually taped to a finger provides the individual with information on how to reduce constriction of blood vessels in hands and feet. This treatment method may be most useful for those who suffer from Raynaud's disease, migraines, hypertension and anxiety.
- Electrodermal Activity (EDA). EDA measures changes in sweat activity. Sensors are attached to the palm side of the fingers or hand and detect moisture. Increased sweat can be an indication of

stressful thoughts, rapid breathing or activation of part of the autonomic nervous system. EDA is often used for anxiety.

- Finger Pulse. This particular method of biofeedback measures pulse rate and force. It is one method for measuring heart activity and arousal of the autonomic nervous system. It is most often used for hypertension, anxiety and some cardiac arrhythmia's.

- Breathing. This method uses breath rate to provide feedback for the individual in treatment. Sensors may be placed around the chest, abdomen, or air flow may be measured from the nose or mouth. Feedback helps the individual learn how to control their breathing. Breathing may be used most often for individuals with asthma. (Schwartz and Schwartz, 1993)

Research results with biofeedback appear to be variable. According to Schwartz and Schwartz (1993) biofeedback and relaxation training are similarly effective in the treatment of headaches. It appears that a number of controlled evaluations dating back to 1973 have shown the efficacy of EMG in treating tension headaches. The data examining the effectiveness of the standard treatment of migraines, thermal biofeedback, appears to not be as clear and it has not been shown to be superior to a attention-placebo condition.

Research suggests that a number of illnesses have been successfully treated using biofeedback. The data support symptom relief for those suffering from diabetes mellitus, insomnia, urinary incontinence, fecal incontinence, hypertension, anxiety, and myofascial pain syndromes. Specifically, Blanchard (1994) found that thermal biofeedback treatment was helpful for reducing medication usage and also reduced blood pressure in hypertensive individuals. Others, however, have suggested that biofeedback has not lived up to its promise as a treatment technique or as a coping procedure (Rice, 1992) and it does not have specific value for treatment of those with generalized anxiety disorders since other forms of relaxation seem to yield comparable clinical effects (Emmelkamp, 1994).

Most of the research done on biofeedback and its effectiveness has been done with children and adults under the age of 65. Many of the studies done using elderly participants have focused on the treatment of incontinence. There have been reports of pelvic muscle exercises combined with biofeedback to successfully treat stress incontinence in older women. There were, however, no reports on the use of these techniques in persons with cognitive impairment. It is simply very unlikely that demented individuals could either comply or master the required procedures (Skelly & Flint, 1995). Behavioral treatment consisting of biofeedback, pelvic floor exercises, scheduled voiding, and other strategies for preventing accidental urine loss has also been provided to a group of non-demented outpatients aged 56 to 90 years old who suffer from urinary incontinence. The authors concluded that behavioral treatment was an effective and well tolerated treatment for urinary incontinence in the non-demented elderly (McDowell et al., 1992).

Overall, it appears that biofeedback has been shown to be reasonably effective as an adjunct therapy for a number of diseases that effect elderly people. There does however need to be continued study examining elderly participants in order to better understand the conditions that increase the likelihood of success.

Mindfulness Meditation

Mindfulness (Kabat-Zinn) Meditation was developed as a method for enhancing an individual's moment-to-moment awareness. When thoughts come up individuals are taught to review them in a non-judgmental intentional manner. The aim of the program is to develop a stable and nonreactive present moment awareness. "If you are experiencing a distressing thought or feeling or actual physical pain in any moment, you resist the impulse to try to escape the unpleasantness; instead, you attempt to see it clearly as it is and accept it because it is already present in the moment" (Kabat-Zinn, 1993, p. 263).

Acceptance does not imply that one simply learns to live with whatever concern or pain has come into awareness. It is not a passive or resigned response. According to Kabat-Zinn (1993) acceptance means opening yourself up to the moment making it more likely that you will be able to respond effectively to any situation. The goal of this form of meditation is not to stop stress but to make mindful intentional decisions on how to respond. Or as Kabat-Zinn (1993) illustrated by describing a poster of a 70ish yogi Swami atop a surfboard, riding the waves off a Hawaiian beach. The caption read "You can't stop the waves, but you can learn to surf" (p. 263).

According to Kabat-Zinn (1993) individuals can perform mindfulness either through informal practice or formal meditation. "Ultimately, mindfulness is best thought of as a way of being, rather than as a technique" (p. 264). During formal practice the three most basic meditation tools used are body scan, sitting meditation, and hatha yoga postures. Individuals are exposed to all three methods and are then asked to determine which one suits them best. Practice is not meant to mean rehearsing to get better but implies an effort by the individual to be present in the moment.

The body scan is done while lying flat on your back and involves systematically becoming aware of any physical sensations as you move your attention throughout your entire body. Lying down makes this activity easier for individuals who struggle with chronic pain or other physical difficulties. Sitting meditation involves finding a comfortable position, then concentrating on a single object.

Informal practice involves reminding yourself to live in the present moment. Since it is difficult for individuals to learn the skills necessary to practice mindfulness as a regular part of their life from a tape or book alone it becomes important for people to initially participate in some type of formal training. This might include a structured workshop or meeting with a group of like minded individuals who are interested in enhancing the quality of their lives. Once an individual has developed a more mindful way of living it becomes easier for them to integrate those skills and beliefs into their daily lives. At that point any living activity becomes an opportunity to practice mindfulness. Other materials on this subject can be ordered from Stress Reduction Tapes, P.O. Box 547, Lexington, MA 02173.

In summary, Mindfulness Meditation is not simply a skill people use to overcome particular health problems. It is a lifestyle change requiring people to practice living in the moment. The outcome of these efforts includes an increased calmness and a heightened awareness of everyday living experiences.

The research examining the effectiveness of Mindfulness Meditation suggests its efficacy in reducing the physical symptoms of chronic pain (Kabat-Zinn, Lipworth, Burney, & Sellers, 1986; Kabat-Zinn, Lipworth, & Burney, 1985; Kabat-Zinn, 1982), and stress (Tate, 1994). A recent study examining patients with anxiety disorders (Miller, Fletcher, & Kabat-Zinn, 1995) indicated maintenance of the original clinical improvements at a three-year follow-up. According to the authors, the intervention was not focused on simply treating individuals with anxiety disorders or any specific diagnosis but rather on teaching participants "a way of being rather then a technique" (p. 198). In another recent study examining the relationship between the practice of meditation and melatonin, Massion et. al. (1995) found that meditation was associated with hormonal changes. The results of this small pilot study comparing eight women who meditated to eight who did not found that the meditation group did have higher melatonin levels. This study has considerable implications for medical treatment since others have found that increasing melatonin levels was predictive of a favorable response to chemotherapy in a group of cancer patients (Lissoni, Tisi, & Barni, 1992).

While the research examining the effectiveness of Mindfulness Meditation is just beginning to get developed, others are suggesting its use with individuals struggling with other diseases. For example, in a recent paper Teasdale, Segal, and Williams (1995) present a model therapy which includes the use of Mindfulness Meditation as a method for preventing relapse in depressed individuals. They suggest that mindfulness is a skill that can be practiced on a wide range of thoughts, feelings, and experiences. It appears that the activity is intrinsically positive and practice is likely to continue. In addition, since mindfulness training encourages people to live in the moment it would be difficult for them to preseverate on thoughts that were associated with thinking about one's "problems."

According to Hawks, Hull, Thallman, and Richins (1995) one weakness of some of the research examining Mindfulness Meditation has been the use of nonrandomly selected comparison groups. While that limitation must be recognized, those authors go on to state that replication studies done in many parts of the country with a number of dissimilar populations have shown consistent results. Thus, there appears to be strong support for the usefulness of Mindfulness Meditation (Hawks, Hull, Thalman & Richins, 1995).

A review of the literature specifically focused on the use of Mindfulness Meditation with elderly populations, however, suggests that much still needs to be done. A Medline search found no papers examining either the use or effectiveness of Mindfulness Meditation with older adults. While the assumption can be made that modifying one's behavior as dramatically as suggested by Kabat-Zinn will also enhance the quality of life for elderly persons, it is still important to better understand the effective components of the program with a variety of populations. For example, will elderly individuals be more or less compliant than other groups with the concept of disciplined practice? Will the positive effects of fewer doctor visits and use of less medication also occur in elderly groups? It must be understood that studying "a way of being" using empirical evidence is not an oxymoronic exercise. The current research being done by the Stress Reduction Clinic (Kabat-Zinn) indicates that continued research is necessary to better understand the effectiveness of these methods with all people.

Social Support

As individuals age the chances of suffering from some type of illness dramatically increases. The increased likelihood of physical impairment may disrupt one's support system leaving them feeling lonely and at risk for depressive symptoms. These changes may be a result of not being able to use the phone, public transportation, or your own car. Individuals may also feel cut off from their friends, family and community. One's quality of life is disrupted as they feel less in control of their ability to meet others, reducing their social interactions (Newsom & Schulz, 1996).

Many elderly individuals suffer from a reduction in their ability to meet with others due to their own physical limitations. They are also faced with the stress of losing significant friends through death, limiting their ability to find support when needed. Thus, unless support groups are developed for elderly individuals they are unable to utilize a health promotion activity that has been shown to have positive psychological consequences.

It appears that participation in support groups may have life-sustaining consequences. Studies done in Alameda County (Berkman, 1985) and Techumseh, Michigan (House, Robbins, & Metzner, 1982), seem to suggest that there is a causal relationship between social support and mortality risk (Kahn, 1994). Specifically, Berkman and Syme (1979) found that those individuals who were least socially connected were twice as likely to die when compared to those who had strong social ties. Other studies indicate a relationship exists between a lack of connectedness and heart disease (Seeman and Syme, 1987).

In addition to the relationship between increased social contacts and health it seems that participation in formal support groups is a positive health promoting activity. For example, a support group for women with breast cancer at Stanford University seemed to help patients live better, with less anxiety, depression, and pain (Spiegel, 1993). Rapheal (1977) found that women who participated in a support group following the death of a spouse showed lower overall morbidity than those in a control group. Support groups seem to have a positive impact in cases as diverse as rheumatoid arthritis (Lorig & Holman, 1989) and heart disease (Ornish, Brown, Sherwitz, et. al., 1990; Ornish, 1991; and Ornish, 1992). In the first setting, educational support groups were developed to help individuals better cope with their illness. The heart disease project run by Ornish used programs incorporating group support to lower the risk of heart attack for people at risk. According to the research all of these activities which enhance connectedness are ultimately health promoting and could potentially reduce the cost of health care.

Structure of a Support Group

Support groups and opportunities for social connection appear to be available for anyone interested in participating. From groups focusing on chronic illness to bands playing at your local senior citizens center, all of these groups have therapeutic value. What they all have in common is an opportunity for social contact.

While support groups can be social gatherings or leader-led therapy groups, they need to be structured in a way that will encourage community participation. Formal social support groups are often lead by professionals. Many of these groups focus on dealing with difficult problems, cognitive restructuring, and/or education. For this to occur they need to follow a number of specific guidelines.

First do a community needs assessment. This first step involves gathering information to assess what type of groups will be well attended in your area. Setting up community focus groups of elderly individuals will provide the leaders information necessary about what topics should be discussed to encourage maximum community participation. Second, try to hold the support group in a community setting. Again the goal is to maximize participation and it appears that holding the group in a given community will only enhance the opportunity to participate. Third, utilize respected community leaders to help advertise the group. This step will enhance the credibility of the group leaders particularly if they do not live within the community. And, finally, make sure the group has a specific focus.

Groups can be for cancer patients, spouses whose significant other has died, arthritis sufferers, or elderly caregivers. The goal is to enhance the participants' sense of social connectedness. For those who are ill, increasing social contact may have an impact on the quality and length of their lives. Those who are living with an ill person or who have just had a loved one die will find that the increased social contacts may result in their staying healthier longer. Overall, according to Spiegel (1993) social support groups seem to enhance participants sense of control over their lives and increase their ability to cope with illness.

CHAPTER SUMMARY

The cost of health care in the United States is skyrocketing. One reason for the increase in health care costs is that Americans do not participate in health promotion activities which have been found to be effective in reducing their levels of stress. Increasingly, evidence suggests a strong link between stress and physical illness. It appears that when individuals struggle with chronic stress they place their immune systems at risk and ultimately suffer from a number of diseases. Current evidence seems to also suggest that there are a number of strategies that are effective for reducing stress. Health promotion programs need to be accessible so people can learn these stress reduction methods, enhance the quality of their lives, and reduce the overall cost of health care.

CHAPTER 10

SPIRITUAL HEALTH AND AGING

Spiritual well-being parallels the concepts of happiness and life satisfaction--it refers to the intangible aspects of a person's quality of life. Viktor Frankl, in his book *Man's Search for Meaning* (1984), uses the concept of "geist" to build an understanding of spirituality. Frankl suggests that to define the word "spirit" requires an understanding as to what type of spirit is at issue. The German root word for geist (spirit) contains several forms. For our purposes, geistig (ability of the individual to transcend beyond self) and gestlich (relationship with God) are the principal forms applied under spiritual health. Unfortunately, the integration of geist and geistig forms of spiritual health into health promotion programs has made sparse progress.

Many health promotion professionals are too embarrassed or uneasy to embrace the basic concepts of spiritual health that emphasize love, joy, peace, sense of purpose, and achieving one's full potential. Despite this uneasiness, spiritual health is a vital program component deserving attention and commitment. Chapman (1986) writes that "spirituality is an illusive issue lying at the heart of an examined and well-managed lifestyle. Skip it and your wellness program will have to fuel itself on the intellectual equivalent of wonder bread" (p. 38). Our purpose in Chapter 10 is to address the inclusion of spiritual health under the health promotion umbrella for older adults. This discussion will include defining program parameters for spiritual health.

SPIRITUALITY: THE SEARCH FOR THE HOLY GRAIL OF WELLNESS

Don Ardell (1986) describes the search for spirituality as the pursuit for the "Holy Grail of Wellness." His solution for integrating spirituality into wellness programs is simply to call it something else--ethics, values, or life purpose. Chapman (1986) argues that Ardell's solution is less than optimal because it undervalues or removes the integral elements of the human condition; the body, soul, and spirit. Yet both Ardell and Chapman agree that spiritual wellness should be a vital part in health promotion programming. This inclusion, however, will require definitive parameters.

Defining Spiritual Health/Wellness

The difficulty in addressing and including spiritual health under health promotion programs is related to its association with denominational religion and our cultural emphasis on materialism. Chapman (1987) acknowledges this dilemma as a preconceived notion by participants as to the meaning of the term spiritual. Some may associate spiritual with "God" or a "Creator" and immediately feel that they are becoming indoctrinated into a religious experience. Or the term spiritual may refer to Eastern meditation, Yoga, or "New Age" activities. Confusing spiritual with New Ageism may lead its association to a "cult" mentality. Additionally, there may be a perception that "spiritual health" is an end result rather than a process. In our Western society, where we tend to be result-oriented rather than process-oriented, the journey approach to spiritual health may be difficult to grasp. Some scholars are attempting to resolve this dilemma by associating spiritual health with the development of the human consciousness beyond the ego level. Fahlberg and Fahlberg (1991) write:

> efforts have recently been made to differentiate spirituality and religion. Because a person may be spiritual but not identify with any religious group or organization, the terms "spiritual" and "religious" are not synonymous. Religion has been characterized as that which is concerned with the social activities of a church group, cult, or occult. Spirituality on the other hand, has been defined by Banks as a unifying force within individuals; meaning in life; a common bond between individuals; and individual perceptions or faith. (p. 274)

Fahlberg and Fahlberg prefer to define spirituality as "contacting the divine within the self" (p.274). "Self" is used here to refer to realms of consciousness beyond the ego. Chapman (1986) provides a more elaborate definition of spiritual health:

> Optimal spiritual health may be considered as the ability to develop our spiritual nature to its fullest potential. This would include our ability to discover and articulate our own basic purpose in life, learn how to experience love, joy, peace and fulfillment and how to help ourselves and others achieve their full potential. (p. 32)

The phrase "optimal spiritual health" implies an individual or absolute point of reference for spiritual health. To develop one's fullest potential is an ultimate goal that requires the development and application of skills in such areas as self-awareness, self-inquiry, cognitive restructuring, life goal planning, and lifestyle management. Chapman also assumes that each of us has an intrinsic curiosity for exploring life meaning and that there is a fundamental value that governs life patterns, specifically such core values as serving others, serving God, and acquiring wealth. The use of the word "learn" in the definition implies that the spiritual skills of love, joy, peace, and fulfillment can only be attained through effort. A more complex implication underlying Chapman's view of spiritual health is that health promotion professionals must first experience spiritual feelings and values in order to teach such "exemplary" health habits and behaviors. Or the question may be raised as to whether health promotion professionals need to define their own parameters for spiritual health before subjecting participants to health profession biases.

Connectedness and Spiritual Health

The self-transcendent definition for spiritual health of Fahlberg and Fahlberg (1986) and Chapman (1986) is closely tied to Maslow's (1959) theory of the hierarchy of needs. Maslow's hierarchy of needs theory emphasizes that human development beyond the ego deserves careful attention. Underlying self-transcendence and human development are the concepts of connectedness and consciousness-modifying behaviors.

The concepts of connectedness and spiritual health are vitally and integrally related. According to the Merriam-Webster's New World Dictionary (1969), "connectedness" means to join together. Bellingham, Cohen, Jones, and Spaniel (1989) explore the relationship between connectedness and spiritual health by using the term spiritual health to mean the ability to live in the wholeness of life. This definition fits well with the views of Fahlberg and Fahlberg (1986) and Chapman (1986). Bellingham et al.'s use of the word connectedness implies that one can grow through and toward relationships, or relational mutuality. Relational mutuality may provide purpose and meaning to an individual's life. Failure to establish relationship mutuality may also lead to disconnectedness and dire consequences, such as self-alienation, loneliness, and lack of meaning or purpose. As Bellingham et al. (1989) write:

- Self-alienation results from losing connectedness with oneself. People who are self-alienated are out of touch with their life goals, their values, and their feelings in the present moment: they do not experience directly any of their emotions. (p. 19)
- People who experience loneliness normally desire to be connected to others, but lack the ability to fulfill this desire. There are three very important points for agreement in the way scholars view loneliness. First, loneliness is a result of deficiencies in a person's social relationships. Second, loneliness is a subjective state; it is not synonymous with social isolation, but reflects a loss of "place"-- social as well as physical. Third, loneliness is an unpleasant and distressing experience which has a proven negative effect on one's health.
- A lack of meaning or purpose comes from losing connectedness with any set of guiding principles. This type of disconnectedness usually brings on a spiritual crisis accompanied by either a feeling of pervasive dread or a feeling of pervasive boredom. (p. 19-20)

The consequences of disconnectedness on physical and spiritual health can be devastating. Books by Scott Peck, *The Road Less Traveled* (1978), Robert Bellah, *Habits of the Heart* (1989), and Bernie Siegel, *Love, Medicine and Miracles* (1986), provide scientific evidence for the conviction that disconnectedness in life impairs both the mind and the body. People can learn, however, skills in life that lead to connectedness. Bellingham et al. (1989) present three levels of connectedness: connecting with oneself, connecting with others, and connecting with a larger meaning or purpose.

Connecting with Oneself. To be connected means that we must be congruent with our own feelings and values. The ability to become in touch with the inner self is a difficult process because it involves passing through layers of anxiety and fear. Achievement of connectedness with oneself can only be done in solitude, a time to pay attention and reflect on inner feelings and thoughts. Solitude is a difficult time for many people, however, because they are caught in the trap of wanting immediate answers. Bellingham et al. present three skills that can help promote the search for the inner self: exploring feelings, understanding values, and achieving congruence.

Exploring feelings is the ability to connect with one's own emotional experience. To take charge of emotions, we need to be able to express how we actually feel at a particular moment. Feelings control the person when he or she does not understand the emotional basis for such feelings. The hostile reaction to stress associated with the Type A personality (time-oriented, aggressive) is a good example. Another example common to older adults is the fear of losing cognitive capacity (memory, dementia) and becoming a burden to one's family. The fear of becoming demented or losing one's memory can become so dominant that such conditions may actually occur in consequence.

Understanding values is the ability to sense what is truly important and to understand what motivates our behavior. Values formed over time are an extension of our attitude toward life. Our hopes, dreams, desires, and ambitions are tied to personal values. As values play such a critical role, it follows that we should be able to clearly articulate the values that form the foundation for our attitudes. Unfortunately, most of us have a vague and imprecise understanding of our own values. Inner conflict is often caused by our inability to identify personal values.

Achieving congruence is the ability to live a life that consistently fits with our feelings and values. Anthony Campolo, in his book *Who Switched the Price Tags* (1986), writes "Sometimes I have the feeling that somebody has gone through our world and switched the price tag on everything. People work and slave and spend their money on things that really don't matter and ignore the things that do. How did we get so far off-base?" (quoted in Bellingham et al., 1989, p. 21). This quotation by Campolo illustrates the tremendous impact that culture has on our values; congruence is placing the right price tags on things we really value, not the tag dictated by culture.

Connecting with Others. Bellingham et al. emphasize that connecting with others requires that we create a space that people can visit and that we have a willingness to leave that space to visit others. Creating such a space obviously makes us very vulnerable. Three skills that help us to accept vulnerability by reaching out to others are assessing connectedness, sharing who we are, and enriching our connectedness.

Assessing connectedness is a measurement of how we are connected to others physically, emotionally, and intellectually. Physical connection is shared space, shared time, and shared actions. Emotional connection is shared feelings. And intellectual connection is shared values and goals.

Sharing who we are is letting other people know about our life and the values that are important to us. Sharing openly with others carries risks; in doing so, we become vulnerable. Yet connecting significant others with one's life can only be done when values and feelings are openly shared. Finding one's balance between needed solitude and solidarity is a difficult task.

Enriching connectedness is creating a space for relations to be dynamic. Growth in relationships should include physical, emotional, and intellectual dimensions. Unfortunately, enriching connectedness is probably the most challenging of the skills needed to connect with others. The mobility of Americans, prevalence of extended families, and changing cultural values are viable obstacles.

Connecting with a Larger Meaning or Purpose. Each of us needs something outside ourselves to anchor and give meaning to our life. The word "purpose" actually means to have a sense of direction or duty or larger goal. Without a life purpose, we experience the anxiety of emptiness and meaninglessness which impairs our spiritual well-being. Paul Tillich, in his book *The Courage to Be* (1952), writes:

> The anxiety of meaninglessness is anxiety about the loss of an ultimate concern, of a meaning which gives meaning to all meanings. This anxiety is aroused by the loss of a spiritual center, of an answer, however symbolic and indirect, to the question of the meaning of existence. (quoted in Bellingham et al., 1989, pp. 22-23)

The anxiety of emptiness and meaninglessness was explored in the 1991 movie *City Slickers* that starred Billy Crystal as a man encountering a mid-age crisis. Crystal was intrigued by the life of an old cowboy, played by Jack Palance. According to the old cowboy, the secret to life is comprised in one thing that is particular to each individual. This one thing, or purpose in life, can only be captured after deep reflection. An intriguing sociological study paralleling this search for the elusive "one thing in life" was conducted with a group of older adults aged 95 years or older. These older adults were asked the question: "If you could live your life over again, what would you do differently?" Although a multiplicity of answers were given by the older adults to this question, Campolo (1986) noted that three answers consistently emerged and dominated the study results. The three answers were (1) I would reflect more, (2) I would risk more, and (3) I would do more things that would live on after I am dead. The underlying theme for these answers is connection to a larger meaning or purpose in life.

Spiritual Health and Older Adults

Plato once said that "spiritual eyesight improves, as physical eyesight declines." Spiritual health embraces both the "profane world of experience as well as the sacred world of the transcendent" (McFadden & Gerl, 1990, p. 35). For older adults, life is a series of role transformations; the loss of loved ones, physical changes, and a myriad of environmental events cause a continual reassessment and restructuring of life priorities. Approaches to understanding the reassessment and restructuring of life priorities require that we look at aging from a spiritual side of health and not just from a technical problem perspective.

Why do we grow old? How should we grow old? What does it mean to grow old? Maddox (1991) argues that American culture has paid very little attention to such questions. Instead, the dominant cultural voice has focused more on how we age, "in order to understand and control the aging process" (p. 30). Modern gerontology and geriatrics have certainly elevated the physical health of older Americans. But this perception of old age as a technical problem has overshadowed the spiritual side of health. As Maddox notes,

> focusing narrowly on a retried "problem of old age," apart from the actual lives and cultural representations of people growing older, the scientific management of aging denies our universal participation and solidarity in the most human experience. But homo sapiens are spiritual animals; we need love and meaning no less than food, clothing, shelter, and health care. (1991, p. 30)

Ebersole and Hess (1990) suggest that the crux of spiritual health is captured in Maslow's concept of self-actualization. Maslow (1959) defines self-actualization as the highest level of human function as an inner motivation that is free to express one's most unique self. Maslow also suggests that young persons are not capable of achieving a self-actualized state because it requires wisdom and maturity acquired through facing life's realities and trials and then choosing to be fully oneself. Sperry and Springman (1983) add that in old age most growth is an internal, personal matter that is independent of physical attributes or observable actions. Maslow believes few people of any age ever truly reach a self-actualized state.

The later years do present a tremendous challenge to the human spirit. An older adult's ability to successfully confront this challenge can be a valuable lesson to younger adults. Unfortunately, gerontological research over the past six decades has emphasized the impoverishment of meaning or purpose in later life rather than the spiritual successes. For example, researchers such as Rosow (1974), and Atchley (1977) have claimed that American culture provides limited norms to govern the lives of older adults. The meaning of old age has largely been tied to two archetypal themes: the division of life into ages or stages, and a lifespan approach that uses the metaphor of life as a journey.

The division of life into stages has been approached from two directions. Mechanistic theorists view the individual as a passive reactor to the environment, and organismic theorists view the individual as an active rather than a passive reactor. The lifespan approach combines the elements of both the organismic and mechanistic theories. This approach which has been called contextualism, emphasizes ongoing reciprocal transactions between the individual and the environment. The contextual model recognizes both the normative events of aging (events that virtually affect all adults of the same age) and non-normative events. McFadden and Gerl (1990) suggest that the contextual model offers a vehicle for addressing spiritual health issues:

> Although it emphasizes the increasing differentiation produced by aging, the contextual model also recognizes the role of "normative age-graded influences" on development. This means that certain biological and environmental events affect nearly all persons at approximately the same age. Toward an understanding of adult spirituality, this model encourages us to examine the effects of the normative physical changes of aging on individuals' dynamic sense of spiritual integration. What challenges are presented to this sense of integration when physical disability means one can no longer hike beloved trails, visit with friends, or even attend religious services? Likewise, this model would explore the impact of the deaths of friends and relatives on spirituality in late life, for this is an experience that all aging persons undergo. (1990, p. 36)

Non-normative events may also influence the lives of older adults and thus need to be addressed as part of spiritual health. For example, why do some older adults elect to be political activists in later life while others choose to be uninvolved? Normative history influences experienced by age-cohort groups are also important. For example, a person who reached age 85 years in 1990 was born in 1905. At that time, the United States was not heavily industrialized and was reliant on a resource-based economy. Those who grew up in the early 1900s had less access to education and work opportunities than those born 10 to 20 years later. Their lives were tied to the community in which they were born, and their value systems were based on survival. Thus the spiritual journey of those age 85 or older may be quite different from that of adults age 65 to 75.

Summary: Embeddedness and Dynamic Interactionism

Contexualism includes two related assumptions, "embeddedness" and "dynamic interactionism," that are important for addressing spiritual health in late life. Embeddedness states that the most important aspects of human life may be experienced at different levels. Biological, psychological, social, cultural, and historical events do not function independently but instead operate in dynamic interaction with one another. For example, the older adult who feels void of personal meaning may also feel a related lack of connection with other people. This lack of personal ties may actually be the result of an environment that devalues old age.

The contextual model contains three important implications for spiritual health in the later years. First, the model emphasizes plasticity, the potential for change. Plasticity is not limitless, but an older adult's sense of spirituality is also not immutable. The vast amount of interacting changes and reorganization in late life conspire to weaken or strengthen spiritual bonds. For example, the impact of chronic illness may bring suffering, but it can also lead to reintegration and a renewed sense of spirituality. Religious faith as a response to suffering may guide the reintegrative process.

Second, the contextual approach assumes that one may influence his or her own development. Despite varying degrees of biological and environmental constraint, older adults can actively enhance their own spiritual development. McFadden and Gerl (1990) note that "aging is not like a train one passively rides until one reaches the station called 'wisdom' or 'spiritual integration.' Aging alone does not automatically confer integration within the self or with others, the natural world, and the transcendent realm" (p. 37).

Finally, plasticity means that interventions for spiritual development can be implemented even in very late life. Life review or autobiographical tapes, for example, are used to enable older adults to examine the course of their lifelong spiritual development. The multiple influences in spiritual development and ways to enhance spiritual integration may also be addressed. Normative age-graded events, non-normative events, and normative history-graded events should all be included. As an older adult addresses these events, he or she may understand how spiritual integration can motivate one to pursue the cultural aims of life.

SPIRITUAL HEALTH PROMOTION: A SENSE OF COHERENCE

Antonovsky (1987) views health or well-being as a product of three principal functions: (1) the capacity to understand ourselves and the expectations we and others share of ourselves; (2) the resources needed to meet the expectable challenges, even the extraordinary challenges, of life in personally satisfying and socially acceptable ways; and (3) the attachment of meaning to life that makes pursuit of "aging well" seem relevant and compelling. These three principal functions represent a sense of coherence that falls under the spiritual dimension of health promotion.

The challenge to health promotion professionals is to develop programs whereby spiritual wellness is perceived as an important personal and social task that stimulates the older adult to pursue a consensus about a deserved future and a gratifying past. Although some older adults may find life less satisfying, they can still find it meaningful and purposeful. Three major spiritual wellness programs pertain to this objective: Life Reminiscence, consciousness-modifying techniques, and learning and growing in later life.

Life Reminiscence

Journal, diary, life review, and oral biography are all terms that have been used to designate a body of material, genre of writing, or personal exploration that older adults may use to record information about their lives. Each of these techniques documents personal experiences of aging and constitutes a distinct and personal form of creativity.

Personal Journal. The personal journal as a literary form has evolved over the past three centuries. One of the most noted personal diaries was that of Samuel Pepys written between 1660 and 1669. By the 19th century, the journal was accepted both by experienced and inexperienced writers as an authentic creative and literary endeavor. For women in particular, the journal once signified one of the only available means of creative literary expression. "The journal form was and continues to be an important creative outlet partly because it mirrors the possibilities for living that have been historically available to women: emotional, fragmentary, interrupted, modest, not to be taken seriously, private, restricted, daily, trivial, formless, concerned with self, as endless as their tasks" (Moffat & Painter, 1974, p. 5). In general, women still dominate the art of personal journals and diaries and seem more interested in chronicling their life history.

Journal Writing. Journal writing is a creative venture that is not only for experienced writers, but also for those inexperienced writers who may want to write as a hobby and have no intentions of publishing their works. It is a vehicle for self-understanding and for a creative outlet. Because the main topic of the personal journal is oneself, the form of creativity is solely dependent on the author's vantage point of what "creativity" means to him or herself. Cohler (1982) writes that the self is understood to be a coherent narrative, a story that integrates the culturally available meanings attached to separate life experiences and provides continuity in response to anticipated and unanticipated life changes. Ricoeur (1981) further elaborates by stating that the personal journal is a quintessentially human product because it reflects a fundamental aspect of human nature. Czikszentmihalyi (1990) has termed the experience of personal journal writing "flow" because it describes not only how one is in control of psychic energy but also a mental state in which people feel intrinsically motivated, alert, able to concentrate, unselfconscious, and not monitoring others' perceptions of them.

Life Review. Wolf (1985) recommends the use of life review and reminiscence for older adults in classroom settings. She found that older learners could connect their current educational experience with the past. Helpful techniques include (1) initial taped interviews that focus on childhood and early experiences in school, (2) development of a "lifeline" in which each decade is marked and important events placed at appropriate times, and (3) mapping of neighborhoods and marking of important places in the world of childhood.

Personal journals, journal writing, and life review provide rich descriptions of the interior lives of their authors. Each may serve as a vehicle for self-understanding, self-guidance, and expanded creativity. Life review strategies may also be used as a medium to purge one's soul and to close a chapter in life in order to move on to a different life stage. Health care professionals, for example, are recognizing the value of tapping into the past to bring the individual into contact with feelings and motivations of the present. Oral biographies have been quite effective for clinical purposes.

Life reminiscence can play a significant role in the spiritual growth of older adults. The inner exploration required by life reminiscence, however, requires considerable effort and can be a trying experience. Scott Peck, in his book *The Road Less Traveled* (1978), views our struggle for truth and reality as a map that we use to negotiate the terrain of life. We know where we are in life when the map is true and accurate. We also know how to get to where we want to go. A map that is false or inaccurate, however, will cause us to be lost. Although this is obvious, some people choose to ignore life maps because the route to reality is difficult. Peck (1978) explains as follows:

> First of all, we are not born with maps; we have to make them, and the making requires effort. The more effort we make to appreciate and perceive reality, the larger and more accurate our maps will be. But many do not want to make this effort. Some stop making it by the end of adolescence. Their maps are small and sketchy, their views of the world narrow and misleading. By the end of middle age most people have given up the effort. They feel certain that their maps are complete and their Weltanschaung is correct (indeed, even sacrosanct), and they are no longer interested in new information. It is as if they are tired. Only a relative and fortunate few continue until the moment of death exploring the mystery of reality, ever enlarging and refining and redefining their understanding of the world and what is true. (pp. 44-45)

The biggest challenge for "life map-making" is not to start from scratch but to continually revise. Major revising in life maps can be terribly stressful and frightening. If an older adult has worked diligently to construct a viable view of his or her world, encountering or confronting new information that suggests the life-map is no longer valid can be overwhelming. The tendency is to cling to the outmoded map by ignoring and denouncing new information. This process of clinging to an outmoded map or view of one's world is called "transference" by psychologists and psychiatrists. Life reminiscence techniques can be effectively employed to overcome the problem of transference. The reader is encouraged to consult Peck (1978) for an excellent discussion of how life reminiscence techniques can be effectively employed for both clinical and nonclinical purposes.

Consciousness-Modifying Techniques

The early 1990s has experienced a dramatic surge of interest in the nature of consciousness and in consciousness-modifying techniques. Consciousness techniques experiencing popularity include meditation, biofeedback, and Yoga to name but a few. The trend toward consciousness-modifying techniques goes far beyond what we once thought were the limits to human potential. New discoveries linking the brain to the immune system suggest that the mind has a powerful influence on the body.

Many scientists find it hard to believe that such mental abstractions as loneliness and sadness can have a physical impact on a person's body. This skepticism may be tied to questionable claims by New Age psychic healers (e.g., transcendental meditation and body levitation). But lately solid evidence is accumulating to support the belief that good thoughts are tied to good health and bad thoughts are tied to bad health. Sophisticated laboratories have enabled researchers to demonstrate that emotional states can translate into altered responses in the immune system. Sheldon Cohen's investigation of the question of whether we catch a cold more readily when feeling threatened and alone is a good example. Gelman (1990), in a Newsweek article entitled "Body and Soul," examines current research:

> That direct linkage--of state of mind, altered immune response and illness--is the "hard science" that researchers like Cohen are now tackling. Scores of studies have already found suggestive correlations. Some show higher rates of illness among people who have recently lost a spouse, indicating that bereavement significantly affects their immunity. The same is true of people who feel socially isolated. In one of the largest of these studies, researchers found that for all age and sex groups, mortality was three times higher among those with the fewest close relationships. Having good friends and relatives seemed to afford a measure of protection from stressful life events. Scientists at the University of Michigan reviewed some of the research and agreed that social isolation alone is "a major risk factor" for mortality, perhaps as much as that of cigarette smoking. Similar correlations turn up among nursing home patients who sense no "control" over their daily lives, breast cancer patients who are pessimistic about recovering and partners locked in strife-torn marriages.

> The reverse is also true: positive mental states seem to bear favorably on health and longevity. One study headed by psychologist Sandra Levy at the Pittsburgh Cancer Institute this year found that a factor called "joy"--meaning mental residence and vigor--was the second strongest predictor of survival time for a group of patients with recurring breast cancer. (pp. 88, 89)

The whole field of body-mind research has been mushrooming with excitement since the mid-1970s. Research by Martin Seligman on learned helplessness, Friedman and Rosenman on Type A and Type B personalities, Herbert Benson on the relaxation response, Neil Miller on training individual responses to the autonomic nervous system, Candace Pert on neuropeptides, Theodore Barker on the ability of hypnosis to alter body conditions, and Gerald Epstein's research on medicine and imagery head the list (Dienstfrey, 1991). The most serious research, however, is coming from a new hybrid discipline called psychoneuroimmunology (PNI).

Robert Ader's research on conditioning immune system responses lies at the heart of PNI research. Dienstfrey (1991) does not believe disease is a product of a single physiological or psychological cause. He sees disease as psychosomatic and arising from a constellation of physiological and psychological elements. PNI involves the complex communication between the central nervous system and the immune system.

Recent research suggests that the immune system produces chemicals that feed information back to the brain, forming an intricate feedback loop between the brain and the immune system. Candace Pert calls this intricate feedback loop a shared consciousness where it is sometimes difficult to know who is in charge (Dienstfrey, 1991). Gelman (1990) adds:

> Brain to Immune System: Although the immune system reacts to infection on its own, the brain may influence the response with hormones and nerve signals to the main immune organs.

> Immune System to Brain: Immune activity may affect the brain, "talking back" to it with hormones apparently identical to the brain's own neurotransmitters. The hormones can affect states of mind, even bringing on depression. (p. 90)

Shared-consciousness is a force that most of us undervalue. Doctors are especially uneasy about body-mind medicine; they see it more as a concept than a true discipline. For many scientists, the anecdotes of mind-over-body cures advocated by New Age healers are unconvincing. It is important to remember that PNI is a cross-disciplinary science still in its infancy. Dramatic research breakthroughs of late, however, are beginning to unlock the mystery of the mind-body connection. As this mystery is unlocked, the consciousness development techniques of Eastern culture and the New Age movement will filter more actively into the spiritual components of health promotion programming. Examples of such programming include meditation, visual imagery, acupressure, and environmental devices.

Meditation. Meditation has been used in Eastern cultures for thousands of years. However, many types of meditation have become popular in Western cultures only in the past two decades. Researchers investigating neuropsychological benefits of meditation have found consistent results. Benefits have included a decrease in oxygen consumption, changes in skin conductivity, increased perceptual awareness, pain control, decreased or stabilized blood pressure, and renewed energy. Zen meditation (Yoga) and Transcendental Meditation are two of the more common meditations used in Western culture. Both Zen meditation and Transcendental Meditation are characterized by a pattern of low arousal and a predominance of alpha waves in the EEG pattern. A decline in psychosomatic disorders such as headaches, backaches, insomnia, digestive problems, and colds has also been reported. Reduced reliance on alcohol, cigarettes, coffee, and other drugs may be additional benefits.

The term "meditation" is often met with mixed feelings. Meditation is defined by Pelletier (1981) as an experiential exercise that involves an individual's actual attention, not just his or her belief system or cognitive process. But many people mistakenly believe that a total lifestyle change must be adopted in order to successfully practice meditation-- vegetarianism, or some quasi-religious mind-control system. Despite this reticence, meditation is slowly being accepted by older adults as a viable method to quiet the mind, relax the body, or to "center oneself." Some older adults use meditation as a stress management technique or as an aid to better sleeping patterns. More adventuresome older adults have used meditation to explore the inner consciousness and to attain a higher level of self-actualization.

Other popular forms of meditation techniques include autogenic training, progressive deep-muscle relaxation, biofeedback, and visual imagery. Many meditation disciples declare that their techniques are very different and are the best method for attaining "inner calm." In truth, the meditation techniques may be classified into two categories: (1) those that use the mind to relax the body (e.g., Transcendental Meditation) and (2) those that use the body to relax the mind (e.g., progressive deep-muscle relaxation). All of the meditation techniques have been found to benefit inner calm.

Acupressure. Acupressure may be described as a relaxing and natural form of touch therapy that uses slow and gradual finger pressure applied to the same points that acupuncturists treat with needles. According to the Chinese theory of acupuncture, a basic energy, or Chi, flows throughout the body along 12 different meridians or pathways. Pain and disease are a result of imbalances along those pathways. The application of needles to specific points in the meridians alter and balance the Chi energy, which alleviates pain and disease. Thus, touch rather than needles is applied to the meridian points to relieve distress.

Touch therapy strategies such as acupressure have been shown to relieve muscle tension and to increase blood circulation. David Bright, director of the Pain Control Unit at UCLA, found that pressing neural receptors also affects heart rate and endocrine function. The release of pain-killing hormones as endorphins may occur. Moreover, acupressure has been found to ease back pain and tension, fatigue, headaches, insect stings, colds, toothaches, and irritation from poison ivy (Bauer, 1991).

Touch therapies are usually done in conjunction with other types of therapies such as massage, herbalism, and conventional medical treatment. Older adults may especially find touch therapy useful because they can easily administer it to themselves or others. Touch is also an excellent therapy for older adults experiencing a void in physical contact due to the death of a spouse or close friends. For an excellent review of touch therapy, the reader is encouraged to consult Cathryn Bauer (1991).

Environmental Devices. Flotation tanks and sound and light machines have recently been introduced as stress management techniques. A flotation tank is a technological variation of an age-old meditative technique used by monks. Flotation tanks were popularized by Dr. John Lilly in the 1970s and were found to decrease stress-related neurochemicals in the body. The flotation suspension coupled with total darkness, which removes all sensory input, fosters relaxation and rejuvenates body energy.

Sound and light machines were marketed in the 1980s but have been slow to catch on. These machines use sensory overload in the form of flashing lights and synchronized pulsating sounds. Theoretically, the rhythmic interplay between the flashing lights and pulsating sounds moves the individual from a normal thinking state (beta waves) into a more composed or relaxed state (alpha waves).

Visual Imagery. Imagery has become an increasingly popular form of therapy that serves as a complement to medical intervention. Patients using visual imagery are asked to visualize what their problem may look like, clarify the problem, and then to actually process through the problem. For example, when visual imagery is used for cancer treatment, patients may be asked to imagine that the medicine entering the body is a healing balm that weakens and destroys cancer cells. This form of visual therapy is conducted several times a day. Most therapists employing visual imagery prefer that patients are drug-free for the duration of the treatment as the body seems to respond more effectively when not influenced by medications.

Gerald Epstein, in his book Waking Dream Therapy (1981), discusses the potential of using visual imagery during sleep. Dreams are used to help the patient move through troublesome events and the emotions associated with those events. Epstein maintains that under most conditions, the mind is the central tool for healing. For an interesting discussion of visual imagery used with older adults, the reader is encouraged to consult Jean Houston's *The Possible Human*. Noted therapists from European, Asian, and Eastern Indian cultures have long been believers of mind-body approaches for healing physical and psychological ills. Scientific documentation for these claims, however, remains rather questionable.

Learning and Growing in Later Life

Many gerontologists believe that most educators and professionals do not facilitate the self-actualization of older learners (Ebersole & Hess, 1990). This omission is largely due to the mistaken belief that education does not remain an integral part of healthy aging in the later years. Distorted myths assume that older adults are no longer capable or interested in educational opportunities. Today's societal views are changing and we are now beginning to understand that older adults have unique gifts and needs. In fact, older adults are actually books of "walking history" that can be used as peer educators in all kinds of educational settings.

Brockett (1987) investigated the relationship between life satisfaction and self-direction in learning programs used with older adults. His series of studies found a positive correlation between self-directed learning and the perception of meaningful life, self-concept, and the self-perception of one's health. Due to these benefits, community colleges, elderhostels, and peer education programs for older adults are now flourishing. Community colleges have been instrumental in offering courses that develop specific skills or knowledge bases. Elderhostels are unique international education programs developed in the early 1970s to provide academic courses with a low-cost room and board program on university and college campuses. Peer education programs are a life-long learning opportunity provided at low cost and sponsored as an international, ecumenical program in senior centers. For an excellent review of learning and education as a spiritual wellness component, the reader is encouraged to consult Ebersole and Hess (1990).

Summary: Integrating Spiritual Wellness Components

Chapman's (1987) "optimal spiritual health" definition for spiritual wellness is suggestive of a highly standardized reference point that can be used to produce "cookbook" approaches to spiritual health programs. Certainly there are well-defined programs that can provide such structure. Examples of such structural programs were presented in this section. Chapman, however, recommends that spiritual health be addressed from three basic program levels: (1) the overall program, (2) the programs dedicated exclusively to spiritual health, and (3) the existing programs. Table 10-1 provides an overview of activity ideas that pertain to these three program levels.

Standardized approaches including spiritual dimensions in health preparation programs are likely to remain controversial. The underlying concept of spiritual wellness as an "inner journey" is a very difficult perception to grasp in Western society. Inner journeys are likely to be very personal and individualized. Ideally, the ideas and concepts presented in this section and the preceding section will encourage dialogue among health promotion professionals as to how to integrate spiritual wellness into health promotion programs.

CHAPTER SUMMARY

A notion addressed in the first chapter of this book suggested that aging is seen as a disease; aging is seen as a process of continual physiological and cognitive decline with the passage of time that sets up older adults for a self-fulfilling prophecy. Pictured as rusted physical and cognitive machines, it is not difficult to imagine that spiritual wellness can significantly sag in the later years. This degrading picture can be very difficult to challenge. Aging has been mistakenly used to describe life in the older years from a "dark side" perspective; rarely has the term development been applied to the changes that occur in late life. The "growth of wisdom" referred to by Langer lies at the heart of spiritual wellness programs. As Langer (1989) notes,

> cognitive skills and psychological and physical health are presumed to be curvilinearly related to age. In this view, the individual grows to maturity and then lives out the adult years of life adjusting to diminishing capacities. Some cultures incorporate the growth of wisdom into their accounts of human aging. However, this continuing growth of wisdom is usually seen as a stream of development that is either independent of, or occurs in reaction to, a process of decline that is taking place in other areas. (p. 96)

Table 10-1. Programs concerning spiritual health.

Overall Program	Existing Programs
• Incorporating spiritual health into a definition for health promotion efforts	• Including spiritual health as part of the health assessment process
• Including spiritual health in program descriptive brochures	• Providing spiritual health related publications and "door prizes"
• Incorporating spiritual health into the program logo	• Developing spiritual themes as part of communication programs
• Using a program theme that incorporates spiritual health issues	• Integrating spiritual health issues into management and organization retreats and meetings
• Including spiritual health references in general program material	• Integrating spiritual health issues into other intervention programs such as physical fitness, stress management, substance dependency
• Using symbolic gestures as part of program efforts	
Programs Dedicated Exclusively to Spiritual Health	• Including spiritual health issues in health behavior change workshops
• Conducting lifegoal planning seminars for career, family, recreation, retirement and education	• Integrating spiritual health issues into outdoor recreation programs
• Providing personal awareness workshops that address connectivity	• Integrating spiritual health issues into pre-retirement planning programs
• Sponsoring spiritual renewal retreats	
• Developing spiritual health support groups	
• Establishing a spiritual health-oriented lending library	
• Conducting spiritual health workshops	

From L. S. Chapman, "Developing a Useful Perspective on Spiritual Health: Love, Joy, Peace and Fulfillment" in *American Journal of Health Promotion,* 2(2), 12-17, fall 1987. Michael P. O' Donnell Publishers, Rochester Hills, MI. Reprinted by permission.

Our negative images of aging are largely a product of mindset assumptions as to what it is supposed to be like as we grow old, rather than what it should or could be like. Langer (1989) adds "if we didn't feel compelled to carry out these limiting mindsets, we might have a greater chance of replacing years of decline with years of growth and purpose" (p. 113). Replacing mindsets through spiritual wellness programs will require the development of new life endpoints and creative alternatives for exploring continued growth and wellness. Life reminiscence, consciousness-modifying practices, religion, and educational opportunities are serving as a viable foundation for this objective.

CHAPTER 11

COMMON CHRONIC DISEASES, INJURY, AND AIDS IN LATE LIFE

Chronic health problems are a fact of life in mid-to-late old age. Special chronic diseases such as hypertension, diabetes, osteoporosis, breast cancer, and arthritis are especially prevalent. Moreover, accidents and injury problems are much more frequent and serious in later life. One can assume that this propensity to injury and accidents is associated not only with age-related psychomotor and cognitive changes but also with chronic diseases. Our purpose in this chapter is to address the attendant problems of physical disorders and the older adults potential to adopt lifestyle strategies that prevent and manage chronic disease conditions. The key is that physical deterioration associated with chronic disorders does not mandate psychological deterioration and dependency. Our discussion begins with a look at accidents and injuries in late life.

INJURY CONTROL PROGRAMS

Unintentional injury ranks fourth as a leading cause of death in the United States. Although the death rate due to injuries in the 1980s has actually declined, the death rate remains higher among the elderly than younger populations (Table 11-1).

Common Injury Problems

Falls, motor vehicle accidents, thermal stress, and pedestrian injuries account for many of the hospitalizations of persons over the age of 60. The mortality rate for various types of accidents rises dramatically for older adults. The overall mortality rate is 20%. Moreover, 88% of older adults suffering from accidents do not return to their previous level of independence (Ebersole & Hess, 1990). Health status before these injuries surprisingly has little to do with the survival rate after an accident.

Motor Vehicles. The death rates due to motor vehicle accidents vary dramatically by age and sex. The peak years for motor vehicle accidents are in the late teenage years, then decline until age 65 before abruptly rising again. Older adults as a group drive fewer miles than the younger population and have fewer collision rates. But the collision rate for miles driven is higher for older adults. Factors contributing to motor vehicle accidents include vision, alcohol intoxication, experience and judgment, amount of travel, seat belt use, osteoporosis, age, and physical condition (Dible, Pardini, & Bogart-Tullis, 1985).

Falls. Injury and death rates from falls are the highest among the elderly. Hip fractures particularly account for the high death rate and increased hospital admissions; 84% of hip fractures are sustained by people over age 65. Thirty percent of all deaths from

Table 11-1. Death rates from accidents and violence (1970–1985)*.

Cause of Death & Age	WHITE Male			WHITE Female			BLACK Male			BLACK Female		
	1970	1980	1985	1970	1980	1985	1970	1980	1985	1970	1980	1985
Total[1]	101.9	97.1	84.1	42.4	36.3	32.8	183.2	154.0	123.2	51.7	42.6	35.8
Vehicle Accidents	39.1	35.9	28.2	14.8	11.4	11.4	44.3	31.1	26.7	13.4	8.3	8.3
Other Accidents	38.2	30.4	26.2	18.3	14.4	12.9	63.3	46.0	37.2	22.5	18.6	14.5
Suicide	18.0	19.9	21.5	7.1	5.9	5.6	8.0	10.3	10.8	2.6	2.2	2.1
Homicide	6.8	10.9	8.2	2.1	3.2	2.9	67.6	66.6	48.4	13.3	13.5	11.0
15-24 years	130.7	138.6	111.8	34.9	37.3	32.3	234.3	162.0	132.8	45.5	35.0	29.4
25-34 years	96.6	118.4	98.8	23.8	29.0	25.1	384.4	256.9	186.5	76.0	49.4	40.4
35-44 years	85.7	94.1	80.6	25.8	29.2	25.3	345.2	218.1	175.1	77.2	43.2	36.5
45-54 years	87.5	90.8	77.1	30.4	31.8	17.4	303.3	207.3	147.9	65.6	40.2	33.1
55-64 years	101.5	92.3	85.4	36.3	33.8	30.6	242.4	188.5	145.5	56.0	47.3	36.3
65 and over	216.9	163.9	155.3	122.4	87.2	81.4	220.0	215.8	186.9	107.9	102.9	84.7
65-74 years	128.0	116.7	104.2	57.7	46.4	45.4	217.4	182.2	151.5	81.5	68.7	53.4
75-84 years	229.3	209.2	207.2	149.0	101.5	92.3	236.0	261.4	232.8	140.1	137.5	110.7
85 years & older	446.7	438.5	427.3	391.4	268.1	223.4	271.8	379.2	344.6	214.3	235.7	197.1

*Per 100,000 population. Excludes deaths of nonresidents of the United States. Beginning 1979, deaths classified according to the 9th revision of International Classification of Diseases. For earlier years, classified according to the revision in use at the time.
[1]Persons under 15 years of age not shown separately.

Source: Data from U. S. National Center for Health Statistics: Vital Statistics of the United States, annual.

falls occur in the age-85-and-over population and half of all fall deaths are incurred by people 75 years or older. Older adults are more likely to suffer serious injury from falls than younger populations for several reasons, including various medical problems, changes in skeletal composition, and decreases in posture and gait control (Dible et al., 1985). For people over 75, falls are more likely to be caused by organic failure than by accident. Tideisaar (1989) acknowledged this concern: "For example, a patient with poor balance and declining vision may trip over a carpet edge simply because it is unseen" (p. 57).

As the American population continues to age, we can fully expect falls to occur at an alarming rate. Excessive mortality and morbidity will be a result. To reduce this trend, primary and secondary prevention strategies will need to focus on the intrinsic and extrinsic factors that underlie the geriatric fall. Tideisaar (1989) provided an excellent synopsis of these factors:

> One third of persons 65 and older residing in the community experience one or more falls per year. Studies of institutionalized elderly reveal an even higher prevalence of falls. In hospitals, the elderly are victims of up to 40% of all falling episodes, and in nursing homes approximately 45% of residents can be expected to fall annually. The U.S. Public Health Service estimates that two thirds of falls by the elderly are potentially preventable. Determining the reasons behind these data is the key to initiating effective prevention.
>
> Within the community, hospital, and nursing home settings, a number of factors have been identified that place older people at risk for falling. These factors can be categorized into intrinsic (pathological disease states and medications) or extrinsic (environmental obstacles), and they often act in combination to cause a fall.
>
> Intrinsic factors include cardiovascular disease, orthostatic hypotension, arrhythmia, syncope, vertigo, drop attack, hemiplegia, impaired balance, impaired gait, parkinsonism, impaired neck turning and extension, decreased vision, poor muscle strength, bladder dysfunction, cognitive impairment, and use of sedatives, hypnotics, and diuretics.
>
> Extrinsic factors include the stairway, bedroom, bathroom, bedrails, assistive devices, improper shoes, poor lighting, room location, decreased nursing staff, and the first week of institutionalization.
>
> Common activities implicated in intrinsically and extrinsically induced falls include transferring on and off beds, chairs and toilets, tripping over objects or floor coverings, such as carpets, rugs, and door thresholds, slipping on wet surfaces or linoleum-tiled floors, and descending stairs. (p. 61)

Within the context of health promotion programs, primary prevention strategy would include an assessment of persons age 65 and older at least once a year to determine the risk for falling. The purpose of this assessment would be to identify intrinsic and extrinsic fall factors. Secondary prevention (after a fall has already led to injury) would require even closer monitoring of extrinsic and intrinsic factors. This assessment should include four thorough examinations: (1) physical examination, (2) mobility testing, (3) fall history, and (4) environmental assessment (Tideisaar, 1989).

The physical examination should consist of an assessment of specific organ systems responsible for preserving vertical stability--musculoskeletal, neurological, vision, cardiovascular, and pediatric. Mobility assessment will focus on the ability of the older adult to maintain functional stability while walking and transferring. Assessment examinations pertinent to this concern were addressed in Chapter 3. Walking or transferring dysfunction should be evaluated as to whether it is caused by organic dysfunction. Finally, a fall history should be constructed based on symptoms, previous falls, fall location, activity at the time, and time of the incident. If the physical examination and the mobility and fall history assessments rule out intrinsic fall factors, then an environment assessment should be performed for such areas as ground surface, lighting, and stairs. The goal of environmental assessment is not to correct all potential hazards in the older adult's living environment, but to "observe the person's function and to modify only those hazards or obstacles that interfere with safe walking and transferring activity" (Tideisaar, 1989, p. 58).

Thermal Stress. Ability to respond to thermal stress (heat and cold) decreases with age. For example, an older adult requires twice the time to return to core body temperature following exposure to extreme heat or cold than does a younger adult. This difference is especially pronounced after age 70. Dible et al. (1985) acknowledge this point:

> The aging process increases the risk of injury by burns or fires, since aging is often accompanied by a decreasing ability to detect and escape from fires, smoke, or scalding liquids. Scalding burns from liquids, for example, like excessively hot tap water and hot beverages are the main cause of nonfatal, but hospitalized burn injuries in the elderly and small children. Burns from scalds and other contact with hot substances result in about 200 deaths each year, or 3 percent of all deaths from fires and burns. Eighty percent are caused by hot liquids or steam, and scalds from hot liquids cause about 30 percent of all hospital admissions. (pp. 1-3)

The mortality rate for older adults due to fire is almost twice that of any other age group except children ages 1 to 4 (Ebersole & Hess, 1990). Cigarettes smoldering in upholstery and mattresses, and heating equipment rank first and second as leading causes of fatal house fires. Deaths from clothing ignition account for only 5% of all fire and burn related deaths, but 75% of such deaths are incurred by people age 65 and older. Interestingly, older men are twice as likely to incur fatality by fire than older women.

This may be due to their greater tendency to smoke and drink alcohol. Death by fire is usually caused by smoke inhalation rather than by flame. Older adults with decreased ventilation capacity are likely to succumb more quickly from inhalation.

Hypothermia (fatally low body temperature) is estimated to kill over 25,000 elderly persons each year. Factors making the elderly vulnerable to hypothermia include physiological body changes, prescription drugs that interfere with the body's ability to sustain core temperature, and a wide range of chronic diseases that damage the body's defense against cold (Ebersole & Hess, 1990). Alcohol consumption is especially dangerous because it blocks the vasoconstrictive response to cold. Older adults begin to experience hypothermia problems indoors when temperatures hover between 50° F and 65° F. The prevalence of death due to hypothermia has sharply increased with rising energy costs. Median oral temperature for the elderly is 96.8° F. Thus, an environmental temperature below 65° F can be quite serious as it may cause a drop in core body temperature to 95° F. Factors complicating the problems of hypothermia for older adults include reduced perception of cold, impaired shivering and peripheral vasoconstrictive mechanisms, medications, decreased activity, insufficient clothing, inadequate heating systems, lack of subcutaneous fat, and disease conditions (Ebersole & Hess, 1990).

Hyperthermia risks contributing to heat illness in older adults include cardiovascular disease, infection, dehydration, stroke, agitation, hyperthyroidism, and drugs. Alcohol consumption is dangerous in hyperthermia as it impairs the autonomic response and dulls skin sensation. Debilitated, functionally impaired elderly are at great risk to heat illness when environmental temperatures and humidity are high. Table 11-2 provides an overview of pathophysiology temperature dysregulation in the elderly.

Risk factors for developing temperature regulating disorders include (1) age, (2) chronic mental illness, (3) depression, (4) impaired mental status, (5) poor nutrition and fluid intake, (6) drugs and alcohol, (7) low socioeconomic status, (8) impaired functional status, (9) poor social supports, and (10) extreme environmental temperature. Despite these factors, Robbins (1989) emphasizes that mortality and morbidity are primarily due to serious medical conditions during environmental stress and not hypothermia and hyperthermia:

> during the prolonged heat spells, elderly patients more frequently manifest cardiovascular and cerebrovascular disease. Increased blood flow to the periphery (through vasodilation) to increase body heat transfer to the environment creates an increase in cardiac demand which may precipitate cardiac failure or myocardial infarction. During cold periods, there are more deaths due to pneumonia, myocardial infarction, and stroke. (p. 73)

The many symptoms of temperature disorders in the elderly are nonspecific. Thus diagnosis depends on a high degree of suspicion rather than concrete facts. Differential diagnosis in the early stages of hypothermia can include a variety of disorders. To

Table 11-2. Pathophysiology of temperature dysregulation in the elderly.

Hypothermia	Hyperthermia
-- Diminished sensation to cold	-- Higher threshold of central temperature to sweating
-- Impaired sensation to change in temperature	-- Diminished or absent sweating
-- Abnormal autonomic vasoconstrictor response to cold	-- Impaired warmth perception
	-- Abnormal peripheral blood flow response to warming
-- Impaired shiver response	
-- Diminished thermogensis	-- Compromised cardiovascular reserve

Reproduced with permission from A. S. Robbins, "Hypothermia and Heat Stroke: Protecting the Elderly Patient" in *Geriatrics,* Vol. 44, No. 1, 1989. Copyright by Avanstar Communications, Inc.

offset this problem, it is imperative to have a high index of symptomatic conditions that lead one to suspect different types of temperature disorders. Table 11-3 provides an overview of a temperature disorder index.

Once an older adult develops a temperature disorder, the prognosis is very poor. Therefore primary prevention strategies are extremely important. Older adults at high risk should be identified; for example, persons over age 80 who have multiple chronic diseases, impaired functional status, and poor social support networks are considered high risk. Primary prevention strategies for hypothermia and hyperthermia are then introduced. Hypothermia strategies include education, careful medical supervision for the chronically ill, and adequate heating of the living environment; they also include avoiding the outdoors, wearing heavy clothes, ingesting hot foods and drinks, observing adequate nutrition, and using extra blankets. Hyperthermia strategies might include education, avoiding activity, wearing light and loose fitting clothes, maintaining adequate sodium and water intake, keeping proper ventilation, taking cool baths, and avoiding direct sun. The chronically ill in nursing homes should be carefully monitored for hyperthermia conditions (Robbins, 1989).

Tertiary treatment of mild hypothermia includes moving the patient to a warm environment. Individuals with mild hyperthermia illness require fluid therapy and movement to a cool environment. Heat stroke requires rapid cooling with ice water or evaporative techniques (Robbins, 1989). The key, however, is that temperature disorders are preventable, and health promotion programs can play a key role by including educational strategies under primary prevention.

Pedestrian Deaths. Pedestrian deaths make up almost one-sixth of all traffic-related deaths for the general population. However, such deaths are almost one-third for those age 70 and older. Pedestrian death rates are most likely to occur at intersections for

Table 11-3. Diagnosis and treatment of temperature disorders in the elderly.

Condition	Diagnosis	Treatment
Mild hypothermia	Fatigue, weakness, cool skin, impaired mental status, slowed movement, may not shiver	Passive rewarming: move to warm environment > 70°, insulate, check for predisposing conditions
Moderate-severe hypothermia	Delirium or coma, muscle rigidity, cold skin, edema, hypoventilation, hypotension, arrhythmia	Active core rewarming: inhalation, peritoneal dialysis, warmed IV solutions, intragastric or colonic irrigation, other
Mild hyperthermia	Lethargy, mild confusion, cramps, sweating, dehydration	Passive cooling: move patient to cool environment and give fluids
Moderate-severe hyperthermia	Temperature > 105°F; delirium or coma; hot, dry skin	Active cooling: sponge immediately with cold water and use fans, vigorous fluid and support therapy

Reproduced with permission from A. S. Robbins, "Hypothermia and Heat Stroke: Protecting the Elderly Patient" in *Geriatrics*, Vol. 44, Number 1, 1989. Copyright by Avanstar Communications, Inc.

older adults in contrast to child pedestrian fatalities which tend to occur along the roadway. The peak time for pedestrian fatality of older adults is about one hour after sunset. Inadequate safety islands and inadequate light duration are notable factors contributing to pedestrian deaths of older adults.

Injury Control and Older Adults

Unintentional injuries due to accidents are not random events but are predictable results of environmental variables. Thus, prevention strategies that focus specifically on environmental protection can dramatically reduce accidental deaths in the later years. In a publication by the U.S. Department of Health and Human Services entitled A Resource Guide for Injury Control Programs for Older Persons (Dible et al., 1985), three conceptual program modules were developed for older adults. They are Home Safety Audits, Community Safety Audits, and Fitness for Injury Prevention.

The guide consists of five sections. The first two sections focus on injury control for the elderly and on community organizations and strategies for developing and utilizing community resources. The remaining three sections describe program models that can be used at the local community level. At the end of each program module, a brief list of program resources is provided. Additionally, the guide provides material for training staff, encouraging the participation of key individuals and agencies in the program, and marketing and public relations material.

BLOOD PRESSURE

No part of the body escapes the aging process. This fact is particularly true for the cardiovascular system. As discussed earlier in this book, stroke volume decreases with age, maximum heart rate decreases, and blood vessels thicken and become elastic. A by-product of all of these concerns is that blood pressure tends to rise with age. This natural rise in blood pressure may mislead one to assume that higher blood pressure levels are acceptable in later years. Nothing could be further from the truth. There is no threshold level for the increased risk associated with high blood pressure; the higher the blood pressure level, the greater the risk.

Elevated blood pressure levels bombard the artery walls and the heart muscle. Damaged blood vessels become attractive places for blood fats and other undesirable elements to lodge. This repeated bombardment can cause hardening of the arteries (atherosclerosis) and a narrowing of the arteries (arteriosclerosis). Fixed high blood pressure, known as hypertension, can be even more devastating and can result in stroke, heart failure, or kidney failure. Thus, detection and management of high blood pressure and of the prevalence for hypertension is a critical health concern in the later years.

Postural Hypotension

Some older adults experience problems with postural hypotension, a sudden drop in blood pressure when they stand up too quickly. Suddenly rising from sitting or lying down, gravity pulls the blood to the extremities and temporarily deprives the brain of an adequate blood supply Postural hypotension is aggravated in later life due to a decline in cerebral blood flow. Illness and certain medications may also compound postural hypotension. The danger of hypotension is dizziness and loss of balance that may lead to falls and injury. To detect postural hypotension, older adults should have their blood pressure checked while seated and again while standing. A drop in systolic blood pressure of twenty or more mm Hg or a drop of 10 or more mm Hg in diastolic pressure is indicative of postural hypotension. Individuals diagnosed with postural hypotension should be very cautious when rising from a seated or lying down position. They should rise slowly and, if possible, assure that there is support to prevent falling. Elasticized support hose, avoiding alcohol, and drinking plenty of fluids (particularly in hot weather or when flying on an airplane) are also recommended. Hot baths, saunas and whirlpools are not recommended since heat dilates the blood vessels in the skin and lowers blood pressure.

Prevalence of Hypertension

Blood pressure is defined as the force with which blood pushes against the walls of the blood vessels. Systolic pressure is when the pressure rises to a peak as the heart beats and pumps blood into the arteries. Diastolic pressure occurs when the heart relaxes between the beats and the pressure falls to its lowest point. Hypertension is fixed high blood pressure, and people with chronic high blood pressure are called hypertensive.

Two types of high blood pressure are secondary hypertension and essential hypertension. Secondary hypertension affects only 3 to 5% of the population with high blood pressure and has an identifiable cause; such as kidney ailments, or birth control pills. Treatment of this condition through surgery or removal of the underlying condition will usually return the blood pressure to the normal level. Essential hypertension, on the other hand, affects 95 to 97% of people with high blood pressure and does not have an identifiable cause. Several lifestyle risk factors (e.g., obesity, stress, inactivity) are believed to be associated with essential hypertension.

Systolic blood pressure generally varies between 110 and 140 mm Hg, and diastolic pressure between 60 and 85 mm Hg. Abnormally high blood pressure or hypertension was traditionally defined as significantly high systolic blood pressure of 160/95 mm Hg or above. Borderline high blood pressure was defined as blood pressure readings between 140/90 mm Hg and 160/95 mm Hg. Recently, the 1984 Report of the Joint National Committee on Detection, Evaluation and Treatment of High Blood Pressure (U.S. Department of Health and Human Services, 1984) recommended a new classification as outlined in Table 11-4.

Estimates of hypertension prevalence for older adults vary considerably due to different thresholds used for defining systolic and diastolic blood pressure. Prevalence rates are considerably higher when the 140/90 mm Hg definition is used. Unpublished data from the National Health and Nutrition Examination Survey (NHNES) suggests that almost 30 percent of individuals aged 65 to 74 years have isolated systolic hypertension (140/90 mm Hg).

Detection and Evaluation

Resting blood pressure can be measured indirectly by auscultation using a stethoscope and sphygmomanometer which consists of a cuff and either an aneroid or mercury column pressure gauge. Recommendations for blood pressure measurement in the elderly are similar to those for the general population--quiet room, proper cuff size, and multiple readings to take into account blood pressure fluctuations. However, due to the possible presence of orthostatic hypertension, a strong recommendation for the elderly is to take measurements while the subject is standing before and during treatment. Additional measurements are taken in the sitting position.

Table 11-4. Blood pressure classification based on confirmed* diastolic and systolic pressures in the same individual 18 years and older.

Diastolic Blood Pressure (mm Hg)	Systolic Blood Pressure (mm Hg)		
	Less than 140	140 to 159	160 or greater
Less than 85	Normal Blood Pressure	Borderline Isolated Systolic Hypertension	Isolated Systolic Hypertension
85 to 89	High Normal Blood Pressure		
90 to 104	MILD HYPERTENSION		
105 to 114	MODERATE HYPERTENSION		
115 or greater	SEVERE HYPERTENSION		

*The average of two or more measurements on two or more occasions.

Source: 1984 Report of the Joint National Committee on Detection, Evaluation, and Treatment of High Blood Pressure. National Heart, Lung, and Blood Institute, National Institutes of Health, U.S. Public Health Service, U.S. Department of Health and Human Services, NIH Publication No. 84-1088, September 1984.

Sources of error in blood pressure readings should be taken into consideration and controlled. The following are general blood pressure measurement errors: inaccurate sphygmomanometer, improper cuff width, auditory acuity of technician, rate of inflation or deflation of the cuff pressure, experience of the technician, reaction time of the technician, improper stethoscope placement and pressure, and background noise. Moreover, many physicians have questioned the accuracy of indirect blood pressure measurements for older adults due to sclerotic changes in the arterial wall. A study of direct and indirect measurements failed to find significant differences between older adults and younger adults (Public Health Service, 1980). But psuedo-hypertension due to severe medical sclerosis of the brachial artery should be suspected if there are no objective signs of organ disease despite significantly high blood pressure. The National High Blood Pressure Education Program Coordinating Committee (Public Health Service, 1980) provides the following screening recommendations for older adults.

- Health care professionals, including physicians (regardless of specialty), dentists, nurses, optometrists, and podiatrists should measure blood pressure at each encounter with a new patient and should inquire about a history of hypertension and any past or present treatment for hypertension.
- Patients aware of their disease but untreated and those found to have elevated readings should be evaluated or if necessary, referred to appropriate sources of medical care for evaluation.
- Blood pressure should be measured in the sitting and standing positions at every visit before and during treatment. If standing blood pressure is consistently much lower than sitting blood pressure, the standing blood pressure should be used to titrate drug dosages during treatment.
- Average systolic blood pressure >160 mm Hg and/or average diastolic pressure >90 mm Hg on three consecutive visits constitute the diagnosis of hypertension, although the 140 to 160 mm Hg range represents borderline isolated systolic hypertension when diastolic pressure is <90 mm Hg. (p. 4)

Treatment for Hypertension

The objective for treatment is to reduce the health risks associated with hypertension. Both pharmacologic and nonpharmacologic modalities are employed for this purpose. Diuretics are usually the preferred pharmacologic approach for diastolic hypertension and isolated systolic hypertension. The initial goal is to reduce the systolic blood pressure to an acceptable range (140 to 160 mm Hg) rather than to normalize the blood pressure. Unfortunately, the side-effects of blood pressure drugs has led many older adults not to adhere to prescribed regimens.

The concept of "quality of life" has received increasing attention in hypertension programs. The patient's functional capacity, self-perception of general health status, and life satisfaction are at issue. Of particular concern are potential drug side-effects, excessive drug cost, and unfavorable alteration of serum lipid levels, glucose, and electrolyte levels. Potential side-effects from diuretics and beta-blockers have included sexual dysfunction and breast enlargement and tenderness. Statson's (1989) report from the Gallup Poll indicated that only 49% of all persons have health insurance for medication. Only 44% had health insurance for medication in families with income less than $15,000. The fiscal pressures of today are likely to play even more havoc in health insurance coverage for medication.

The potential barriers to "quality of life" by an exclusive pharmacologic approach to hypertension have led to nonpharmacologic strategies. Table 11-5 summarizes many of these strategies. The wisdom, however, appears to be a step-care therapy approach as recommended from the 1988 report of the Joint National Committee on Detection, Evaluation, and Treatment of High Blood Pressure. For some patients, nonpharmacologic approaches should be tried first. Pharmacologic approaches would be initiated if the blood pressure goal is not attained.

Although both pharmacologic and nonpharmacologic intervention play an important role in hypertension, it is unfortunate that the emphasis is still placed on tertiary prevention rather than on primary and secondary prevention. Primary and secondary prevention of hypertension are especially missing in health promotion programs directed toward older adults. As the prevalence of hypertension is so high and its treatment places a tremendous burden on the health care system, it would seem advantageous to focus on behavioral risk factor alteration.

Exercise programs for CHD patients are especially important. Empirical research has clearly established that physical activity programs help CHD patients improve cardiovascular function and better adjust to their disease (Neiman). In the not to distant past, CHD patients were prescribed bed rest for a two- to three-week period. Today, patients are prescribed activity of a low-level ambulation nature within the first 24 to 48 hours after a heart attack. Low-level ambulation exercises consist primarily of passive exercises, standing, stairclimbing and stationary bike exercise. These exercises are prescribed and monitored by the medical staff.

As the CHD patient moves from a convalescent to a post-convalescent period, more progressive exercise forms will be avoided. Physical activity programs of a competitive nature are also avoided. Early convalescent usually consists of a 12- to 20-week period and consists of walking, stationary cycle use, and possibly, low-level bench step exercises. The convalescent phase is supervised and patients are evaluated by multi-stage exercise stress tests. The unsupervised post-convalescent phase generally maintains exercise intensity programs of 65 to 85% of peak heart rate determined by the most recent multi-stage exercise stress test. Exercise duration is kept between 30 to 60 minutes and frequency is four to five times per week (Hanawalt, 1992). A prolonged warm-up period of 10-15 minutes and cooldown of 5 to 10 minutes are recommended.

Table 11-5. Reducing risk for hypertension

Recommendations for Reducing Risk for Hypertension

Inform everyone about non-behavioral and behavioral risk factors, and provide opportunities to develop personal competencies necessary to modify behavioral HT risk factors as follows:

1. Minimize consumption of sodium by limiting intake of highly processed and salt-cured foods, and develop a preference for foods without the addition of extra salt.

2. Reduce consumption of foods high in total fat and saturated fat, including beef, pork, cheese, ice cream, butter, and foods made with coconut, palm, and hydrogenated oils.

3. Ensure adequate intake of potassium and magnesium by eating the majority of daily calories from foods high in complex carbohydrates including fresh fruits, vegetables, dry beans and peas, and whole grains.

4. Ensure calcium intake by consuming low-fat dairy products such as nonfat milk and green leafy vegetables on a daily basis.

5. Ensure adequate intake of polyunsaturated fatty acids by eating a diet rich in legumes, vegetables, and whole grains,   and by consuming moderate amounts of nuts, seeds, and cold water fish.

6. Engage in regular aerobic physical activity at least every other day.

7. Seek to incorporate regular periods of relaxation in the daily routine and develop constructive means of coping with stress.

8. Use alcohol in moderation, if consumed at all.

From C. L. Melby, " Beyond Blood Pressure Screening: A Rationale for Promoting the Primary Prevention of Hypertension" in *American Journal of Health Promotion,* 3(2), fall 1988. Michael P. O' Donnell Publishers, Rochester Hills, MI. Reprinted by permission.

The CHD exercise program includes education about over-exercise exertion symptoms, orthopedic problems, and environmental condition (heat, cold) concerns. The potential intervention between physical activity and medication are also closely monitored. Digitalis and beta-adrenergic drugs are known to alter heart rate and alter ECG responses. For an excellent review of exercise programs for CHD patients, the reader is encouraged to consult Page, Schweder, and Coghlan (1996), Miller (1995), and Pollack and Schmidt (1995). Dean Ornish (1990) has also devised a CHD intervention program consisting of diet, exercise, and stress management worthy of review.

STROKE

A stroke occurs when an artery or vein in the blood becomes occluded or bursts. As a result, a lack of blood to the brain causes a loss of sufficient oxygen and nutrients reaching the brain. In a very short period of time, brain cells die. Recovery from a stroke: (1) Ischemic strokes and (2) Hemorrhagic strokes.

Ischemic strokes are defined as a deprivation of blood supply to any part of the brain which causes the brain to stop functioning properly. The cause of ischemic strokes is similar to CHD; a build-up of plaque in the arteries. This atherosclerotic plaque build-up, however, occurs in the arteries of the neck and head instead of the coronary arteries of the heart. An ischemic stroke may occur by the compete blocking off of blood flow in the artery, by the formation of a blood clot (called a thrombus) that forms a temporary plug in the artery, or by a fragment of a thrombus (called an embolism) that breaks off and lodges in one of the smaller blood vessels of the brain (American Heart Association, 1995).

Hemorrhagic strokes occur when an artery leading to the brain bursts. This hemorrhaging causes the spilling of blood into the brain or into the cavity between the outer surface of the brain and skull (Gordon, 1993). People with advanced athero-sclerosis and long-term high blood pressure are at risk for hemorrhagic strokes. These strokes are more fatal than ischemic strokes.

Role of Exercise

Rehabilitation for stroke patients follows a three-phase process: (1) Acute, (2) Post-acute, and (3) Rehabilitation. The acute phase normally lasts between 4 to 7 days and contains the sole objective of survival. The post-acute phase usually lasts 2 to 4 weeks and emphasizes the objective to relearn old motor skills and new motor skills that may compensate for the loss of old motor skills that cannot be recaptured. Rehabilitation, the third phase, covers an indeterminate time period. But, the body is most receptive to the beneficial impact of physical therapy during the first six months after a stroke. The objective of the rehabilitation phase is to attain full recovery of physical, social, vocational and economic function. It is important to emphasize, however, that rehabili-tation does not stop after this six-month period.

The role of exercise for the stroke patient is to assist in the transition between these three phases. Although full recapturing of neurological functioning is not practical in a six-month period, exercise programs play a significant role in helping the client to re-duce the degree of disability. The value of exercise programs extends beyond disability. Gordon (1993) writes:

> The one benefit of long-term, regular exercise that can almost always be
> guaranteed—even in elderly patients and those with chronic condi-tions
> such as heart and brain disorders—is an increase in physical fitness.
> With a higher fitness level, you can exert yourself more strenuously for

longer periods of time. With more energy, you'll have more reserve for participating in new activities—or in old ones that you mistakenly thought you didn't care about anymore. The result is an increase in functional capacity and a decrease in disability. (p. 14)

Stroke patients are classified according to a 5-grade scale continuum developed by Rankin (1957).
- Grade 1 Disability (none or almost none)
- Grade 2 Disability (slight)
- Grade 3 Disability (moderate)
- Grade 4 Disability (moderately severe)
- Grade 5 Disability (severe)

Patients classified in Grades 1-2 are still able to exercise without limitations. Grade 3 disabilities require a close supervision of exercise by a qualified health professional. Grades 4 and 5 disability will require a more detailed prescriptive exercise program developed and supervised by health professionals. Range of motion, muscle strengthening, and aerobic exercise programs provide the foundation for stroke patients.

Recommendations

The recommendations discussed for CHD clients apply as well to stroke patients. Basic components of an exercise sequence will generally follow a 10 to 20 minute warm-up consisting of stretching and strengthening muscle groups and a 5-minute aerobic routine. The foundation of the exercise program consists of 15 to 60 minutes of aerobic exercise at prescriptive intensity levels. A 10-minute cooldown period contains 5 minutes of aerobic cooldown and 5-minutes of stretching. For an excellent review of an exercise routine for stroke patients consult Gordon (1993).

Precautions

Emphasis is placed on exercise education according to the disability level classification. Similar to CHD patients, exercise interactions with medication are of concern. The patients physician should be consulted as to potential interaction.

DIABETES

Diabetes is the third leading cause of death by disease in the United States, surpassed only by heart disease and cancer. Approximately 12 million Americans--about 1 in 20--have diabetes. Over 90% of diabetics have a form of the disease called noninsulin-dependent diabetes (Type II). Type II diabetes is considered adult-onset and occurs as the body continues to produce insulin, but not in sufficient quantities to prevent the blood sugar's level from soaring. Type I is child-onset diabetes and occurs when the body completely loses its ability to produce insulin.

Unglamorous Disease

Diabetes, as compared to such diseases as cancer and Alzheimer's, is generally not viewed as one of the principal "dreaded" diseases. Because it appears to be non-life-threatening and somewhat manageable, diabetes has often been miscast as a nonserious disease. Nothing could be further from the truth. People with diabetes may lead active and productive lives for quite some time, but they later find that this insidious disease will erupt with brutal savagery. The case of Arthur Hettler III, a high school principal from San Antonio, Texas, exposes diabetes as a dormant volcano waiting to erupt.

> At first Hettler thought he had just a mild case of diabetes. He required no medication to control the excess blood sugar caused by the disease; instead, he watched his diet as carefully as he could. Then, two summers ago, Hettler strolled barefoot across some sun-scorched pavement and blistered his foot. Ominously, the blisters on his right foot refused to heal. A few months later the foot was so badly infected that it had to be amputated. Shortly before Christmas, Hettler, 47, suffered a paralyzing stroke. The infection and the stroke were complications resulting directly from the slow progression of diabetes. "The disease," observes Hettler, "can really creep up on you." (Nash, 1990, p. 52)

Treatment and control of Type II diabetes can reduce the chances that the harmful changes or complications will impair health. But this treatment is not a cure. Eventually the disease will creep up on its victim. Because the symptoms of diabetes are mild (fatigue, frequent urination), half the 12 million Americans with diabetes are unaware that they have this disease. Myocardial ischemia (angina) is frequently silent in Type II diabetic patients. Because diabetics experience less angina, their coronary disease is likely to be more advanced before it can be detected as compared to patients who are symptomatic. Given this reduced sensitivity to pain, Davidson (1991) emphasizes that noninvasive testing is of critical importance for diabetic patients. Moreover, many of the victims are unaware of its potentially devastating impact; diabetes doubles the risk of a disabling heart attack or stroke, is the leading cause of blindness in adults, accounts for 33% of kidney failures, ranks just behind traumatic injuries as a cause for amputation, and is the seventh leading cause of death in the United States.

Diabetes: How It Impairs Health

Both Type I and Type II diabetes impair the body's ability to use digested food for energy. Although diabetes does not interfere with digestion, it prevents the body from using glucose for energy. Glucose is a form of sugar that is broken down from food during digestion. Circulating blood carries the glucose throughout the body. When some part of the body requires energy, it metabolizes (burns) the glucose for fuel. This process of metabolizing glucose for energy needs a hormone called insulin to convert glucose into energy.

Insulin, produced by the pancreas, responds to the amount of glucose in the blood. Glucose in the blood is normally quite high after a meal. The presence of blood glucose leads the pancreas to secrete insulin, which enables the body to convert glucose to energy and to store what is left for future use. Glucose can be stored in the liver, or as glycogen in the muscle, or in the form of fat. For the Type II diabetic, this conversion process does not work properly. Excess glucose accumulates in the bloodstream rather than being stored, and is cleared by the kidney for excretion in urine. The loss of so many calories through the urine usually causes a loss of weight. Extreme cases of diabetes create sugar-starved cells. Deprived of glucose, the sugar-starved cells will switch to burning fatty acids, a process than can poison the bloodstream with its toxic by-products. The blood fat level rises when blood sugar levels exceed the normal range. This elevation in blood fat is believed to cause the higher risk for cardiovascular disease in diabetics.

Insulin resistance at the cell receptor site may lead to organ damage. Insulin receptors are surface locations on cells to which insulin must bind in order to have an effect. Several things may go wrong at the receptor site. There may not be enough receptor sites or there may be a defect in the receptors preventing insulin from binding. In some cases insulin may bind to the receptor, but the cells do not carry out the job of metabolizing glucose.

How Diabetes Creates Havoc in the Body

Possible long-term complications of diabetes include the following: (1) damage to the retina and lens in the eye, leading to blindness; (2) acceleration of atherosclerosis, increasing the risk of heart attack or stroke; (3) destruction of the kidney filtration system; (4) destruction of nerve cells; (5) wounds healing slowly, with danger of serious infections; (6) children born with congenital defects to pregnant diabetics; (7) potential impotence; and (8) loss of sensation in feet that can lead to injury. Just how excess glucose in the bloodstream causes such long-term damage remains a hot topic of debate.

One plausible mechanism is called the "biological super-glue" theory. Sugar is chemically active and combines with protein in the blood and blood vessel walls. These sticky fragments aggregate over time (i.e., like super-glue) and become a constant source of irritation. This source of irritation signals the body of damage in need of repair. The repair preparations cause a spurt of new growth that thickens blood vessel walls and thus constricts blood flow. Restricted blood flow will eventually damage critical organs (Nash, 1990).

The second plausible theory is elevated levels of sorbitol. Sorbitol is a sugary alcohol. Certain cells, particularly those in the lens of the eye, continue to absorb glucose even in the absence of insulin, however, without insulin glucose cannot be metabolized in the usual way. Instead, the cell converts glucose to sorbitol which, in abnormal amounts, causes cell membranes to swell and leak. The sorbitol conversion may also interfere with vital biochemical processes (Nash, 1990).

Diagnosing Diabetes

A doctor may diagnose diabetes by noting such symptoms as excessive urination, excessive thirst, excessive hunger, weight loss, fatigue and weakness, blurred vision, and slow healing of wounds. When these symptoms are present, tests are administered to measure the amount of glucose in urine or blood. A urine test can detect diabetes because the kidneys eliminate excess blood glucose levels as urine. However, urine analysis is prone to false positive errors as it reflects blood sugar content in the hours urine is being formed. The real threshold for glucose also varies from one individual to another; a variation that can be quite large. People with high renal thresholds may actually receive negative urinalysis results when blood sugar is fairly high.

Berg (1986) is a strong supporter of blood glucose monitoring kits for home use. In addition to being convenient, blood glucose monitoring kits may be more accurate than urinalysis tests. The cost for electronic monitoring blood kits has dropped considerably in recent years. Kits that formerly cost $300 are now available for less than $150. Insurance companies may pick up the bill for this purchase if the diabetic's physician writes a supporting purchase letter.

Blood glucose tests are done in the morning before breakfast (fasting glucose test) or after a meal (postprandial glucose test). Fasting blood glucose levels between 140 mg/dl and 160 mg/dl are considered borderline diabetes. Blood glucose levels of 160 mg/dl or higher are diagnosed as defined diabetes. The postprandial (oral glucose tolerance test) is used to measure how the body responds to an increase in blood glucose after eating. Normally the amount of blood glucose will rise quickly in response to a meal and then fall gradually again as insulin functions to convert glucose to energy and store the excess as glycogen. But with diabetes blood glucose levels will continue to remain high after a meal thus indicating that insulin is not functioning properly.

Management of Diabetes

The goals of diabetic treatment are twofold: to keep blood glucose levels within a normal range and to prevent the long-term complications of diabetes. Three major management factors are used to regulate blood glucose levels: (1) oral diabetic drugs or insulin injections, (2) diet, and (3) exercise. The sum of the effects of each factor in this three-prong strategy determines blood glucose level. Proper diet and weight loss should serve as the principal foundation for keeping diabetes under control (Vranic & Wasserman, 1990). Presently, a diet with 20 to 30% of calories from fat, 55 to 65% from complex carbohydrates, and 15% from protein with high fiber content is recommended (Davidson, 1991). But when diet and exercise (weight loss) fail to control diabetes, both oral diabetic drugs or insulin injections become the treatment of choice. The actual choice of treatment or combination of treatments is based on the person's age, lifestyle, and the degree of disease severity. Optimal treatment usually is a balance between lifestyle and medication strategies.

Obesity is an especially important factor in Type II diabetes. In the United States, 90% of those who develop Type II diabetes are obese (Nash, 1990). The tendency to increase body fat composition with age partially explains why Type II diabetes becomes more prevalent after age 40. The cells of obese people become more sluggish and sated which reduces their sensitivity to insulin. This reduction in sensitivity causes the pancreas to secrete more insulin but with little effect.

Despite the attention to weight loss, Type II diabetes is linked more to genetics than obesity. If both parents have diabetes, the chance a child will contract diabetes before middle-adulthood is almost 80%. Moreover, diabetes is endemic among many American Indian tribes and Hispanics. Unfortunately, awareness of this ethnic impact on diabetes has not received sufficient attention. The risk of cardiovascular mortality from smoking should also not be ignored. Sixty-five percent of cardiovascular disease deaths in diabetes are attributed to smoking. Smoking also accelerates atherosclerosis in peripheral arteries (Davidson, 1991).

Simple methods for monitoring blood glucose levels, proper nutritional practices (e.g., avoid high glucose foods and alcohol), aerobic exercise, and adherence to prescribed medication are all critical for managing and controlling diabetes. The common foundation between these management strategies is education. Unfortunately, our health care system does not pay for education through third party reimbursement. Many experts vehemently argue that this needs to change because diabetes already costs the nation $20 billion a year. Moreover, rising affluence and obesity tend to go hand-in-hand. We can expect diabetes, therefore, to flourish even more in the coming decade. Dollar expenditures in education for preventing and managing the long-term complications of diabetes can help curb incalculable suffering (Nash, 1990).

Aerobic and strength building exercise programs are recommended for diabetic patients. The rhythmic and large muscle movements of aerobic programs stimulate weight loss and insulin receptor sites. Exercises involving strength building help regulate glucose metabolism by increasing muscle mass. An increased muscle mass allows more storage capacity for muscle glycogen which helps maintain muscle energy reserve for preventing exercise exhaustion (Rosenberg and Evans, 1991). Walking, bicycling, swimming, and hiking are excellent exercise programs for diabetic patients. Gordon (1993) and Campagne and Lampman (1994) are excellent resources for exercise and diabetes. The reader is also encouraged to consult Hanawalt (1992) for special exercise precautions with diabetic patients.

BREAST CANCER

Fifty years ago breast tumors were rarely detected until they had reached the size of golf balls. This delay in detection meant that the cancerous cells had infiltrated the lymph nodes and were actively invading the lungs, bones, liver, and brain. Physicians had but one treatment weapon at their disposal--radical mastectomy. Today, better screening technology now enables physicians to detect and remove tumors two to three years before they can even be felt. Yet the news about breast cancer still remains grim. As Cowley (1990) writes,

> Surgery for more advanced tumors has become less barbaric. And advances in cell analysis promise to make today's drug treatments far more effective in the future. The problem is that scientific knowledge accrues slowly, and people are still dying fast. Breast cancer remains the second leading cause of cancer deaths among women. The best treatments still fail thousands of people every year, and prevention is still a dream. (p. 66)

There has been almost a 30% rise in breast cancer incidence since the 1970s. Despite the initial impression of an epidemic rise, some experts are more optimistic, suggesting that this rise is due to earlier detection which improves the odds of successful treatment. Dr. Vincent Devita, Jr., former head of the National Cancer Institute, states "combine the gains from mammography screening with advances in treatment, and you can predict a substantial decline in breast-cancer mortality in the 1990s" (quoted in Cowley, 1990, p. 66). In a study by Seattle's Fred Hutchinson Cancer Research Center, an analysis showed that early detection accounted totally for the rise in breast cancer among the 45- to 64-year-old women group. But early detection explained only 50% of the increased breast cancer rate for the under 44 or over age 65 group (Cowley, 1990).

Risk Factors and Breast Cancer

Breast cancer, unlike lung cancer, has few known avoidable causes. Epidemiologists have identified a few factors, but they explain only half of the actual cause for breast cancer. Essentially, the average American woman has a one in nine chance of developing breast cancer over a lifespan of 110 years. But this risk for breast cancer would be only 3.3% for a woman who lacked any of the risk factors. Family history remains the best barometer for predicting breast cancer. A woman whose mother had breast cancer may have a sixfold risk over someone with no risk factor. An afflicted second-degree relative (e.g., aunt, grandmother) may incur 1.5 times the baseline risk.

Despite the genetic link, scientists believe only 5 to 7% of all breast cancer is strictly hereditary. Other suspects include diet (high fat intake, overeating), alcohol consumption, and lifelong exposure to estrogen. Moderate alcohol consumption is believed to increase a woman's risk to 1.5 above the baseline level. Estrogen exposure (e.g., early onset of menstruation, estrogen replacement therapy) may increase breast cancer risks 1.4 times above the baseline level. Smoking and alcohol have also been identified as possible culprits. However, evidence to date does not support a clear connection. Food additives and sunlight are also under suspicion but there is no evidence to convict them (Wallis, 1991a).

The Fat Factor

Many researchers have identified fat as a principal component in breast cancer. Diets rich in fat promote the growth of mammary tumors in laboratory animals. Additionally, varying rates of breast cancers in different countries have been found to correlate with the amount of fat in a nation's diet. For example, the United States diet is laced heavily with rich fat whereas countries such as Japan maintain a more lean diet; Japan reports lower breast cancer rates than the United States. The possibility that genetic factors in country comparisons may be responsible for different cultural breast cancer rates has been ruled out by studies looking at immigrant groups. For example, Japanese individuals moving to the United States matched the higher breast cancer rate of their adopted country within one to two generations (Wallis, 1991a).

Despite the evidence pointing to fat as a breast cancer risk factor, not everyone shares this conviction. Some fat factor critics argue that correlation studies are not cause and effect. Moreover, the critics suggest that there are probably several risk factors rather than one primary culprit. Dr. Walter Willett, Harvard School of Public Health, believes overall calorie consumption rather than fat is the important factor behind breast cancer. Countries in the "land of plenty" like the United States include women who begin to menstruate at an earlier age, experience menopause later in life, and tend to have children later in life (Wallis, 1991a). Menopause after age 50, delayed childbearing after age 30, and menstruation onset before age 12 are all considered viable breast cancer risk factors. Obesity for older women has also been acknowledged as a risk factor. Mary-Claire King, a cancer geneticist at the University of California, Berkeley, suggests that better education and job opportunities for women advance the trend toward delay in childbearing or childlessness. King adds, "All the things that cause women to be healthy, well-educated and have careers put them at risk for breast cancer" (quoted in Wallis, 1991a, p. 50).

The Estrogen Factor

Many doctors are convinced that women are genetically predisposed to develop breast cancer. The risk is five to six times above the usual risk for a woman whose mother or sister had the disease before menopause. The risk is five times above the norm if the disease was in both breasts (Cowley, 1990). Scientists have not unlocked the secret as to how breast cancer begins, but they have some idea as to how it progresses.

The female hormone estrogen, which is produced in the ovaries and causes a young girl's breasts to develop, also plays an unmistakable role in promoting the growth of tumor cells. Why do childlessness, late menopause, early onset of menstruation, and delayed childbearing all increase the risk of breast cancer? One likely explanation is that all involve a prolonged, uninterrupted presence of high levels of estrogen in the bloodstream. Doctors have also noticed that women whose ovaries were removed before age 40 rarely get breast cancer (Wallis, 1991a, p. 51).

Researchers investigating the role of fat in breast cancer have been viably interested in the estrogen connection. Estrogen is produced in the fat cells as well as the ovaries. Obese women have been found to have higher fat levels than thin women. But the link between estrogen levels and fat in the diet was established only in the last five years. Women consuming a fast food diet (e.g., hamburgers, shakes, french fries) have higher overall levels of estrogen. This higher level of estrogen in large amounts is in a biological active form. A study by David Rose, endocrinologist of the Naylor Dana Institute, found that women switching to a very low fat diet (20% total daily calorie consumption) quickly decreased their estrogen levels by 20% (Wallis, 1991b).

Treatment of Choice

The treatment of choice for breast cancer still remains surgery and drug treatment. The success rate for treatment is up. Today 76.6% of breast cancer patients survive five years after surgery and 63% are alive ten years later. The five-year survival rate in 1970 after surgery was 68%. But for women fighting metastatic breast cancer, the survival rate is no better today than it was 50 years ago (Wallis, 1990b). Thus public health experts argue that screening and dietary practices still play a vital role. Mammogram screening for women above age 40 is especially critical. As Wallis writes,

> Consider these facts. By the time a breast tumor is large enough to be felt as a lump, it is generally more than 1 cm (0.4 in.) in diameter and contains several billion cancer cells, some of which may have broken loose, circulated through the bloodstream and begun to infiltrate other organs. A mammogram can detect pinpoint tumors that are less than 0.5 cm (0.2 in.) across, often well before the process of metastasis has started. This is not to say that a manual exam by a doctor or the woman herself is a waste of time. Such exams can sometimes turn up tumors missed by X-rays. But the early-detection capability of mammography clearly saves lives. A 1987 study found that for women whose tumors were discovered early by mammograms, the five-year survival rate was about 82%, as opposed to 60% for a control group. (1991, p. 51)

Despite the value of mammogram screening, women have been reluctant to follow recommended practices. Less than 33% of women over age 40 have mammograms every one to two years. Lingering fears about radiation, lack of health insurance coverage, and inconsistent professional association recommendations lie behind the inattention of women to mammogram screening. The uneven quality and accuracy of mammograms have also muddled the picture (Beck, 1990). We can expect, however, that recent lobbying efforts to bring breast cancer research to the forefront will lead to better mammography standards and more attention to prevention practices.

CHRONIC OBSTRUCTIVE PULMONARY DISEASE (COPD)

COPD is a breathing disorder involving airflow obstruction caused by several patho-logical and clinical conditions. The term COPD is an umbrella classification of airway obstruction conditions under one disease category. Emphysema, asthma, chronic bronchitis, and bronchiostenosis are the principal COPD conditions. The major symp-tom of breathing disorders is dyspnea which is "labored breathing." Emphysema is an enlargement of the walls of the smallest air passages (bronchioles) and the walls of the small air sacs (alveoli). This enlargement impairs the ability of the pulmonary system to exchange gases, leading to pulmonary recoil. Asthma is the diffusing or narrowing of airways over time. Airflow obstruction is primarily caused by bronchial muscle contrac-tion (Jones, Berman, Barkiewicz, & Oldrige, 1987). When the airways become irritated, bronchospasms occur. This irritation for asthmatic conditions is caused by allergies to certain substances, emotional crises, or a family history of asthma. Narrowed airways caused by irritant conditions make it more difficult for air to be exchanged in and out of the lungs. Chronic bronchitis is excessive mucus in the bronchial trec that causes a persistent cough. This condition is diagnosed when cough and sputum are evident on most days for a minimum of three months for at least two consecutive years or for six months during one year. Bronchiostenosis is an irreversible dilation of the bronchial trec (Jones et. al., 1987).

Consequences of COPD. The health and functional consequences of COPD are determined by the physiological responses to the narrowing and construction of airway passages. The four conditions of COPD are not benign. Emphysema, however, is considered the most deadly. Only 15% of individuals with chronic asthmatic bronchitis are likely to die from this disease or associated complications. But, almost 60% of emphysema patients die within 10 years of diagnosis (Gordon, 1993). In addition to health, one's functional ability decreases due to shortness of breath, wheezing, and chest discomfort. COPD decreases one's ability to use oxygen during exertion. The National Heart, Lung, and Blood Institute (1986) describes the gas exchange problems impacting functional capacity as follows:

- Blood flow and airflow to the alveolar walls where gas exchange takes place are uneven or mismatched. Some alveoli get plenty of blood but little air, while others get a good supply of fresh air but not enough blood. Under these conditions, fresh air cannot reach areas where there is good blood flow and oxygen cannot enter the bloodstream in normal quantities.
- The work of pushing air through narrowed obstructed airways becomes more and more difficult. This tires the respiratory mus-cles and they may not be able to maintain an adequate airflow to the alveoli. The critical step for removal of carbon dioxide from the blood is adequate alveolar airflow. If airflow to the alveoli is insuf-ficient, carbon dioxide builds up in the blood; blood oxygen also diminishes. An inadequate supply of fresh air to the alveoli is called *hypoventilation*. Breathing oxygen can often correct the

blood oxygen levels but this does nothing to help in the removal of carbon dioxide. When carbon dioxide accumulation becomes a severe problem, mechanical breathing machines called respirators or ventilators must be used.   (p. 3)

The gas exchange problem places a large burden on the heart, particularly the right side which functions to pump blood into the lungs. Hanawalt (1992) describes the progressive impact of COPD on the heart:

> . . . the amount of oxygen distributed is diminished and causes impor-
> tant lung blood vessels to constrict. Many other small vessels in the
> lung are also damaged. High pressures must be produced on the right
> side of the heart to force blood through the narrowed blood vessels.
> The right chambers of the heart enlarge and thicken to perform this
> function. Normal rhythms of the heart may be disturbed. This condition
> of an enlarged heart because of lung problems is called corpulmonale.
> (p. 146)

COPD also produces a condition called secondary polycythemia. Secondary polycythemia is an increased production of oxygen-carrying red blood cells. An overpopulation of red blood cells may thicken the blood and cause the small blood vessels to clog. Cyanosis, a blue tinge to the skin, nails, and nailbeds, is a common condition associated with secondary polycythemia.

A number of diagnostic tests are used for detecting COPD. These tests measure lung function by examining lung volumes, the ability to move air into and out of the lung, rate of gas diffusion between the lung and blood, and blood levels of oxygen and carbon dioxide. Unfortunately, these tests do not detect COPD until after irreversible lung damage has occurred. Survival rates for COPD are closely tied to the initial level of lung function impairment and rate of functional decline. The U.S. Department of Health and Human Services (1986) reports a force expiatory volume that is less than one-third of normal functional capacity for a given age has a 67% survival rate of five years or more for people less than age 65. Survival rates for those aged 65 or older are not optimistic. Hanawalt (1992) summarizes the impact of COPD as follows:

> Over 10 million Americans have COPD. Since 1968, it has been the
> fastest rising major cause of death in the United States. Although
> COPD is more common in men than women, this difference is rapidly
> closing. One may surmise that the increased trend in smoking by
> women may be contributing to the increased rate of COPD in women
> (National Heart, Lung, and Blood Institute, 1986). The economic costs
> of the disabling COPDs is staggering. Unfortunately, there is no known
> cure. This prevention is imperative. Smoking cessation, air pollution
> control, postural bronchial drainage, medications, home oxygen thera
> py, and controlled coughing techniques have all been used as

treatment of choice. Exercise training programs have also drawn significant attention.

Role of Exercise. Health professionals once held the beliefs that exercise programs were detrimental to COPD patients since they aggravated negative conditions. Clinical research, however, has substantiated that exercise improves work capacity, decreases the number and frequency of hospitalizations, and improves the patient's sense of well-being (Gordon, 1993).

Management of COPD. Management of COPD includes three components: (1) optimal medical care that uses therapy and supportive measures for airway obstruction; (2) adaptation to disability on a physical, social, and cognitive level by the individual and the family; and (3) an exercise rehabilitation program (Jones et. al., 1987). The latter component, exercise rehabilitation, has received viable attention only in recent years. Regular exercise cannot reverse the impact of COPD on airflow obstruction, lung tissue damage, or air sac damage. But, exercise can help the COPD patient be less bothered by breathlessness during exertion due to beneficial effects on the cardiovascular and musculoskeletal systems. The rationale is that exercise will enable the COPD patient to perform exertion activities that may have been avoided or stopped due to breathlessness and early muscle fatigue (Gordon, 1993). Many of these activities may have been common activity daily living skills.

Exercise programs for COPD patients require a team approach involving the patient's physician, physiotherapist, occupational therapist, social worker, and an exercise instructor. A pre-screening fitness profile sets parameters for a prescriptive exercise program. This pre-screening includes a physical examination, exercise stress test, and fitness tests for range of motion, strength, flexibility, motor agility, balance, and breathing patterns. Pulmonary diagnostic tests are also used. Table 11-6 provides a grading disability profile that is drawn from these tests to prescribe an optimal exercise program.

COPD patients are categorized by four grade levels for exercise recommendations.

> *Grade 1.* Grade 1 patients not limited by impaired pulmonary function can essentially follow the same programming as cardiac patients. Intensity is determined by the heart rate response observed during the exercise test. The exercise session should be 30–60 minutes and should be performed daily, with a minimal frequency of every other day.

> *Grade 2.* Grade 2 patients with moderate impairment will be limited by a reduced ventilatory capacity. An appropriate intensity will not exceed 60 to 80 percent of their ventilature capacity and a frequency of less than 30 breaths per minute. Exercise may be performed more than once a day every day for short periods. Exercise should be terminated before shortness of breath restricts further activity.

Table 11-6. Guide to grading disability (based on 40-year-old man).

Grade	Cause of Dyspnea	FEV (% Pred)	Nax Vo_2 (ml-min^{-1} kg$^{-1)}$	Exercise Max V_E (L • min^{-1})	Blood Gases
1	Fast walking and climbing	>60	>25	Not limiting	Normal $PaCO_2$ SaO_2
2	Walking at normal pace	<60	<25	>50	Normal $PaCO_2$ SaO_2 above 90% at rest and with exercise
3	Slow walking	>40	<15	<50	Normal $PaCO_2$ SaO_2 below 90% at rest and with exercise
4	Walking limited	<40	< 7	<30	Elevated $PaCO_2$ SaO_2 below 90% at rest and with exercise

From N. L. Jones et al., "Chronic Obstructive Respiratory Disorders" in J. S. Skinner, editor, *Exercise Testing and Exercise Prescription for Special Cases.* Copyright c 1987 Lea & Febiger. Reprinted by permission of Williams and Wilkins, a Waverly Company.

Grade 3. Grade 3 patients are often difficult to prescribe exercise to because the intensity may be extremely low; so low that it is unlikely to produce a training effect. Consideration should be given to oxygen supplementation, interval training, and specific muscle group training (i.e., one leg at a time). Breathing exercises are recommended along with the guidelines stated for Grade 2 patients.

Grade 4. The emphasis for the patients is on adaptation to their disability. Activity is guided toward efficiency and energy conservation in daily tasks. Exercise at this level may be extremely taxing. Dyspnea, fatigue, anxiety and headaches may occur. Rating of perceived exertion may be a better indicator of intensity than heart rate. (Jones et al., 1988)

Three major types of exercise programs are conducted based on the four COPD levels: (1) in-hospital programs for Grade 3 and 4; (2) day-time outpatient clinics Grades 1 and 2; and (3) evening programs for patients who are employed and cannot afford time away from work. Aerobic training programs are emphasized for Grades 1 and 2. Optimal aerobic modalities include swimming, cycling, and walking. The more disabled COPD patients, upper Grade 2 and Grade 3, are prescribed interval training exercise programs. Grade 4 patients are bed-bound and committed to oxygen therapy and passive exercise programs to maintain range of motion. Regardless of grade level classification, extended warm-up and cooldowns are required for COPD patients. For a thorough review of exercise programs for COPD, consult Gordon (1993). Precaution is also required for medication and exercise interaction. Bronchadilator aerosols, oral aninophylline products, oral steroids, and inhaled steroid preparations are common medications used with COPD patients. Medication for fluid retention and cardiac dysfunction may also be prescribed. Close cooperation between the COPD patient's physician and exercise leader is imperative.

OSTEOPOROSIS

Labeled a "silent disease" because it produces no symptoms until a fracture occurs, osteoporosis is virtually invisible to the general public. Osteoporosis is not a disease per se; it is the end result of severe and prolonged bone demineralization that occurs naturally with aging. Demineralization refers to bone loss or gradual thinning and increased bone porosity. The progression of bone demineralization is influenced by multiple factors that will be addressed in this section.

Fractures of the spinal vertebrae, wrist, and hip are quite common. Every year 200,000 women over the age of 45 fracture one or more bones. Complications from these fractures can lead to death. For example, 15% of women who fracture their hip die shortly after their injury, and another 30% die within one year (Dibble et al., 1985). The monetary and emotional costs are also staggering. In 1990, the annual national expense for osteoporosis was projected to exceed $3 billion. The pain, deformity, and disability profoundly affect emotional and spiritual health.

How Age Affects the Bones

Normal reduction in bone mass is called osteopenia. A person is said to have osteoporosis if the loss of bone is excessive or prolonged to the point of microscopic fractures. The two identified types of osteoporosis are primary and secondary. Primary, sometimes called postmenopausal osteoporosis, is attributed to multiple causes (e.g., heredity, hormones). Secondary osteoporosis is attributed to a single cause, usually some drug, or disease, or alcoholism.

The skeleton changes as we age. New bone tissue is produced until early adulthood then bone begins to break down. Estrogen and progesterone stimulate bone growth for females, and androgens stimulate it for males. The process of bone remodeling and breakdown is described by Notelovitz and Ware (1984):

> Throughout childhood, new bone formation occurs on the [outer] periosteal envelope, and a lesser amount of breakdown occurs on the [inner] endosteal envelope. During adolescence, bone formation occurs on both surfaces, leading to large overall gains in bone mass.

During early adulthood, bone breakdown begins again on the endoste-al [inner] envelope, heralding the beginning of the age-related decline in bone mass. (p. 25)

All bones undergo age-related changes but are not affected in exactly the same way. The structural makeup of the two basic kinds of bone tissue determines age-related changes. Cortical bone is solid and dense and trabecular bone is more porous. Every bone is composed of both cortical and trabecular tissue. Trabecular is inside bone tissue surrounded by cortical tissue. The relative proportions of cortical and trabecular tissue differ for each bone. The vertebrae and spine are mostly trabecular bone and the long bones of the arms and leg are principally cortical tissue. Trabecular bone is very strong, but its latticework structure creates an enormous amount of exposed area that leads to excessive bone loss.

How Women and Men Differ in Bone Loss

Men and women both experience bone loss as they age. However, the rate of bone demineralization is more accelerated for women than men. Bone demineralization commences in the early 20s for both sexes with the loss of trabecular bone in the spine. But by the time a woman reaches age 80, she will have experienced a 47% loss of trabecular bone whereas men only lose 14%. Cortical bone, on the other hand, reaches its peak around age 30 to 35. Both men and women experience a slight cortical bone loss until age 50, primarily from both the arm and leg bones (Notelovitz & Ware, 1984). But after age 50 a woman will begin to lose cortical bone at twice the rate of a man (Figure 11-1).

Following menopause, the rate of bone loss in the first five to six years greatly accelerates. This loss of bone is almost six times as rapid as a man's demineralization rate. Notelovitz and Ware (1985) add ". . . if a woman does nothing to prevent it, it is estimated that by age 55 the bone loss may be equivalent to that gained during her adolescent years" (p. 27). By the age of 65, the rate of bone loss will slow down so that it is similar to the demineralization rate of men. But it is important to remember that women had less bone density than men to begin with and that they have already lost more mass than men at this point.

How Hormones Affect Bone

Figure 11-2 provides an overview of the hormones that affect bone growth and demineralization. Essentially, the key is calcium as it regulates many vital body functions. Calcium is not only vital to bone physiology, it is also essential for muscle contraction, blood clotting, and bond functioning. To monitor these functions, the body uses hormones as chemical messengers to increase calcium levels in the blood. The body may acquire this calcium by breaking bones down. Thus hormones may serve a good purpose (preventing bone breakdown) or a bad purpose (breaking bone down).

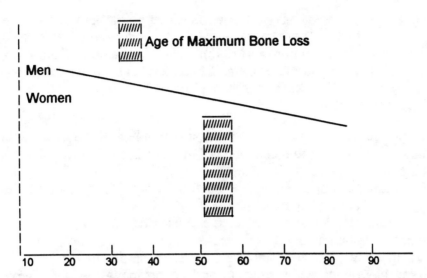

Figure 11-1. Bone loss with age: A comparison of men and women. Source: M. Notchvitz and M. Ware, *Stand Tall!* NY: Bantam Books, 1985, p. 49.

Vitamin D is considered to be a hormone because it increases the absorption of calcium from food in the intestines and reabsorbs calcium through the kidneys. But if the need for calcium is very great, or if Vitamin D is present at very high levels, it can withdraw calcium from bones as activated Vitamin D.

The functions of calcitonin and estrogen are to prevent the dissolving effects of Vitamin D. Estrogen normally stimulates the release of calcitonin which is a bone-protecting hormone. The ability of estrogen to stimulate the release of calcitonin stops with the loss of estrogen during the early menopause years. Moreover, men have more calcitonin than women, thus partially explaining the accelerated bone demineralization difference between men and women.

The parathyroid hormone also plays a key role. This hormone signals the kidneys to put calcium that would otherwise be excreted in urine back into the bloodstream. It also stimulates the breakdown of bone to produce calcium and converts Vitamin D into an active form. A normal function of estrogen is to block these bone dissolving effects of the parathyroid hormone. The loss of estrogen levels after menopause thus makes the body's bones more vulnerable to the parathyroid hormone.

Bone Density Tests

Screening tests for bone density include the following: (1) Dual-Energy X-ray Absorptiometry (DEXA); (2) Singe-Photon Absorptiometry (SPA); and (3) Radiographic Densitometry (RD). If bone screening tests indicate a low bone mass, the patient will be advised to undergo additional diagnostic tests that can pinpoint specific problem areas. Diagnostic tests include the DEXA of specific sites (e.g., lumbar and hip) and Quantitative Computerized Tomography (QCT). Blood and urine tests have also been used to detect bone demineralization. Urine tests include calcium to creatine ratio and urinary hydroxpolene tests. The alkaline phosphostic activity test has been used as a blood test. Notelovitz and Tonnessen (1993) provide a critique of bone density test. Experts agree that bone-mass measurement is a significant factor for preventing and treating osteoporosis. The National Osteoporosis Foundation recommends bone density testing for four situations:

1. following a natural menopause, surgical removal of the ovaries, or prolonged amenorrhea (cessation of menstruation) — regardless of the cause
2. if you have spinal abnormalities such as collapsed vertebrae, edging, or "ballooning" of spinal plates
3. if you take steroids to control such diseases as rheumatoid arthritis, hepatitis, inflammatory bowel disease, asthma, or chronic obstructive pulmonary disease (steroids can cause rapid bone loss)
4. if you have hyperparathyroidism and do not have the parathyroid gland surgically removed, an overactive parathyroid gland can lead to decreased bone mass.

Other women who should consider bone-density testing include women with osteopenia or osteoporosis who are taking medication to prevent further bone loss. Bone-density tests can help monitor the efficacy of your treatment.

For more information and referrals to physicians and organizations that perform bone-density testing, contact the National Osteoporosis Foundation, Suite 500, 1150 17th Street, NW, Washington, DC 20036.

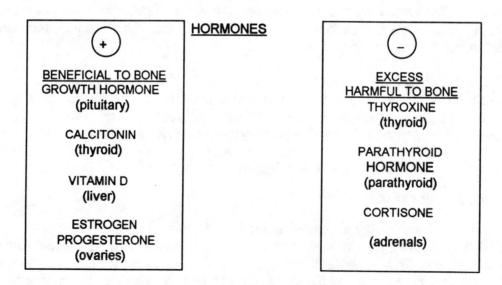

Figure 11-2. Hormones involved in calcium and bone metabolism. Source: M. Notchvitz and M. Ware. *Stand Tall!* NY: Bantam Books, 1985, p. 49.

Risk Factors: Treatment of Choice

Osteoporosis has often been described as a pediatric disorder that presents itself to the geriatrician. Despite the prevalence of osteoporosis, we still have sparse information on the effects of lifestyle risk factors during the formative years on bone mass in adult life. It is generally assumed that the genetic predisposition to osteoporosis is heavily influenced by a variety of uncontrollable and controllable risk factors.

Risk factors associated with osteoporosis that cannot be controlled include age at menopause, genetic factors, ethnic differences, bone structure, and diseases (e.g., endocrine disorders). Critical risk factors that affect osteoporosis that can be controlled include exercise, diets that include adequate amounts of calcium and less phosphorous food, smoking cessation, abstention or moderate alcohol consumption, flouridated water, calcium, vitamin supplements, a monitoring of medications that cause severe bone loss (e.g., corticosteroids, anticonvulsent drugs, diuretics), and restricted salt diets. The reader is encouraged to consult Notelovitz and Ware (1985) for an excellent discussion of these risk factors.

Identifying those at risk for osteoporosis, however, is still a major problem. Risk factor assessment and bone mass measurement used in combination are still the closest approximation for diagnosing osteoporosis. The effects of each risk factor in an individual patient cannot be quantified. How much bone density one has at maturity, one's bone demineralization rate, and how long one lives are all vital factors. In other words, if a person lives long enough, osteoporosis will be a fact of life because bone loss is an inevitable consequence of aging. But the amount of bone at maturity and the bone demineralization rate can be affected by controlling certain risk factors. Table 11-7 provides an overview of pertinent risk factors.

Despite the difficulty in quantifying the contribution of lifestyle modifications for preventing and reducing the risk of osteoporosis, such modifications as increased physical activity and decreased alcohol and cigarette consumption are likely to have a beneficial impact on general health and should be strongly advocated. Moreover, although osteoporosis is considered a female disease, it may also occur among men. Approximately 20% of men age 80 and older are suspected to be osteoporotic. The risk factors for men are similar to those of women. However, the treatment of men with osteoporosis is more difficult as there are no prevention programs or treatment data pertaining to men. We would still assume that the focal point for treatment, similar to women, would be on disease management. Osteoporosis is not a disease that can be treated and cured. Instead, the strategy is to prevent further bone loss and thus reduce the chances of more fractures. Proper nutrition and exercise again play a critical role. However, drug therapy also becomes the central ingredient. Estrogen therapy, anabolic steroids, calcitonin, fluoride, and Vitamin D are utilized.

Table 11-7. Risk and protective factors associated with osteoporotic fracture.

Established Risk Factors	Proposed Risk Factors	Established Protective Factors
Advanced age	Family history of osteoporosis	Long-term use of estrogens
Female sex	Prior history of Colles' fracture	
White race	Early natural menopause	Black, Latino
Thin	Pregnancies and breast feeding	Obesity
Low bone mass	Low calcium intake	
Previous hip fracture	Caffeine intake	
Bilateral oophorectomy	Moderate use of alcohol	
>2 alcoholic drinks per day	High protein diet	
Chronic corticosteroid use	Thyroid supplements (replacement doses)	
Dementia	Use of antacids	
Disabling rheumatoid arthritis	Use of sedatives with shot half-lives	
Long-acting psychotropic drugs	Type II diabetes	
	Rheumatoid arthritis (with no disability)	
Visual impairment	Sedentary lifestyle	
Parkinson's disease	Scoliosis	
Cigarette smoking		

Reproduced with permission from R. Lindsay, "Osteoporosis: An Updated Approach to Prevention and Management" in *Geriatrics*, Vol. 44, Number 1, 1989. Copyright by Avanstar Communications, Inc.

Hormone Therapy

Estrogen replacement therapy remains the most effective way to off-set bone demineralization. "Arresting or slowing the process of postmenopausal osteoporosis at any stage has benefit, at least up to age seventy-five" (Healy, 1995, p. 434). There is also growing empirical evidence that estrogen may increase bone density and, thus, to some extent, reverse the ravaging impact of osteoporosis. Estrogen is most effective when combined with recommended daily calcium intakes. Postmenopausal women with osteoporosis should take minimally 1,000 mg calcium daily and, ideally, 1,500 mg. Calcium intakes for all ages should not exceed 2,500 mg. Benefits of estrogen therapy for women eighty and older are not known. It is important to remember that estrogen has a beneficial impact on bone only when it is being taken. Long-term use of estrogen, unfortunately, has been associated with increased risk for breast cancer after 10 years of use. Adding complexity to the issue is that hormone replacement therapy may also be beneficial for preventing heart disease. The pros and cons of estrogen therapy were summarized by Cole, Park, and Smilges (1995).

For a detailed discussion of the pros and cons of estrogen therapy, the reader is encouraged to consult Lita Nachtisall's *Estrogen: The Facts Can Change Your Life*. The prevailing medical review remains that most women should stay on estrogen for a long period of time since its "preventive" wonders occur only if taken for many years. For example, to prevent osteoporosis a woman must use estrogen continually for at least seven years (Cole et. al., 1995). But, presently, 95% of women are on HRT for three years or less--not long enough to attain a beneficial impact on bones. Research suggests similar long-term use for preventing heart disease. Estrogen functions to keep LDL levels low and HDL levels high. Without HRT, a woman's risk of heart disease 15 years after menopause is the same as the risk for men. The long-term benefits and risks of HRT, however, are woefully inadequate. Recent research initiatives such as the Estrogen/Progesterone Intervention Trial and the women's Health Initiative Study will, hopefully, provide much needed answers to these questions.

Exercise and Osteoporosis

Evans and Rosenberg (1991) provide convincing empirical evidence that exercise programs are essential for osteoporatic patients and for preventing osteoporosis. Non-gravity support exercises such as walking and weight training are recommended. The principal objective is to improve muscle strength. Additional benefits of exercise include postural stability, reduced risk of bone and joint injury, mobility, increased self-confidence and reduced depression. An excellent resource for exercise programs and osteoporosis is *A Fitness Leader's Guide to Osteoporosis* (1986). Precautionary concerns of exercise and medication similarly apply to osteoporosis.

ARTHRITIS: THE NATION'S PRIMARY CRIPPLER

Holly Wallace was on a college trip to London in 1974 when she noticed the first troubling changes in her body. "My feet just hurt all the time," recalls the once athletic tomboy who was then 20 years old. Back home a few weeks later, she told a doctor, "I know it's just a coincidence, but my fingers are swelling too." Within days, the pain had spread throughout her body. Even the weight of a nightgown was unbearable to her aching joints. Her doctor diagnosed arthritis, but Holly didn't believe him. "I lay in a dark room, naked, crying, knowing that they were lying to me," she says. "I thought everybody knows arthritis--it's when you can't pick up a pencil from a table. It doesn't make you feel like this." (Beck, 1989, p. 64)

Holly Wallace was later diagnosed as suffering from rheumatoid arthritis. A healthy young woman, she turned into an 85-year-old invalid in a few short weeks. Holly Wallace consulted numerous physicians and was placed on a battery of prescription drugs, such as steroids, penicillamine, and Advil. Despite this medication, she succumbed to the persistent inflammation that leads to scar tissue. This scar tissue formed between the pads of her bones until the joints in her wrist and right foot gradually fused together.

Holly Wallace's case is certainly startling and alarming. And yet we too often forget that arthritis is the nation's primary crippling disease, particularly for older adults. It is the most common chronic disease of the aged and afflicts more than 37 million Americans. Moreover, many older adults suffering from arthritis may have osteoporosis. Despite the dramatic impact of arthritis on the lives of its victims and on society in general, it remains a mysterious disease.

The Many Faces of Arthritis

Scientists believe that there are more than 100 forms of arthritis. However, osteoarthritis (OA) and rheumatoid arthritis (RA) remain the most common forms. OA has usually been considered a wear and tear disease, a natural part of the aging process. However, this conventional wisdom of wear and tear is changing. Some scientists now theorize that enzymes are released when joints are used. These enzymes digest cartilage while the cells, at the same time, are busy repairing loss. OA may develop when the enzymes break cartilage down ahead of the cells' efforts to repair cartilage. This discrepancy between breakdown and repair may be caused by an excessive enzyme release, a slowing of the cell repair process, or both (Beck, 1989).

Scientists remain puzzled as to why the breakdown and repair cycle is imbalanced, but the culprit may be a body misalignment that places excess stress on the joints. Accidents, injury, or childhood defects are also capable of producing body misalignment problems leading to serious problems in the later years. An important point, however, is that simple use on wear of the joint is not a factor in causing arthritis. Genetics may play a key role. For example, OA in the hands is thought to have a particularly strong genetic relationship. Hormone imbalance may be the reason why women are more commonly afflicted by OA than men; OA usually appears after menopause, thus there may be a link to estrogen. Obesity is also a factor, as it places excessive loads on weight-bearing joints (Ekblom & Nordemar, 1987). RA is an inflammation of the synovial tissue which causes destruction of the articular cartilage and subchondral bone. This inflammatory process leads to the gradual destruction of the joint surface.

Eventually, the joint capsule and ligaments are weakened. Tendons and tendon sheaths can also become inflamed. Pathological changes may actually occur in the skeletal muscles due to this generalized inflammation.

Scientists have demonstrated a genetic tendency for RA. But the primary suspect is thought to be tied to the immune system. The body's natural defenses from the immune system may actually turn on bone and cartilage as if they were foreign invaders. Scientists remain puzzled as to what triggers this effect in the immune system, but the recent discovery of Lyme's disease may turn up some of the answers as the symptoms of Lyme disease are very similar to RA. Because Lyme disease is caused by bacteria spread by ticks, the thought is that infectious agents may trigger the immune system to turn on cartilage and bone. Viruses may actually produce proteins that are near mirror copies of joint tissue. This similarity may trick the immune defenses into attacking healthy joint tissue (Beck, 1989).

Despite the attention paid to the immune system, it is important to remember that RA is a systemic disease, meaning it is body-wide. The cardiovascular, pulmonary, gastrointestinal, and nervous system may all be implicated. In fact, researchers at the University of California, San Francisco, are convinced that the nervous system plays a viable role. The basis for the nervous system contention is that stroke victims who develop arthritis at a later date are free from symptoms on the side of the body that has been impaired by the stroke.

Diagnosing Rheumatoid Arthritis

Diagnosing RA has been difficult. Recently, the American Rheumatoid Association classified RA according to seven criteria (Table 11-8). The first five criteria identified in Table 11-8 must be continuous for a minimum of six weeks. Definitive diagnosis for RA requires the presence of at least five symptoms, probable RA requires three symptoms, and possible RA two symptoms. Total duration of the symptoms must be present for at least three weeks (Ekblom & Nordemar, 1987).

The pain, swelling, and stiffness from RA is usually experienced as a gradual onset. Although the onset of RA may occur at any age, the most common age is between 25 and 60 years of age. Females suffer from RA three times more than men. The impact of RA on the individual's functional capacity is used to determine the severity of RA. The American Rheumatism Association (ARA) uses four classifications:

Class 1: Complete ability to carry on all usual duties without handicaps.

Class 2: Adequate ability for normal activities despite handicap, discomfort, or limited motion at one or more joints.

Class 3: Ability limited to little or none of the duties of usual occupation or to self-care.

Table 11-8. Diagnostic criteria of rheumatoid arthritis (RA) (American Rheumatism Association).

1. Morning stiffness.

2. Pain on motion or tenderness* in at least one joint.

3. Swelling* (soft tissue thickening or fluid, not bony overgrowth alone) in at least one joint.

4. Swelling* of at least one other joint (any interval free of joint symptoms between the two joint involvements may not be more than 3 months).

5. Symmetric joint swelling,* with simultaneous involvement of the same joint bilaterally (bilateral involvement of midphalangeal, metacarpophalangeal, or metatarsophalangeal joints is acceptable without absolute symmetry). Terminal phalangeal joint involvement does not satisfy this criterion.

6. Subcutaneous nodules* over bony prominences, on extensor surfaces, or in juxta-articular regions.

7. Radiographic changes typical of RA (which must include at least bony decalcification localized to or around the involved joints and not just degenerative changes). Degenerative changes do not exclude patients from any group classified as RA.

8. Positive agglutination test (demonstration of the "rheumatoid factor" by any method that in the laboratories has been positive in not more than 4% of normal control subjects) or positive streptococcal agglutination test.

9. Poor mucin precipitate from synovial fluid (with shreds and cloudy solution).

10. Characteristic histologic changes in synovial membrane with three or more of the following: marked villous hypothrophy; proliferation of superficial cells, often with palisading; marked infiltration of chronic inflammatory cells (predominantly lymphocytes or plasma cells) with a tendency to form "lymphoid nodules"; deposition of compact fibrin, either on surface or interstitially; or foci of cell necrosis.

11. Characteristic histologic changes in nodules showing granulomatosis foci with central zones of cell necrosis, surrounded by proliferated fixed cells; peripheral fibrosis; and chronic inflammatory cell infiltration, predominantly perivascular.

*Observed by a physician.

From B. Ekblom and R. Nordemar, "Rheumatoid Arthritis" in J. S. Skinner, editor, *Exercise Testing and Exercise Prescription for Special Cases.* Copyright 1987 Lea & Febiger. Reprinted by permission of Williams and Wilkins, a Waverly Company.

> Class 4: Incapacitated, largely or wholly bedridden or confined to a
> wheelchair; little or no self-care. (Ekblom & Nordemar, 1987,
> p. 103)

This classification by the ARA may be too crude to detect minor improvements or deterioration. For that reason, Schoening and Iverson (1968) advocate a functional capacity scoring system of 50 to 100 for separate activity daily living skills (ADL). The ability of the individual to perform each ADL is worth one point. The optimal functional capacity is the highest score total for the ADL. This scoring system, however, has proven to be cumbersome and time consuming.

Diagnosing Osteoarthritis

Pathological and radiological criteria for diagnosing OA have recently been clarified and standardized by the ARA. Pathological criteria include painful range of motion, morning stiffness not exceeding 30 minutes, bony enlargements, and cripitance. Criteria for radiological diagnosis include osteophytes, subchondral cysts or sclerosis, joint-space narrowing, and attrition and misalignment of normal bone formation (Smith, Smith, & Gilligan, 1990, p. 517).

OA most often occurs in the weight-bearing joints, such as the knee, hip, and spine. Non-weight-bearing joints such as the distal intraphalangeal and first carpal-metacarpal joints are also commonly affected. Different from RA, the OA symptoms are characterized as nonsystemic. OA affliction is common for both men and women, primarily affecting people over age 40. However, more males have OA in the pre-45 age group and more females are affected in the past-55 age group (Piscopo, 1985). An excellent resource for OA intervention is Greslamer and Loeble (1996).

Dubious Treatments

The pain associated with RA and OA can have a devastating impact on the personality of its victims. Depression, feelings of helplessness, guilt, and anxiety are common. The emotional cost, decreased functional capacity, and general inactivity lead to the isolation of the individual from his or her environment and from society. Beck (1989) describes the impact for OA victims:

> for many of the 16 million osteoarthritis sufferers, walking across a
> room, turning a doorknob or making a cup of coffee can require a
> supreme effort of will. The pain is not necessarily visible, so employers
> and loved ones often don't sympathize. Divorce is three times more
> common in couples where one spouse has the disease. (1989, p. 65)

The impact on the life of the RA victim may be even more devastating. Ten percent of RA individuals are dependent on another person for daily activities (Ekblom & Nordemar, 1987). Muscular weakness and low endurance are not only common but cyclical because inactivity further aggravates the condition. This inactivity leads to bone decalcification, which in turn contributes to osteoporosis concerns. Body weight may also fall as appetite is usually reduced during the active inflammation periods of RA.

RA and OA victims have consulted a gamut of rheumatologists, neurologists, orthopedists, and chiropractors. They have also chosen to pursue such dubious cures as copper bracelets, injections of turtle blood (because turtles live long lives without getting arthritis), wonder salad dressings (garlic oil and cider), and the spraying of the household lubricant WD-40 on affected joints.

Equipment that vibrates the body limbs has also been a hot item. Vibrating equipment may provide interesting sensations but is likely to do more harm than good as it aggravates inflamed joints. Special diets have also joined the inventory of special quackery tricks. Cod liver oil, alfalfa, pokeberries, and blackstrap molasses are but a few of the items sold for arthritic diets. Even snake venom has been tried as a rheumatoid arthritis cure.

Management of Arthritis

The dubious cures for arthritis amount to an expenditure in excess of $1 billion every year. This expenditure represents $25 for every $1 spent on legitimate arthritis research. Arthritis quackery is likely to persist because of a quirk of the disease called spontaneous remission. The pain and swelling of arthritis can literally disappear for days, weeks, or months leading the victim to believe that a quackery device actually works. In time, however, remission occurs and the victim realizes the dubiousness of the device. The gloomy point is that arthritis cannot be cured--it can only be managed. Yet there is good news. The modes for arthritis treatment have greatly advanced in recent years. This management treatment is broad and usually includes medication, surgery, heat, rest, support groups, and exercise. (The role of exercise was discussed in Chapter 4.)

The management concepts for arthritis therapy contain three goals: (1) relief of pain, (2) maintenance and improvement of joint range of motion, and (3) delaying further damage of joints. Pharmacologic agents are directed at the first and third goals. When pain is present, anti-inflammatory agents containing salicylic acid compounds are initially used. Later drug therapy may include such drugs as naproxine, ibuprofen, and motrin (non-steroidal anti-inflammatory drugs). In severe cases, cortisone (steroids) is used. These drugs have an effect on symptoms but do not alter the disease course.

Some anti-rheumatic drugs (e.g., penicillamine, levamisol) are slow-acting drugs that may introduce remission of RA for brief or prolonged periods. Unfortunately, all anti-rheumatic drugs have multiple side-effects. For example, ibuprofen has been linked to ulcers, and corticosteroids, the most effective anti-inflammatory drugs used, lead to bone demineralization, gastric disturbance, thin skin, and elevated blood pressure (Ekblom & Nordemar, 1987).

Surgery may be used in the early phase of RA. The purpose of surgery is to reduce the symptoms and arrest the disease process. Application of heat (e.g., hot packs, hot baths, and heat lamps) has been used to soothe the muscles and relax and lessen muscle spasm. Whirlpool baths are effective for loosening stiff joints and decreasing pain. Rest therapy may be advisable during active arthritic flare-ups. The effectiveness of rest therapy, however, is not empirically documented. Support groups are also a key component in arthritis management programs.

Despite the army of available symptom-relief methods for RA and OA, all the therapies confront the same problem: most forms of arthritis are so variable that health experts cannot delineate whether the disease's ups and downs occur naturally or as a result of treatment. Arthritis victims are left at the mercy of quack remedies, overuse of drugs that lead to serious side-effects, or general indifference by health care providers. One of the principal goals of RA and OA therapy should be the encouragement to stay active and undefeated. Navigating that line to maintain activity and independence may not be easy but it remains the central strategy for offsetting the psychosocial damage that often accompanies arthritis.

Both RA and OA are associated with joint pain, muscle weakness, loss of motion, and reduced working capacity. Exercise programs are, therefore, an important intervention program. Aerobic range of motion exercises and nonstress muscle strengthening exercises are of primary importance. Hanawalt (1992) writes:

> Prescribing aerobic and strengthening exercises will ultimately depend on each individual's functional ability. Smooth, repetitive motions such as walking, ice skating, cross-country skiing, and bicycling are recommended. Most activities, as long as they are comfortable, are encouraged. However, some weight-bearing activities should be avoided because they may aggravate arthritic joints. For example, activities that involve jumping up and down may do more harm than good; thus basketball, volleyball, and high-impact aerobic dance should be avoided . . . (p. 135)

Class 1 RA patients may perform any type of exercise. Patients classified under a 2 or 3 level may perform most types of exercises during nonflare-up phases of the arthritic joint. Swimming, and bicycling are common exercises. During a flare-up phase, no-load or very low-load exercises are recommended.

Patients classified under level 4 are advised not to perform complicated exercise movements. Passive range of motion exercises are advised. The reader is encouraged to consult Gordon (1993) and Ekblom and Nordemor (1987) for a detailed description of exercise programs for arthritis.

A precautionary note is added as to exercise and medication for arthritic patients. Most arthritis drugs are employed to relieve pain and stiffness. This relief enables the patient to exercise but also reduces pain signals associated with ongoing tissue damage.

Exercise programs should be carefully prescribed due to the loss of pain sensation with exercise. Moreover, the drugs gold, penicillamine, and cryostatics have potential side-effects that may interact with exercise. The patient's physician should be consulted.

AIDS: PEOPLE AGE 50 AND OLDER

We live in an aging society--approximately 25% of the American population is age 50 and older. As our demographic profile continues to tilt toward aging, we have learned a great deal about the characteristics and problems of older adults. But escaping our attention is how AIDS is infecting millions of Americans age 50 and older. Our purpose in this section is to explore this oversight.

Hidden for Years

Nadine Brozan writes, "Hidden for years by secrecy, shame, and in some cases the assumption that their symptoms were simply those of aging, a growing number of older people are emerging as victims of AIDS" (1990, p. A1). In fact, AIDS now occurs more frequently among adults over age 50 than among children younger than age 13 (Table 11-9). Adults age 50 and older account for 10% of the more than 150,000 AIDS cases.

Table 11-9. Age distribution of AIDS cases reported in the United States pre-1981 to September, 1988.

Age	Number	Percent
Under 5	977	1
5-12	194	*
13-19	295	*
20-29	15,163	21
30-39	33,951	46
40-49	15,287	21
Over 49	7,527	10
Total Cases	73,394[a]	100

* = less than 1%

[a]Includes 9,720 patients who meet only the 1987 revised surveillance definition for AIDS; thus not directly comparable with data for earlier years.

Note: Of the 73,394 cases, 41,393 (56%) are known to have died.

Source: Data from the Centers for Disease Control (CDC) Weekly Surveillance Report - cumulative totals.

Table 11-10 presents the percentage of AIDS distribution according to the modes of transmission. Federal statistics indicate that the majority of adults over age 50 who have AIDS are homosexual or bisexual men who contracted the disease through sexual intercourse. But older women may be even more vulnerable to AIDS through transmissions passed on by spouses through sexual intercourse. Vaginal changes in postmenopause may develop fissures in the vaginal wall. These fissures may become sites for the HIV infection. Many older adults are unaware of this vulnerability. Arlene Kochran, program director of Senior Action in a Gay Environment, notes, "We talk about sex in the schools but not among our seniors, and that is based on erroneous assumptions" (Brozan, 1990, p. A10).

The reader should pay particular attention to the similarity between adults age 50 to 64 (column 1) and the total for all age groups (column 4). Homosexual and bisexual males represent the primary mode of AIDS transmission (70%) for both groups. But intravenous (IV) drug abusers (second ranking factor at 12% for adults age 50 and older) is considerably less important than for younger-aged groups (26%). The largest source of AIDS transmission for older adults was blood transfusions (55%) before the introduction of routine blood screening in 1985.

AIDS Progression in Later Years

The past and projected trends of HIV infection and AIDS are largely influenced by the underlying dynamic process of AIDS as a protracted disease. Riley (1989) writes,

> AIDS is not an isolated event that occurs at a single moment of time in a body that is changeless. AIDS is, rather, a protracted disease, which coincides with a major segment of the individual's life course. While the HIV virus is developing, the infected individuals--until they die--are growing older. Thus those now infected who are in their forties may have passed age 50 before being diagnosed with AIDS, and those now infected who are in their sixties may have passed age 70. Thus two sets of dynamic processes, AIDS and aging, running concurrently over a person's lifetime, are continually interacting with one another. In addition, they share an important common feature: both sets of processes are marked by heterogeneity, as individuals differ widely both in expression of the disease and in the ways they grow old. (p. 13)

Scientists know a great deal about the processes of aging. Every day more is learned about the links between aging processes and the many forms of chronic diseases and disability. Knowledge is also accumulating as to the progression of HIV infection from initial exposure up until death (Riley, 1989). It is known, for example, that the majority of HIV-infected people experience progressive immunodeficiency and, without effective treatment, will likely develop AIDS. This period between initial infection, onset of symptoms, and eventual death may be very long. Some scientists, however, believe that the AIDS disease progresses more rapidly in older adults. Symptoms are also thought to be more severe. Dr. William Adler, chief of the National Institute on Aging's Clinical

Table 11–10. AIDS cases in the United States, older people and all ages (percent distribution by age and transmission category).

| | Age 50+[a] | | | |
Transmission Category	50-64 %	65+ %	Total 50+ %	All Ages[b] %
Homosexual/bisexual male	68	26	62	62
Intravenous (IV) drug user	10	2	8	19
Homosexual male & IV drug user	2	1	2	7
(Total homosexual/bisexual)	(70)	(27)	(64)	(70)
(Total IV drug user)	(12)	(3)	(10)	(26)
Hemophilia	1	4	2	1
Heterosexual cases	3	4	3	4
Transfusion, blood components	9	55	16	3
Undetermined	7	8	7	4
Total cases = 100%	6,167	1,008	7,175	72,223

[a]Pre-1981 to August, 1988.
[b]Pre-1981 to September, 1988. Excludes children under 13.

Source: Data from the Centers for Disease Control (CDC) Weekly Surveillance Report - cumulative totals.

Immunology Section, suggests that older adults who contracted AIDS through blood transfusions experience the ravaging consequences of the disease at twice the rate of children (Brozen, 1990). Patients age 60 and older tend to survive less than two years after being infected while children survive between five to seven years.

The actual interaction between aging processes and HIV infection is not known. Scientists conjecture that the interaction may be due to declining immune function. This decline in function may be connected with the increased susceptibility to HIV infection and the rapid progression of the disease. As we age, there is a loss of T-cell function. Confounding this relationship is that older adults appear likely to attribute the symptoms of HIV infection to their age rather than to the disease (Riley, 1989). Dementia in later life is especially vulnerable to this confusion.

AIDS and Dementia

Clinicians and pathologists are being increasingly challenged to consider HIV infection as a possible cause for dementia in older adults who are initially not known to be at high risk for AIDS. Infections of the central nervous system by HIV have been found. However, AIDS development in the elderly may be problematic as the risk factors of AIDS and dementia (fatigue, muscle weakness, rashes, coughs, memory loss) are often confused. Weiler (1989) writes,

Although AIDS may have a variety of manifestations in the elderly, including Kaposi's sarcoma and atypical presentations of pneumocystis corini pneumonia, the neurological complications may be of particular relevance to those in geriatrics. Three major neurological complications include subacute encephalitis (brain inflammation), vascular myelopathy (spinal cord disease), and psychiatric disorders and dementia. Patients with dementia deteriorate rapidly over a period of months or weeks, sometimes years, develop myoclonus (muscle spasms), and eventually become bed-bound and incontinent. These symptoms can mimic a degenerative dementia, but usually the clinical course is more rapid and is atypical of the normal degenerative dementias. The differentiating points of AIDS dementia include early behavioral manifestation and memory difficulties, but with profound physical signs and fatigue as well. There may be some insight into the cognitive problems, but the patient may be more aware of his physical problems than the fact that he is also cognitively impaired. (p. 17)

The confusion between AIDS and Alzheimer's has been especially pronounced. Alzheimer's dementia includes the symptoms of irritability, euphoric apathy, nominal aphasia with word-finding difficulty, and frequent use of circumlocutory phrases. These early physical symptoms and manifestations are more severe in AIDS dementia than they are in Alzheimer's disease. The AIDS victim is likely to have the same mental and memory difficulties of the Alzheimer's victim but also feel very weak and sick and suffer from fatigue and weight loss. Weiler (1989, p. 17) suggests that these types of physical symptoms relatively early in the course of the disease should raise a warning flag. In early Alzheimer's disease there are no neurological findings, but AIDS dementia is often accompanied by ambulation problems, leg weakness, myclonus, nonspecific tremors, or signs of peripheral neuropathy. Loss of sensation reflex reactions, abnormal reflex functions, and urinary incontinence may accompany the AIDS myolopathy. The patient develops early depressive symptoms that may be confused with depression, but the progression results in definite apathy, chronic confusion, and severe memory loss.

The growing cohort of HIV-infected older adults will undoubtedly lead gerontologists to be more concerned about AIDS in the later years. Serious dementia may appear before any evidence of an opportunistic infection. The misdiagnosis prevalency between Alzheimer's disease and AIDS dementia is still largely unrecognized; there are so many other plausible explanations of cognitive decline and disability in the elderly that prevent clinicians from thinking of AIDS as readily as they would for a younger adult. The lack of good research data on the current problem of AIDS dementia in the elderly warrants a closer look at this issue.

AIDS and Long-Term Care

The American health care system is vast and spreading. In the past, health care resources have existed to meet new needs. But rising health care costs now threaten to seriously dampen this flexibility. For example, HIV-related health care has accounted for only 1% of total national health care costs (Crystal, 1986b). But the impact in the 1990s will be much more substantial and will place additional pressure on a system that is already cracking at the seams. Thus new health needs are presenting themselves to a system that is already in a crisis. Crystal (1986b) explains how the American health care system is not just a crisis of cost but of organizational structure:

> Unlike almost all the rest of the developed world, the United States lacks a national health system. It depends on a uniquely diversified and uniquely fragmented health care structure, which is a source both of strengths and glaring weaknesses. The system's special strengths include the widespread availability of high technology diagnostic and treatment methods, the relatively fast diffusion of such methods, the access to capital that speeds this diffusion, and the concomitant highly trained cadre of specialist physicians and other health personnel oriented to the maximal use of technology.
>
> The mirror image of these strengths is the system's weaknesses in providing coordination and continuity of care in meeting "lower-tech" needs, particularly in supportive and long term care. Perhaps the most obvious weakness of our system from the patient's point of view is the wide disparity in financial access to care. These strengths and weaknesses have marked sharply the health care experience both of the elderly and of persons with AIDS. While the elderly have some protection from financial catastrophe with respect to hospitalized physician care, this is not true for long term care. Both for the elderly and for persons with AIDS, the system's shortfalls are particularly glaring in this area; both encounter a long term care system that is fragmented and to which access is highly variable as a function of geography and socioeconomic status. (p. 27)

Crystal (1986b) goes on to argue that developments in the AIDS epidemic mandate a shift toward a more coordinated and complete health care system, particularly an emphasis of the impact of this epidemic on the elderly. He presents three cogent arguments. First, there is not likely to be a "quick-fix" vaccine or other technological advances that will prevent or cure AIDS in the near future. Second, behavioral change to reduce the risk for AIDS has not been prevalent among heterosexual populations thus increasing the second-wave impact of the AIDS epidemic (first wave was impact on homosexuals). Third, antiviral, antibiotics, and other treatments are increasing the lifespan of those infected by HIV and the AIDS virus. These advances shift the clinical picture of the AIDS virus from an acute care system to a chronic one, resulting in a dire need to care for a much larger population of chronically ill individuals.

The three arguments presented by Crystal (1989b) suggest that it is inevitable that the elderly and AIDS victims will crash head-long into a health care resource system that is limited. Bed shortage is already being experienced in urban cities that have been hard hit by the AIDS virus. Persons with AIDS have not infrequently received more than

50% of the beds in some large public hospitals--hospital services that had previously been occupied mostly by the frail elderly.

The impact of AIDS on the long-term care industry has been less obvious than the impact on hospitals but just as real. This impact has been diluted in the traditional nursing home because AIDS has not yet been primarily included in this industry. Most nursing home operators have been reluctant to admit AIDS victims. However, the increasing number of HIV and AIDS victims and the pressure to minimize hospital stays due to cost containment provisions will place increasing pressure to allocate nursing home beds. These new demands will spell significant competition for resources as nursing homes, unlike hospitals, are already near 100% occupancy. Many nursing home operators, previously reluctant to admit people with AIDS, now perceive that the future will demand a more active role.

Nursing home operators cite the following reasons for rejecting persons with AIDS: lack of isolation areas in the facility, concern that staff and other clients will be infected, staff not properly trained to take care of AIDS persons, families of current residents would not accept admissions of people with AIDS, and insufficient reimbursement (Crystal, 1989b). Moreover, conventional nursing home environments are viewed by many persons with AIDS as unsatisfactory care environments: the elderly and AIDS persons tend to have incompatible needs (Crystal & Jackson, 1988).

Many policy-makers consider the development of specialized residential treatment facilities for AIDS persons as a more satisfactory solution. Development of such facilities poses a major challenge for existing long-term care providers because it moves away from conventional facility care. Despite this call for specialized facilities, Crystal and Jackson's survey of the AIDS population indicated that isolation and loneliness are the chief complaints of AIDS persons (Crystal, 1989b). Nursing home facilities that emphasize socialization and recreation as well as health care may help counter isolation and loneliness. Crystal (1989a) adds,

> It therefore appears likely that many long term care facilities will need to address the issue of AIDS care in the near future. A proactive rather than reactive stance on the part of the long term care community will help in the development of creative and financially feasible solutions. Long term care planners and operators, in implementing such projects, should take into account the differences as well as the similarities in the needs of the two populations. (p. 25)

The most likely approach to satisfy all concerned will be the development of specialized AIDS facilities that can serve on a free-standing basis or as a special wing of a larger facility. Ideally these specialized facilities would be developed in conjunction with both community organizations and the long-term care industry. Development of such facilities certainly involves special costs, but Crystal (1989b) emphasizes that they may prevent unnecessary hospital expenses. This latter point needs to draw special attention from third party payers.

Health Promotion and Aids

A basic question is whether there is a need for new prevention programs specifically targeted to older adults. Or can we rely on the existing AIDS-prevention efforts that are targeted to the general population? Recent evidence (Catania, Turner, Kegeles, et al., 1989) suggests that older adults are less knowledgeable than younger people about AIDS prevention. It appears that existing prevention methods have not effectively reached the older population. Thus prevention efforts specifically tailored to older adults appear to make the most sense.

Program Content

As earlier discussed, three main groups of people age 50 and older are at risk for HIV infection: (1) people who received HIV-infected blood transfusions, (2) sexual partners of those initially infected by HIV blood transfusions, and (3) people having unprotected sexual activity outside of a monogamous relationship. Although these three groups cut across sexual orientation groups, the largest at-risk group consists of older homosexual and bisexual men. The AIDS prevention program, however, must still be comprehensive enough to reach the heterosexual population--both male and female.

Catania et al. (1989) provide a risk reduction model, Figure 11-3, that serves as a conceptual framework for understanding the processes by which at-risk people may come to label their behaviors as putting themselves or others at risk, make a personal commitment to reduce risk behaviors, and initiate activities that encourage desired behavior change. The authors of this model hypothesize that each process requires different kinds of knowledge and belief systems, and increasing levels of social skills:

> Stage one--labeling--may require basic knowledge of the condition associated with HIV risk and routes of HIV transmission, while stage two requires knowledge of alternative behaviors (date activities) and an understanding of their costs and benefits. Step three may require a higher degree of social skills than that needed for traversing earlier stages--for instance, for negotiating changes in sexual behavior with one's sexual partner or for eliciting help from others with the change process. (p. 51)

The schematic diagram in Figure 11-3 is broken into three primary stages: (1) recognizing and labeling the person's sexual behavior for contracting HIV; (2) making a behavioral commitment to reduce high-risk social contacts and adopt low-risk activities; and (3) enact strategies to obtain these goals. In brief, the AIDS Risk Reduction Model (ARRM) suggests that to avoid high-risk HIV activity, a person must perceive that his or her behavior is placing the self at risk. After this perception, the person must make a strong commitment to alter his or her at-risk activities. Assessing the benefits and costs of certain behaviors apply under the commitment stage. Finally, enacting change usually requires the support from informal and formal sources. The process of enactment may also require complex negotiations between the person and his or her sexual partner(s).

The three stages are not necessarily unidirectional or nonreversible. For example, Catania et al. (1989) acknowledge that some people will experience considerable difficulty in changing their behavior and, eventually, relabel their activities as nonproblematic. They also may choose to reduce their commitment to change. Moreover, some compliant individuals may unknowingly skip the labeling stage and commitment stage and change their behavior (enactment) due to the urgings of a highly motivated sexual partner. For our purposes, however, we will focus on the likely influences of each stage.

Labeling. The actual influences of the labeling stage attempt to expose one to the susceptibility of high-risk activity. This susceptibility is largely dependent on the attitudes, knowledge, and behavior of older adults in relationship to AIDS. The reader is cautioned that the research in this area is very weak because AIDS has been a contemporary topic only in the past decade. Public opinion polls pertaining to public knowledge about transmission of the HIV virus, attitudes toward people with AIDS, opinion issues on public policy, and personal fear of AIDS represent the principal research efforts that apply to the labeling stage. Much of this research fails to address results by age categories. However, recent analysis of the 1985 National Health Interview Survey (NHIS) specifically addressed these age categories: 18 to 29, 30 to 49, and 50 and older. Levy and Albrecht (1989) summarize the NHIS findings:

> Adults over the age of 50 are more likely than younger people to state that they "know nothing" about AIDs, and fewer older people than young reported knowing "a lot." People over 50 were also somewhat more likely than younger people to perceive that AIDS could be transmitted through casual contact (such as eating in restaurants where the cook has AIDS; sharing food implements; working near or kissing someone who has the disease; or using public toilets).

> Conversely, people over 50 were less likely than the younger segments of the sample to associate the transmission of the AIDS virus with the practice of sharing needles during illegal drug use. They were less likely to have heard of the blood test for HIV-specific antibodies or to indicate willingness to be tested. Moreover, they appeared less well informed about the efficacy of various prophylactics, including condoms, in preventing transmission of the virus. (p. 45)

Albrecht, Levy, and Sugrue's study about AIDS-related behavior found no age differences in the probability of hearing about AIDS (Levi & Albrecht, 1989). However, more people in the age group 40 to 60, when compared to younger adults, were less likely to perceive themselves at risk for AIDS. The older age group was also less likely to adopt AIDS prevention behaviors. A more exhaustive study of AIDS-related behavior is presently being completed by the National Opinion Research Center at the University of

Chicago. Still, much of the AIDS-related behavior research continues to ignore older adults (Levy & Albrecht, 1989).

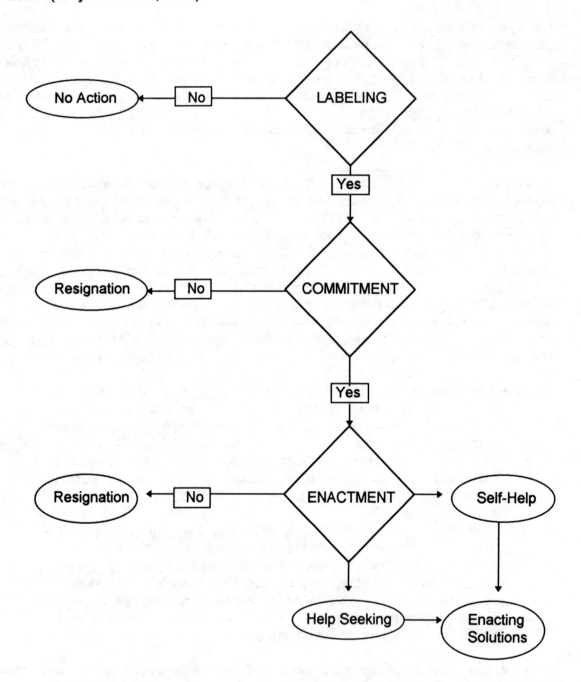

Figure 11-3. HIV transmission risks of older heterosexuals and gays. J. A. Catania, H. Turner, S. M. Kegeles, R. Stall, L. Pollack, S. E. Spitzer, and T. J. Coates. In M. W. Riley, M. G. Ory, and D. Zablotsky, AIDS in an Aging Society, (1989), Springer Publishing Company, Inc., New York, 10012. Used by permission.

Risk for HIV infection is also affected by the number and character of relationships with sex partners. The level of multiple sex partners among older heterosexuals may becoming a more common trend (Catania, Turner, & Kegeles et al., 1989). Even if older adults maintained monogamous relationships, the lack of safe sex practices would expose them to HIV infection. Answers to these questions need further study.

Commitment. The actual location of people in the change process dictates the program content and type of intervention. Stage one in the ARRM supports the use of mass media campaigns to build awareness of the AIDS issue for older adults. This awareness approach is used to address the susceptibility issue of AIDS as it applies to the labeling stage. However, building commitment to change may be a much more difficult process. Drawing from stage one, the commitment stage entertains more controversial topics by addressing such sexual issues as condom protection. Prevention-oriented sexual practices need to focus on what is presently known about older adults' sexual behavior and knowledge.

In Table 11-10, blood transfusions were identified as a major source of transmitting AIDS among people age 50 and older. The 1985 blood supply screening procedures have effectively dampened the blood transmission route for AIDS. However, many people who are already infected by blood transfusion form a nucleus for additional HIV transmission. For example, Peterman, Stoneburner, Allen, et al. (1988) found 8% of the older male and 18% of the older female sexual partners of seropositive blood recipients to be HIV infected. This continuous exposure to HIV transmission places tremendous importance on prevention-oriented sexual practices for older adults.

The sexual practices and knowledge of older transfusers has received only recent attention. Early studies, however, are producing rather startling results. One very important study, supported by the National Institute of Mental Health, was conducted by Coates, Kegeles, and Catania. The sample size for the Coates et al. study contained 57 older participants age 50 to 78 years. Forty percent of the respondents sought HIV testing due to their fear of blood transfusion contamination. Although the sample size was quite small, the preliminary findings have produced important and consistent results in respect to sexual practices and knowledge. Catania, Turner, Kegeles, et al. (1989) summarized some of the pertinent study findings:

> Among those older transfusers who answered questions about condom use (n = 10), none were using condoms during intercourse with their primary or secondary partners over the 6-month period prior to seeking testing. Consistent with this observation, the study by Peterman and associates (1988) found that none of the older heterosexual transfusers with HIV-positive sexual partners (median age for men was 72 and for women 62) had been using condoms since receiving their blood transfusions. In our sample, we also found that over half of older transfusers did not know that latex condoms can prevent HIV transmission. (1989, p. 80)

Additional findings by Catania et al. are that older transfusers were less likely to believe they could infect a sexual partner with HIV. Thus, older transfusers tended to neither be aware of the implications of their sexual behavior for HIV transmission nor of the importance of protective measures. Catania et al. theorize that many of the older transfusers were unaware of their risk for infection and, therefore, did not adopt prevention sexual practices leading to unintentional HIV transmission. This unintentional HIV transmission may account for the increase in heterosexual AIDS cases among older adults. The failure of public health and news media messages to effectively reach at-risk older individuals may underlie the unawareness of older adults as to HIV infection through blood transfusions.

Health promoting behaviors may also play a key role by protecting the immune system. Some estimates suggest that approximately 35% of HIV-positive persons will manifest formal AIDS symptoms within eight years after infection. This latency period is likely to be strongly affected by a variety of host characteristics, such as recreational drug use, stress, and co-morbid infectious processes. Many of the physiological and behavioral host factors may stimulate the immune system which, in turn, produces biochemical effects that activate the latent AIDS virus (Manton & Singer, 1989). It has been suggested, therefore, that adoption of health promoting behaviors (e.g., better nutrition) delays the triggering phenomena in the manifestation of AIDS. By protecting the immune system, the latent period of AIDS may be significantly delayed.

Enactment. To be labeled as having AIDS not only causes upheaval in the lives of patients but also impacts the lives of their family, extended kin, and friends. The perception that people with AIDS are "different" from the rest of the population certainly contributes to self-denial--"AIDS does not apply to me"-- that is often associated with stigma. Despite this perception, the trend toward AIDS in heterogeneous populations has led to a clinical diagnosis that distinguishes between HIV serapositive, ARC, and full-blown AIDS. These labeling distinctions have potentially serious implications. They affect both the self-definitions of patients and the definitions ascribed to patients by others. The labels assigned are certain to affect an entire range of feelings, attitudes, and behaviors for AIDS patients and their relationships with others.

The ARRM supports the contention that seeking help from informal or formal support sources is a critical method by which people initiate and reinforce change in high-risk sexual practices. Catania et al. (1989) suggest that the initial enactment strategy should involve joint consultation between sexual partners for meeting sexual behavioral goals. Verbal communication and problem-solving skills serve as the focal point for this initial strategy. But Catania et al. have also found that sexual communication skills may be less developed among older adults than younger adults.

The ARRM is based on the underlying principle that enactment strategies draw from an understanding of existing patterns of help-seeking and of potential determinants of change in these patterns. Studies reviewed by Catania et al. (1989) show that help-seeking behaviors vary by age, but it is not clear whether these differences are age related or cohort related. Early empirical studies indicate that older adults rely more on informal services than formal services. Moreover, younger adults provide more informal support services than older adults. Generalizability of the aforementioned findings, however, must be cautious. Catania et al. (1989) note that, "older people's help-seeking patterns may inhibit rapid dissemination of AIDS-relevant knowledge among this age category. This possibility raises serious concerns about the usefulness of community-level interventions for older persons" (p. 90).

Help-seeking includes a process by which AIDS people may contact formal prevention programs. This process can serve as a catalyst to diffuse intervention effects through-out the community. Catania et al. (1989) state, "Previous research suggests that if a large segment of a community seeks help with addressing safe sex issues, there will be a rapid diffusion of innovations directed at reducing HIV risk." Additionally, older adults seeking help from formal support services may, in turn, become lay helpers. As lay helpers, older adults can identify and train existing informal and formal help sources.

In summary, social support programs are a viable component of enactment strategies. There is considerable evidence that social support (emotional and instrumental aid) can reduce many of the negative consequences of stress. In fact, some studies have shown specific changes in the immune system that help guard against impaired health (McKinlay, Skinner, Riley, & Zablotsky, 1989). The influence of social support networks on the health or quality of life of AIDS patients, however, has received little research attention.

ARRM: Community-Level Intervention

The ARRM has obvious limitations; the stages are overlapping and are not necessarily cognate with one another. However, the stages in the model provide a valuable way to understand how health promotion programs may be used to address the problems of AIDS in later life. A close perusal of the ARRM indicates that both primary prevention (dissuade individuals from at-risk behavior) and secondary prevention (curtail already established at-risk behaviors) strategies are emphasized.

The use of the ARRM as a community-level intervention tool may unfold as follows. In stage one, mass communication (radio, television, mailings, press) would emphasize basic education about AIDS. For example, educational topics might include debunking AIDS myths, emphasizing the sources of AIDS transmission that are prevalent to older adults, and encouraging those at-risk to attain HIV testing. Stage two would focus on more specific sexual practices that lead to HIV infection. For example, topics may include the dangers of multiple sex partners, the use of condoms and lubricants as protection devices, and suggestions for getting a sex partner to commit to prevention practices. The focus of stage two is on helping people to understand how their knowledge, attitudes, and behaviors lead them to engage in at-risk HIV activities. Stage three is likely to be more intense and complicated because the focal point is on the awareness that "something is wrong." The "something is wrong" stage leads to lay consultation, lay referral, and informal care by family and friends.

The influence of cultural and social-psychological factors on health-seeking behaviors is readily apparent throughout the three stages of the ARRM. Investigation as to how these factors apply to AIDS patients, and in particular older adults, has not received sufficient attention. But AIDS research does not need to start from scratch. Cultural and social-psychological research in health-seeking behaviors for other diseases may certainly apply. However, many of the implications of AIDS peculiar to older adults need to be investigated. For example, McKinlay et al. (1989) identify important investigation areas as including the caring and adapting strategies of families with AIDS, the relationship between younger persons with AIDS and their older parents, and how specific behaviors enter into the decision process for seeking help from informal and formal sources.

AIDS: Vulnerability of Older Adults

AIDS and older adults is a subject that can no longer be ignored. As discussed in this chapter, 10% of AIDS cases have been diagnosed among people age 50 and older, including 1% who have attained age 65. These numbers are likely to steadily increase as the number of HIV infected adults grow older and develop AIDS or ARC. Unfortunately, the special vulnerability of older adults to the AIDS epidemic has generally been ignored. Riley (1989) emphasizes two very serious implications of this oversight:

- First, the large and rapidly growing number of people in the middle-aged and older segment of the United States population may well constitute the last major frontier for prevention of AIDS. This presents an early opportunity to begin prevention efforts now, to forestall any possibility that the epidemic may become strongly entrenched among the more than 60 million people aged 50 and over. Here is an opportunity to learn from previous failures with the populations first afflicted with AIDS: homosexual and bisexual males, intravenous drug abusers, and their sexual partners, any one of whom may unwittingly already be infected.
- Second, the head-on competition for long-term care between frail older people and people with AIDS is exacerbating the already heavy care burdens on families, communities, and society as a whole. A great deal is known about the problems of caring for older people, currently the major users of long-term care, and about potential means of helping to alleviate the burdens of care. Here is an opportunity to learn from the experience with the frail elderly, before the emerging demands for care of AIDS patients reach crisis proportions. (p. 4)

The two implications cited by Riley present a very unique challenge for preventing the spread of the AIDS epidemic in late life. But this opportunity requires immediate attention to the social and behavioral implications of AIDS and not just to the biomedical approach which is dedicated to vaccines, treatment, and cures. Solid information about the sexual behavior of older adults and the relationship of that behavior to AIDS is still quite sparse. Myths about sexual activity and scientific disinterest in human sexuality are but two of many barriers contributing to this knowledge void.

The salient point is that the AIDS epidemic is not yet fully entrenched within the older population. Yet we cannot ignore the fact that we have presently failed to educate many older adults about AIDS or to provide facilities that emphasize both prevention and care. Many older adults are unaware of the HIV dangers. Most are not using self-protection devices or pursuing HIV screening. Despite this gloomy picture, there is still time to implement primary and secondary prevention strategies that may deter AIDS from becoming an epidemic crisis in late life.

CHAPTER SUMMARY

Certain conditions and chronic disorders occur more frequently among older adults and deserve special attention. The conditions and disorders addressed in this chapter were accidents, hypertension, diabetes mellitus, breast cancer, osteoporosis, and arthritis. These conditions and disorders become more prevalent in late life due to organ-related changes associated with the aging process. As stated earlier in this book, the estimate is that 80% of older adults have at least one chronic condition and almost 50% are unable to perform some activities of daily living.

Chronic conditions and disorders need not be the end of independence in later life. Primary, secondary, and tertiary prevention strategies are all involved in the management of chronic diseases. Management of existing chronic problems through prevention strategies entails a thorough understanding of the role that lifestyle factors play in disease processes. Additionally, health care professionals must move beyond the belief that chronic conditions and disorders affect older adults only at a biological level. It is quite clear from our chapter discussions that these special conditions and disorders also impinge on the social, psychological, and spiritual lives of older adults. The key is to approach the management of chronic conditions from a more holistic philosophy that encourages self-care and enhances self-esteem. Particular attention was placed on precaution of exercise and drug interactions. An excellent resource for this concern is Groedon and Groedon (1995).

CHAPTER 12

ELDERLY PATIENTS AND THEIR DOCTORS: PARTNERS IN HEALTH PROMOTION

As a group, the elderly come into frequent contact with health professionals. Contacts with their doctors provide opportunities not only for the treatment of specific age-influenced health concerns, but for more general efforts--via ongoing assessment and education--to promote the health of the elderly. This chapter summarizes some of what is known about doctor-patient interaction in general, and the interactions of doctors and elderly patients in particular. Using this information as a backdrop, the chapter concludes with a set of recommendations for enhancing the power of the doctor-patient encounter as a tool for better promoting the health of the elderly.

THE ELDERLY AND THEIR HEALTH

In 1900, 3 million of the people living in the United States, approximately 1 person in 25, was 65 years of age or older. By the late 1970s, these numbers had grown to 22.2 million; 1 person in 10, was 65 years or above. It is estimated that by the year 2000, one in every eight persons will be 65 years or older, for a total of almost 31 million people (Conlin, 1980; Harris, 1978). By the year 2050, nearly 67 million of the estimated 309 million people in the United States will be 65 years or older (McGinnis, 1988).

The statistics summarized above, notwithstanding, the so-called "graying of America" is much more than a basic population issue; it represents an important medical service issue as well. One indisputable fact is that as a person ages, the chances increase that he or she will experience at least one chronic illness or some other disabling condition (Hoenig, 1993; McGinnis, 1988). Persons who are 65 years or older are twice as likely to experience a chronic illness than persons 64 years or younger. Data also indicate that nationally, 27% of the people who are 65 years or over have heart conditions; 38% experience hypertension; 40% have vision or hearing problems (a combined percentage) (U.S. Senate Special Committee on Aging, 1986); and 7% to 12% of those who reside in the community evidence symptoms of mental illness (George, 1992). Dementia is experienced by about 5% of the total elderly population, but by 20% to 30% of those who are 85 years of age or older (U.S. Senate Special Committee on Aging, 1986). Increasing age also significantly influences general functional capabilities. Hoenig (1993) reports, for example, that 11.4% of the noninstitutionalized elderly in the United States evidence difficulties in walking and basic self-care activities. This percentage increases to over 34% by age 85. When activities such as shopping and getting around in the community are considered, reported functional disability rises to approximately 57% for persons over age 85.

With increasing age, there tends to be concurrent increase in health care utilization. For example, in contrast to those who are under age 65, persons who are 65 years or over see their physicians more regularly, get hospitalized more frequently--often for twice as long--and take twice as many medications (U.S. Senate Special Committee on Aging, 1986). Summarizing data compiled by a U.S. Senate Special Committee on Aging (1991), Beisecker & Thompson (1995) indicated that on average, persons 65 years or older make eight visits each year to their doctors, compared to an average of five yearly visits by persons in other age groups. These data, however, are somewhat confusing. They give the impression that all persons over 64 years of age represent a homogeneous group, and that regardless of their actual ages, everyone 65 years or older makes approximately the same number of visits to the doctor each year. A similar impression resulted from initial data collected by Roos and his associates concerning health care utilization in Canada. They found that persons in their sample who were 65 years and over made only .9 more doctor visits each year than those in the 45 to 64 year old group, and on average, only 1.7 more visits than persons in the 25 to 44 age group. However, the authors pointed out that these averaged data in fact masked considerable variations in health care utilization in the 65 and over group (Haug & Ory, 1987; Roos & Shapiro, 1981; Roos, Shapiro, & Roos, 1984). Specifically, 8% of those in the 65 years and over group had made 14 or more visits to their doctor in the previous year. The elderly who constituted this 8% in fact represented 35% of the heaviest users of health care in their sample.

This tendency for a small percentage of the group to utilize a large amount of health care has been documented in the United States as well, following investigations of both ambulatory care and hospital utilization (Haug & Ory, 1987; National Center for Health Services Research, 1985; U.S. Senate Special Committee on Aging, 1985). Collectively, these data underscore the importance of not thinking of the elderly as a homogeneous group (Adelman, Greene, & Charon, 1991; Haug & Ory, 1987; Hoenig, 1993). In combination, the information presented above suggests the following: (1) the elderly will represent a steadily increasing proportion of the general population well into the 21st century; (2) that despite the medical advances that have resulted in people living longer lives, it is very likely that illness and physical decline will continue to be critical components of the aging process; and (3) given 1 and 2 above, health care professionals will have regular contact with increasing numbers of elderly patients in years to come. These points underscore the importance of paying close attention to the intricacies of doctor-elderly patient interaction.

THE DOCTOR-PATIENT RELATIONSHIP

Virtually every area of investigation has at its core one or more early contributions that have organized and stimulated subsequent work in the field. This is certainly true in the now-expansive area of doctor-patient communication. One noteworthy early contribution was a paper by Henderson (1935) that appeared in the *New England Journal of Medicine*. Henderson proposed that the unit that is formed by a doctor and patient should be viewed as a social system. He stressed paying particular attention to the collective sentiments of the doctor and patient, and proposed that "the interaction of the sentiments of the individuals making up the social system is hardly less important than gravitational attraction in the solar system" (p. 820).

Several years later, in a treatise entitled *The Social System*, Talcott Parsons (1951) offered a lengthy sociological account of the intricacies of medical practice. Describing illness as a form of deviant behavior--an occurrence that is both biologically and socially defined--he devoted particular attention to the complementary behaviors of the doctor and the patient that accompany the entry and exit of the latter from his or her "sick role."

Another seminal paper was published by Szasz and Hollender in 1956. They ad-dressed the kinds of interaction that characterize relationships in general, and the dealings of doctors and their patients in particular. Szasz and Hollender (1956) elabor-ated three distinct models of interaction (i.e., activity-passivity; guidance-cooperation; and mutual participation) that link doctors to the patients they treat. The value of this paper, however, extended far beyond the authors' categorization of typical interactional styles. The paper was equally important for Szasz and Hollender's clarification of how particular illness situations in fact seem to demand one model of interaction over the others. For example, the activity-passivity model of interaction is particularly well-suited for situations in which emergency care is needed. Here, by virtue of the situation, the doctor is very much in control while the patient typically assumes a more passive role. Decisions that are intended to alter the health circumstance of the patient are usually made with little or no input from the patient. However, this model may be less desirable in non-emergent health care situations, particularly those in which the patient expects to be a more active participate in the decisions that will guide his or her care. In these situations, the guidance-cooperation or mutual participation models of doctor-patient interaction would likely be more appropriate.

Szasz and Hollender (1956) also argued that although it was possible to categorize the interaction of doctors and patients in very discrete ways, it must be realized that their relationships continuously evolve. This change may occur because of changes in health, or because of the progressive development of the relationships doctors share with their patients. Depending on the illness, more or less participation from the patient may be quite appropriate and desirable. In a statement that presaged many eventual investigations of patient satisfaction with medical encounters, Szasz and Hollender spe-culated that some of the dissatisfactions that arise between doctors and patients may occur when there has been a failure to negotiate (or renegotiate, as the case may be) aspects of their relationship when changes can and should occur. This paper by Szasz and Hollender (1956) was unquestionably instrumental in underscoring some of the interpersonal aspects of medical care (Bloom & Speedling, 1981).

The doctor-patient relationship continues to be a frequent topic of discussion in the professional literature (Cassell, 1985; Mishler, 1984; Quill, 1983; Waitzkin, 1991). Clearly building on the work of Szasz and Hollender (1956), one recent contribution includes a new typology by Emanuel and Emanuel (1992). These authors propose that the categorization of doctor-patient relationships as paternalistic, informative, interpretive, or deliberative. At the heart of the more deliberative model of interaction is a clear effort on the part of the physician to take into account the perspective of the patient, and to engage him or her as an active participant in the planning of care (Laine & Davidoff, 1996). In this regard, it is similar to the model of mutual participation initially proposed by Szasz and Hollender (1956).

DOCTOR-PATIENT COMMUNICATION: GENERAL FINDINGS

An expansive literature has developed that sheds light on some of the specific behaviors that are transacted by doctors and patients during medical encounters (Beisecker & Thompson, 1995; Haug & Ory, 1987; Ong, de Haes, Hoos, & Lammes, et al. 1995). In the following sections, information will be provided regarding some general findings that have been reported in this research-based literature. This will be followed by information that more specifically addresses the interactions of doctors and elderly patients.

Much of this literature contains an important subtext: despite the technology that characterizes both the diagnostic and therapeutic aspects of modern medicine (Fox, 1986; Zola, 1972), the interpersonal communication of doctors and patients undeniably influences both the planning and delivery of medical care (Ong et al. 1995). These interpersonal aspects of medicine have strong implications for the health promotion of all patients, young and old.

Information Giving by Doctors and Patients

Investigations of the verbal behaviors of doctors and patients reveal that during routine medical encounters, doctors tend to contribute approximately 60% of the dialogue, and patients the remaining 40%. On average, about 35% of this doctor-initiated dialogue is in the form of information giving; the remaining 23% involves asking questions of the patient (Roter, Hall, & Katz, 1988). Data from other investigations suggest, however, that doctors may spend much less time giving information to patients. Waitzkin and his colleagues (Waitzkin, 1984), for example, recorded and analyzed a total of 336 doctor-patient encounters that took place in a variety of outpatient settings. They found that the doctors in their study spent comparatively little time dispensing information to patients, barely more than 1 minute during a 20-minute medical encounter. Importantly, doctors tended to overestimate the amount of time they spent giving information to patients, on average, by a factor of nine.

Waitzkin's (1984) research also suggested that information giving by the doctor is influenced by details of the patient's condition. Specifically, when doctors reported being uncertain about the diagnosis and prognosis of patients, there was a weak tendency for them to give more information during the medical encounter. However, greater certainty about an unfavorable patient prognosis was a much stronger predictor of the information giving by the doctor. These patients tended to get more time with the doctor, more total explanations, more multilevel explanations (i.e., technical explanations that then were translated into simpler terms), and more nondiscrepant responses (i.e., answers from doctors that matched the level of technicality of patients' questions).

Information provided by Street (1991) suggests that the amount of information received from doctors is, in part, interactionally determined. He found that the communicative behaviors of doctors were strongly influenced by accompanying behaviors of patients. Specifically, patients who asked more questions, reported more concerns, or were perceived as more anxious, received comparatively more information during their medical encounters. Besides underscoring the inherent complementarity of the typical doctor-patient relationship, this study has particular implication for patients (including the elderly) who may not strongly advocate for their own care during medical encounters (Beisecker, 1988).

A number of patient gender differences have also been reported. Hall, Roter, and Katz (1988) reported that doctors tend to impart more information to female patients than to male patients. This finding has been reported by others as well. Waitzkin (1984), for example, found that women tended to receive more time from their doctors during clinic visits, more explanations in general, more multilevel explanations, and more nondiscrepant responses.

Roter has suggested that more than 50% of a patient's contribution to a medical encounter consists of information giving, typically in response to questions asked by the doctor (Roter, 1989). In terms of question asking, however, patients in general spend as little as 6% of the time asking their doctors questions. Gender differences regarding question asking have also been found, with Waitzkin (1984) reporting, for example, that women tend to ask their doctors more questions. These findings--the tendency for doctors to give more information to women than to men, and for women to ask more questions--are probably interrelated: question asking by the patient is likely to be directly influenced by the amount or clarity of information that has already been provided by the doctor.

Waitzkin (1984) also reported a number of differences directly related to the social class of patients. For example, college-educated patients tended to receive more time, and more (and better) explanations from their doctors than patients from lower socio-economic backgrounds, despite the fact that the patient groups did not differ in terms of their overall desire for information.

Despite the discrepancies in the literature regarding information giving during medical encounters, one very important point remains: scarce information from the doctor about the patient's condition or what he or she specifically needs to do to treat it, can powerfully influence a number of health-related outcomes (Hall et al., 1988; Ong et al., 1995; Roter, 1989).

Patient Outcomes Associated with Doctor Information Giving

Hall et al. (1988) performed a meta-analysis of the results of 41 independent studies in which various behaviors of doctors had been objectively assessed as part of the respective initial investigations. The intent was to obtain an indication of how provider behavior was related (if at all) to three specific outcome variables (i.e., patient satisfaction, compliance, and recall of medical information), and to several patient-specific variables (i.e., social class, age, and gender). Summarizing some of their findings, the meta-analysis revealed that there was a highly significant positive association between patient satisfaction (depending on the study, measured either by questionnaire or post-encounter interview) and the amount of information patients received during the medical encounter (Hall et al., 1988).

Despite a tendency for patients to want more rather than less information about their medical situation (Beisecker & Beisecker, 1990), doctors often underestimate the amount of information that patients would like to receive during medical encounters, particularly when potentially life-threatening diseases are the focus of attention. In a study of the information and decision-making preferences of hospitalized cancer patients, Blanchard, Labrecque, Ruckdeschel, and Blanchard (1988) reported, for example, that 92% of the patients in their sample wanted as much information as possible--good and bad--about their disease, but only 69% wanted to actively participate in decision making that was directly related to their care. Similar findings have been reported by others as well (Sutherland, Llewelyn-Thomas, Lockwood, et al., 1989). These findings suggest that a patient's interest in collaborative medical decision-making may be influenced by the seriousness of his or her disease. A very different process may be operative with reference to patients who are experiencing medical conditions that are not life-threatening (Rolland, 1984).

The meta-analysis by Hall et al. (1988) revealed a weak association between the amount of information given by the doctor during the medical encounter and subsequent patient compliance (i.e., appointment keeping or compliance with treatment recommendations). A significant association was found, however, when the respective probabilities of these two outcomes were combined (Hall et al. 1988). The meta-analysis revealed a stronger (positive) relationship between the amount of information given by doctors and the ability of patients to subsequently recall and demonstrate an understanding of information provided during medical encounters (also see Roter, 1989).

Summarizing particular findings regarding information giving by doctors: (1) patients want a lot of information from their doctors regarding their health circumstances; (2) there is evidence of a positive association between reported patient satisfaction and the amount of information provided by doctors; (3) a weak association has been reported between doctor information and patient compliance; but (4) a strong relationship has been reported between the amount of information given by doctors during patient encounters and the abilities of patients to subsequently recall and demonstrate an understanding of previously provided information.

Patient Outcomes Associated with Doctor Questioning

Questioning by the doctor has also been shown to be associated with particular patient outcomes. In their meta-analysis of associations between provider behaviors and selected outcomes, Hall and her associates (Hall et al., 1988) reported a nonsignificant relationship between information-directed questioning by doctors (including both open and closed questions) and the reported satisfaction of patients with their medical encounters. Questioning by doctors was negatively correlated with eventual patient compliance; specifically, if more questions were asked, patient compliance was less likely. Importantly, however, it was also found if patients were specifically asked about their compliance with medical recommendations, compliance tended to be greater. There is also evidence that too many questions from the doctor may erode a patient's overall satisfaction with the medical encounter. Similarly, too much question asking, particularly after the initial information gathering phase of the encounter, may adversely influence the attributions that patients make regarding the competence of the doctor. Not surprisingly, patients who perceive their doctors as being technically competent tend to report greater satisfaction with the care that is provided (Hall et al., 1988).

Summarizing particular findings regarding doctor questioning: (1) patient satisfaction does not appear to be affected by doctor questioning during the information-seeking phase of the medical encounter; (2) too many questions during the treatment phase of the encounter, however, may reduce patient satisfaction and confidence in the doctor; (3) there is evidence of a negative correlation between the number of questions asked and subsequent patient compliance with treatment recommendations; but (4) questions specific to compliance may actually enhance treatment adherence.

Patient Outcomes Associated with Other Doctor-initiated Behaviors

Smith, Polis, and Hadac (1981) reported positive associations between satisfaction and both the amount of time doctors spend with patients (i.e., longer encounters rated as more satisfactory), and the willingness of the physician to discuss preventive health care with the patient. Buller and Buller (1987) investigated the impact of physician communication style on patient satisfaction. Patients who saw doctors who were perceived as dominant and controlling during their medical encounter were more likely to be dissatisfied with the visit. Increased satisfaction was also reported when doctors exhibited a more affective style of communication during the patient encounter.

Compliance has also been found to be related to other physician behaviors (besides questioning) during the medical encounter (Hall et al., 1988). Specifically, more compliance was associated with more positive talk (e.g., personal remarks, laughter, agreement, empathy, approval, reassurance, supportiveness, etc.) less negative talk (e.g., anger, irritation, disagreement, perceived boredom, speech errors, nervousness, etc.), and more conversation (e.g., casual conversation, words of courtesy at the beginning and end of the encounter, personal remarks, introductions if the doctor doesn't already know the patient, etc.) from the physician.

Behaviors from doctors that suggest a willingness to work in partnership with patients have also been investigated. Partnership building between doctors and patients entails a willingness on the part of the physician to obtain input from the patient that broadens the developing view of the problem, and to assume a less authoritarian position during the medical encounter (Szasz & Hollender, 1956). Perceived partnership building efforts have been shown to be positively associated with patient satisfaction and both the recall and understanding of recommendations made during the medical encounter (Hall et al., 1988).

In contrast to the obvious amount of attention that has been focused on the impact of communication on patient satisfaction and compliance, its influence on health status has been investigated less frequently (Kaplan, Greenfield, & Ware, 1989). The studies that have appeared, however, suggest that the communicative relationship of doctors and patients may also influence health status. Kaplan et al. (1989), summarizing their studies involving patients experiencing chronic ulcer disease, hypertension, and diabetes, found that patients who were more controlling, less forthcoming with information, more skilled in eliciting information from their doctors, and more emotional during the baseline visit, reported fewer functional limitations at follow-up. Patients with fewer functional limitations tended to have doctors who were less controlling during office visits, more willing to demonstrate negative emotion (e.g., frustration, anxiety, apprehension, etc.), and to provide more information during the patient encounter. Specific health status differences were noted as well. Specifically, diabetic patients who exhibited more of the behaviors noted above, had lower blood glucose levels. Accompanying reductions in blood pressure were also reported for previously hypertensive patients. These researchers also demonstrated that patients could be taught particular interpersonal skills that positively influenced a number of health outcomes. When compared to control group patients, those who were taught behaviors that specifically targeted their involvement in the medical encounter--how to negotiate, elicit and weigh care options, choose between competing care options, and state preferences--had better health outcomes at follow-up (Kaplan et al., 1989).

Summarizing particular findings above: (1) positive associations have been reported between patient satisfaction and the amount of time spent with patients, and the willingness of doctors to discuss preventive health care; (2) domineering and controlling behaviors by physicians are associated with reduced patient satisfaction; (3) increased patient satisfaction is associated with more affective communication from doctors; (4) there is a positive association between patient satisfaction and more positive talk and conversation by doctors; (5) efforts at partnership building by doctors are positively associated with satisfaction and subsequent recall and understanding of medical recommendations; and (6) there is evidence that patients can be taught communication skills that appear to be associated with subsequent improvements in health status.

COMMUNICATION BETWEEN DOCTORS AND ELDERLY PATIENTS

Although the communication of doctors and patients in general has received increased attention in the professional literature in recent years, a literature that more specifically addresses issues pertaining to doctors and elderly patients has been slower to develop. A number of studies published during the past decade, however, have underscored the increasingly held belief that although some information from the more general literature regarding doctor-patient interaction may be applicable to all patient groups, quoting Adelman and his colleagues (Adelman, Greene, & Charon, 1987), "There is reason to believe that the doctor-elderly patient relationship differs substantially from the doctor-young patient relationship and must be studied as a unique sub-set of medical encounter" (p. 729). It is assumed, however, that at least portions of the more general information concerning the interaction of doctors and patients may be relevant to discussions of the elderly. Following a discussion of possible constraints to doctor-elderly patient communication, information will be summarized concerning the interactional processes that often link doctors and the elderly patients they treat. Particular attention will be devoted to the research findings that exist at this time that concern the association between interactions during medical encounters and patient outcomes such as satisfaction and compliance.

Potential Constraints to Optimal Doctor-Elderly Patient Communication

A number of factors can influence the encounters that physicians have with elderly patients. Patient-specific factors including possible sensory deficits, and cognitive and functional impairment can significantly constrain the communication process (Adelman, Greene, & Charon, 1991). Problems with mobility, an important issue for the frail elderly, may prevent many from receiving medical attention as frequently as they should (Hoenig, 1993). And when they do come for medical care, the complexity of the issues that must be addressed may add to the length of the encounter. As a result, communication may be truncated in an effort to keep the medical visit as short as possible.

Elderly patients are often accompanied to medical visits by other persons (e.g., spouses, adult children, etc.). Several authors have addressed the range of roles and influences that these additional persons can have on the medical encounter. In some instances, these people can facilitate the communication process (Labrecque et al., 1991), but in others, the dynamics of this more triadic patient care arrangement can in fact have more of a constraining influence on communication (Adelman et al., 1987).

Constraints to communication may also exist at a broader contextual level. This is particularly noteworthy in medical settings with demanding productivity requirements for physicians. Since encounters with elderly patients can be more time consuming, the elderly may be particularly rushed in these settings (Haug & Ory, 1987).

Communication may also be influenced by the general characteristics of elderly patients and their doctors. It is not uncommon for patients and physicians to be mismatched on a large number of factors (i.e., age, gender, social class, race), and particularly in the case of younger doctors treating the elderly, differing expectations of the type of relationship they should have (Adelman et al., 1991; Haug & Ory, 1987). The early experiences of many now-elderly patients were shaped by expectations suggesting that doctors should be dominant and in control of the situation, and the patient passive and essentially uninvolved in the treatment process (Haug & Ory, 1987). Even with progressive changes in the way doctors typically interact with patients (Laine & Davidoff, 1996; Stewart et al., 1995), many elderly patients may remain less communicative and participatory in health care situations simply because they think this is how they should be.

It should also be recognized that despite a rapidly increasing elderly population, in general, geriatric training during medical school has developed at a much slower pace (Barry, 1994). The net effect is that not all physicians are equally skilled in terms of either the often complex health care needs of the elderly, or in terms of communicating with them in an effort to facilitate the best possible care.

But possibly one of the most enduring constraints to communication with the elderly comes in the form of ageism (Butler, 1978). Ageism encompasses a collection of false beliefs, entertained by doctors and patients alike, that have clear implications for the manner in which the elderly may present for medical care, and the kind of assistance that may be provided. When ageism is operative in the medical encounter, it may result in any or all of the following (Adelman et al., 1991): a tendency of physicians to take the problems of the elderly less seriously than they should be, often attributing them simply to the fact that the patient is "getting old" (see Greene, Adelman, Charon, & Friedmann [1989] for a discussion of, in contrast to encounters with younger patients, the reduced concordance that often characterizes doctor-elderly patient encounters--concordance refers to disparities between the doctor and patient about goals, topics, etc.); treating problems less aggressively than may be appropriate, and making fewer recommendations in the area of preventive health care (see Radecki et al. [1988b] for evidence that suggests that appropriate diagnostic testing falls off significantly in patients 75 years of age or over); thinking of or referring to the elderly in a derogatory fashion; spending less time than necessary with older patients (see Radecki, Kane, Solomon, Mendenhall, & Beck [1988a] for a discussion of data documenting a tendency for doctors to spend less time with older patients than younger patients during medical encounters); and, in general, thinking of the elderly as a group that is difficult to deal with (Adelman et al., 1991). Not surprisingly, such ageist views can powerfully influence both the form and content of the communication that occurs between doctors and patients.

Doctors, Elderly Patients, and Outcomes

Patient satisfaction is an important health care outcome. Patients who are not satisfied with the medical care they receive are more likely to disenroll from health insurance plans, seek the care of other doctors, and initiate malpractice suites against physicians. Not surprisingly, dissatisfied patients are also less likely to follow treatment recommendations made by the doctor (Adelman et al., 1991; Beisecker & Thompson, 1995; Kaplan et al., 1989).

The satisfaction of patients with their encounters with doctors appears to be multi-determined. It has been reported that those with less education (Hall et al., 1988) and lower assessed socioeconomic standing (Like & Zyzanski, 1987) tend to report greater satisfaction with medical care. White patients often report more satisfaction than non-Whites (Bertakis, Roter, & Putnam, 1991). And, the elderly, when they are compared to persons who are younger, tend to report greater satisfaction with health care (Bertakis et al., 1991). There is also evidence that satisfaction is influenced at least in part by the health status of patients (Adelman et al., 1991; Snider, 1980). In a longitu-dinal investigation of a large sample of elderly patients, Hall, Milburn, and Epstein (1993) demonstrated that overall self-perceived health was the variable that was most predictive of subsequent satisfaction ratings regarding health care. However, satisfac-tion is also directly or indirectly determined by details of the interactions that patients have with doctors.

Investigating factors that influence the satisfaction of elderly patients with care provided by their doctors, Snider (1980) found that those who rated their own health status as either poor or fair tended to evaluate their doctors on the basis of how interested they were perceived as being in the health circumstance of the elderly. Those who per-ceived their doctors as interested tended to be satisfied with the care they received. Those who viewed their doctors as actually being disinterested in their health situation tended to report overall dissatisfaction with their health care. Elderly persons who rated their health as either good or excellent, however, used a distinctly different set of cri-teria in determining satisfaction. Specifically, those in the healthier categories assessed satisfaction according to whether or not they agreed with the health care recommen-dations made by their doctors. Those who agreed were more satisfied with their health care than those who were in disagreement.

Bertakis et al. (1991) assessed the satisfaction of a large sample of patients treated by family practice and internal medicine physicians. Elderly patients figured prominently in the study sample. Patients' perceptions of the technical competence of their doctors strongly influenced global ratings of satisfaction. Perceived competence and patient satisfaction were positively associated. With more specific reference to communication factors, however, the ratio of doctor to patient talk during the medical encounter was related to satisfaction. Greater satisfaction was reported in those instances where relative to their doctors, patients talked more during the medical encounter. This find-ing was unrelated to either length of visit or the amount of total talk time of each participant.

Studies have also indicated that a number of nonverbal physician behaviors contribute to the increased satisfaction of elderly patients. Specifically, behaviors from doctors that are indicative of nonverbal immediacy (i.e., leaning forward, eye contact, less distance between patient and doctor, etc.) are strongly related to patient satisfaction (Beisecker & Thompson, 1995; Hall et al., 1988).

Increased elderly patient satisfaction has also been found to be positively correlated with factors such as "physician questioning and supportiveness on patient-raised topics; patient information-giving on patient-raised topics; the length of the visit; the physician's use of questions worded in the negative; shared laughter between the physician and the patient; and physician satisfaction" (p. 1279, Greene, Adelman, Friedmann, & Charon, 1994).

Aspects of the doctor-patient communication process that may influence whether or not patients will follow the recommendations of their doctors, have become frequent topics of research in recent years (Kaplan et al., 1989). Haug and Ory (1987) have proposed that a more domineering style by physicians may seriously reduce compliance levels, and possibly create a situation where the patient is dishonest with the doctor about his or her adherence to a prescribed regimen.

Analyzing a number of recordings of interactions between doctors and elderly patients, Coe (1987) investigated the strategies doctors used to ideally enhance patient compliance with prescribed medication regimens. Compliance was improved with efforts to involve family members in the process as medication monitors, match the language used in the medical encounter to the understanding of the patient (and other family members), and to elicit (or entertain) input from the patient about possible modifications in the medication schedule. The strategies discerned by Coe (1987) are important because, as numerous authors have suggested, although noncompliance with prescribed medications is a common problem with the elderly, the elderly are often not willfully noncompliant. Noncompliance often results from factors such as difficulties understanding the recommendations that have been made, vision problems that hinder the reading of instructions, and for some, the confusion that comes with taking multiple medications for multiple illnesses (Adelman et al., 1991; Beisecker & Thompson, 1995; German, 1988). There is also evidence of an age difference regarding the influence of patient satisfaction on patient compliance. Linn, Linn, and Stein (1982) have reported that satisfaction with medical care is positively associated with the compliance of older patients but not younger patients.

Summarizing particular findings regarding the elderly: (1) elderly patients tend to report more general satisfaction with health care than younger patients; (2) satisfaction is influenced by health status (i.e., better health, greater satisfaction); (3) the perceived technical competence of doctors is positively associated with patient satisfaction; (4) there is greater reported satisfaction when, relative to doctors, patients talk more during medical encounters; (5) nonverbal immediacy on the part of the doctor is positively associated with patient satisfaction; (6) satisfaction is positively related to physician questioning and patient information giving on patient-initiated topics, length of interview, and shared laughter with doctors; and (7) compliance is negatively related to doctor dominance and control during medical encounters.

Psychosocial Topics

Psychosocial difficulties are experienced by a number of elderly patients. Quoting Waitzkin (1991), "Such contextual problems derive from bereavement, financial insecurity, isolation and loneliness, declining physical capacity, dependency, inadequate housing, lack of transportation, and a host of other issues" (p. 143). Given the prominence of such concerns in the lives of many elderly patients, a number of studies have been conducted that provide a glimpse of the handling of psychosocial issues during medical encounters.

Researchers have demonstrated that doctors behave differently relative to the psychosocial concerns raised by younger and older patients. Greene, Hoffman, Charon, and Adelman (1987) audiotaped and coded physician encounters with a total of 40 patients; 20 were 45 years of age or younger, 20 were age 65 or over. These authors found that the majority of topics raised by doctors with both younger patients and older patients were medical in nature. However, as had been hypothesized, when doctors raised psychosocial topics, they did so more frequently with younger patients than older patients.

Age-related differences were also found in terms of how doctors responded to patient-raised topics. Although the observed differences were not statistically significant, there was a tendency for doctors to be more responsive (i.e., ask additional questions, provide more information, demonstrate more support) when issues were raised by younger rather than older patients. It should also be noted that physician responsiveness did not differ when they (the physicians) brought up the various psychosocial issues. When patients brought up the issues, however, an age-related difference was found. Doctors were less responsive (i.e., they asked fewer additional questions, and provided less information and support) to older patients than to younger patients. In a subsequent investigation, these researchers found that with reference to both medical and psychosocial topics raised during medical encounters, physicians tended to respond more favorably when they rather than the patients had initiated the topic (Adelman, Greene, Charon, & Friedmann, 1992). The authors suggested that such behaviors by doctors are likely to discourage elderly patients from bringing up crucial topics for discussion during subsequent medical encounters.

Based on extensive analyses of transcribed doctor-patient encounters, Waitzkin (1991) also reported that the psychosocial topics raised by many patients (including the elderly) are often not adequately responded to during medical encounters. Waitzkin highlighted numerous instances where doctors steered the conversation away from the psychosocial domain and back to more medically focused topics. When this happens, the net effect is that critical psychosocial concerns often go unaddressed.

A previously mentioned study by Bertakis and his colleagues (Bertakis et al., 1991) provides an indication, however, of the impact that a discussion of psychosocial topics can have on patient satisfaction. Differential levels of satisfaction were reported relative to the content of the discussion during the medical encounter. In particular, when the medical encounter was restricted to a discussion of medical issues, lower satisfaction was reported by patients. Satisfaction was enhanced, however, in those situations where the doctor was willing to engage in discussions of psychosocial issues.

The apparent reluctance of some doctors to accurately assess and treat the psychosocial concerns of the elderly (and as some have argued, psychosocial concerns in general--see Williamson, Beitman, & Katon [1981]) may ultimately have a detrimental effect on the health of their patients. A growing literature links psychosocial difficulties to stress, and stress to disease (Carroll, 1992; Doherty & Campbell, 1988; Schneiderman, McCabe, & Baum, 1992). Health professionals should target rather than ignore such difficulties.

IMPLICATIONS FOR HEALTH PROMOTION

The information in this chapter is organized around two central themes: first, that health promotion, in its most ideal form, involves contributions from health care professionals *and* patients, and secondly, that the communication that takes place during the medical encounter can powerfully influence a variety of outcomes, including patient satisfaction, compliance, and selected aspects of health status. (It should be remembered, how-ever, that to date, the first two of these outcomes have been the focus of much more research than the third.)

Recommendations

Informed in part by some of the research findings summarized above, the following recommendations are made to persons working to improve the health circumstances of the elderly:

Build a Relationship. Recognize that a critical aspect of the care that is provided involves the relationship that links the doctor (or other health care professional) and the elderly patient. Remember, too, that relationships are built over time. As part of this process, it is imperative that patients come to be appreciated as more than persons simply experiencing a variety of discrete illnesses. Part of relationship building includes getting a broadened appreciation of the life circumstances of the patient (Mishler, 1984). This information is indispensable in efforts that are geared toward treating the whole patient.

Strive for Partnerships with Patients. The early medical care experiences of many elderly patients were organized according to the activity-passivity model of doctor-patient interaction (Szasz & Hollender, 1956). However, many elderly patients respond very favorably (and in fact prefer) a more active involvement in their own care. When-ever possible, encourage active participation (Stewart, 1984; Stewart et al., 1995).

Encourage Assertiveness. Those who are interested in promoting the health of the elderly should teach them to be more assertive in their dealings with doctors (Kaplan et al., 1989). Patients need to be clear and open about the kinds of assistance they need. Health professionals need to appreciate that assertive patients are not necessarily "problem" patients.

Give Time. Health professionals should create opportunities for patients to provide complete, ideally uninterrupted descriptions of their medical problems, their ideas about them, and any accompanying concerns they may have. There is evidence that elderly patients become more participatory during health care visits (e.g., ask more questions, etc.) if they are given time to do so. A hurried medical encounter will not facilitate this process.

Take Time. Realize the optimal patient encounter may not be the shortest patient encounter. The complexity of the health circumstances of many elderly patients (e.g., multiple illnesses, multiple medications, etc.) demands that more time be taken to adequately assess the situation, and to make recommendations that are in concert with their needs. Realize too that shortcuts infrequently work. There is evidence that "attention to overlooked problems and active efforts to treat the whole patient can lead to substantial reductions in subsequent utilization" (Radecki et al., 1988b, p. 718; Rubinstein, Josephson, Wieland et al., 1984). Health professionals should unbalance on the side of giving more rather than less information to patients.

Develop and Use a Range of Interpersonal Skills. In addition to learning to listen to patients, develop teaching skills to better educate them about ways of improving their health circumstances. Demonstrate appropriate affective behavior during the medical encounter (Kaplan et al., 1989). Also, be empathic.

Attend to Differences. Health professionals need to remember that all elderly patients cannot be treated the same way. Factors such as gender, age, cultural, and social class can significantly influence the communication process. The health professional needs to be flexible and capable of adjusting his or her communicative behavior accordingly.

Learn About and from the Families of Elderly Patients. Learn about the support system of the elderly patient. The participation of others (as part of either problem assessment or intervention) is often crucial in efforts to address the health care needs of the elderly. Remember that the absence of a functional support system is a problem for many elderly persons. Recognize that the family may also require assistance, particularly in instances where care demands for the elderly are extreme. Health professionals should know how to intervene with families; the skills to do so are very learnable (McDaniel, Campbell, & Seaburn, 1990; Nichols & Schwartz, 1991).

Don't Ignore Psychosocial Matters. Many elderly patients must confront a number of interrelated medical and psychosocial concerns. Medical encounters should routinely include the opportunity to assess these concerns. Elderly patients should be encouraged to bring these matters to the attention of health professionals. Deciding to not attend to these concerns as part of a medical encounter does not make them go away. Health professionals should recognize that the assistance of a number of allied health professionals (e.g., psychologists, marital and family therapists, social workers, etc.) may be needed to adequately address the psychosocial concerns of the elderly (Waitzkin, 1991).

Show Respect.   When elderly patients receive medical care, they enter a world that is familiar and comfortable for the doctor, but often not for them. Medical encounters can be anxiety provoking, and sometimes very frightening. Health professionals should appreciate the vulnerability of elderly patients and do whatever they can to respect their dignity and self-worth (Haug & Ory, 1987).

CHAPTER SUMMARY

When patients visit their doctors, they generally do so to receive medical assistance. It needs to be recognized, however, that the communication that occurs between doctors and patients actually serves a number of interrelated purposes. To no small degree, it is via the communication process that the doctor and patient negotiate and define the relationship they share with one another (Ong et al., 1995). Similarly, it is through communication that essential information is exchanged by both parties. Ideally, patients are able to communicate openly and clearly with their doctors (and doctors to their patients) about the difficulties that precipitated the medical visit. And finally, it is through communication that the doctor can provide not only details and explanations concerning the difficulty that the patient is experiencing, but ultimately, recommendations that hopefully will solve the problem (Smith & Hope, 1991). The information presented in this chapter suggests that the ways that doctors and patients interact with one another can powerfully influence a number of important health outcomes. The interpersonal aspects of medical care should receive the very careful attention of all professionals who are working to promote the health of the elderly.

CHAPTER 13

PLANNING A HEALTHY RETIREMENT

Retirement should not catch any Americans by surprise. After all, Americans retiring today are the second generation to do so. Retirement has evolved into a normal expectation of life in industrialized nations. Almost all of us have witnessed our parents or another generation experiencing retirement. We all share the cultural expectation that our work lives will one day be over. But retirement does catch many Americans by surprise. Or perhaps it is more accurate to say that Americans are deceptively unprepared for retirement. As you read this chapter, you will come to understand what we mean by the words deceptively unprepared. You will also discover that there is no universal recipe for successful retirement. Different personalities have different retirement needs.

The keys to successful retirement are self-understanding, a feeling of self-worth, and the will and ability to survive emotionally. The will and need to seek new activities that develop integrity and function lie principally within the individual or the couple. But there is much that the organization or company can do to help employees make the self-understanding transition from work to retirement. This enabling process has been termed pre-retirement education or planning, and it is only now beginning to receive the attention it richly deserves.

RETIREMENT: A FLUID PROCESS

Gerontologists are concerned that retirement may sneak up on those aged 60 and above without proper planning or forethought. Retirement has evolved into a normal expectation of life in industrialized nations. We have experienced more than one generation of people having the privilege of retirement, yet, we have not made significant strides in raising pre-retirees' or their employers' awareness of the need for adequate planning for this significant life changing process. Today, each of us has had personal experience with at least one person retiring. We share fantasies about what we will do when we retire such as play golf or fish, travel, sleep late, or complete unfinished projects. But we also realize that the retirement process may look a lot different for the next generation than it did for previous ones because of financial and sociological changes.

On an average, women may anticipate 25 years in retirement and men may average about 16 years. Retirement will be something unique to each person. For example, retirement may mean the following: ceasing work altogether, becoming an entrepreneur and starting a business, finding other employment, trading in their home for a motor home and touring the countryside, spending more time with family and grandchildren, or volunteering more in the community.

When retirees are surveyed to find out their personal viewpoints with regards to "successful retirement," the following factors are commonly mentioned: (1) financial security, (2) health, (3) self-understanding, (4) a feeling of self-worth, (5) leisure interests, and (6) the will and strength to emotionally leave work behind. But, in reality, successful retirement may not be under the individual's control. Demographic changes, employer responses, economics, family dynamics, and disability are but a few key factors that dramatically affect successful retirement.

The Changing Demographics and Retirement

The term "retirement" is viewed very differently today than it was 10 years ago. Some of the changes that have occurred, with respect to retirement, are taking place on a national and policy level and are affecting current retirees as well as future generations. Many of the aforementioned are of concern because of the financial strains the aging population will impose on Social Security, employer pensions, and Medicare. Some of these changes include:

- The population is aging overall with the number of older Americans aged 65 or older projected to double by the year 2030 (U.S. Census, 1989).
- The "baby boom" generation (those born between the years of 1946–1964) is beginning to turn age 50. A group of people 78 million strong will be entering into retirement within 10–12 years.
- The baby boom generation which has altered every conceivable normative pattern, will be playing "financial catch-up" for their retirement, as they have not traditionally been a financial savings generation.
- The birth rates have decreased between the late 1960s and the 1970s, creating a "Birth Dearth" leaving a declining number of qualified entrants in the job market.
- Older workers are continuing to retire before their 65th birthday and, for the most part, have the financial means and physiological capacity to enjoy more years of non-work during retirement.
- An unprecedented amount of minorities will enter retirement age. We will see the percentage of minorities rise from 15% today, to 25% in the year 2030, and 33% in the year 2050 (U.S. Senate, 1991).
- Changes in the Social Security system will increase the age retirees will be eligible to collect benefits.
- The traditional family structure is changing and we are seeing an increase in singles living alone into retirement.
- Many retirees would still like to work part-time or in non-traditional jobs.

In the past two decades, demographics have changed significantly. These changes will greatly impact the process of retirement. The number of older Americans aged 65 or older will account for about 22% of the population in the year 2030 as opposed to 13% today. Most of this increase will occur between the years 2010–2030. Moreover, the number of adults aged 55 to 64 will increase by two-thirds. The number of those under age 55, however, will remain virtually unchanged (U.S. Bureau of the Census, 1989). If we look at retirement in terms of a process for all Americans, instead of a single event for predominately white males, we realize that we cannot separate minorities, labor force activity, economics, and health when predicting the future of retirement.

Our past research on the retirement process has been limited. Much of our past research was formulated by the 1969 work entitled the "Retirement Work Study" (RWS) (Jackson et al., 1996). The last interview for the RWS was conducted in 1979, which encompassed a survey of older Americans aged 58–63, primarily white men. In essence, to date, we have a fairly good understanding of anglo white men with respect to retirement, but we know very little about women and minorities. The 1992 study on retirement, entitled the "Health and Retirement Study" (HRS), is beginning to fill this void. The initial HRS, which is longitudinal in nature, was comprised of 12,000 men and women, aged 51–62, in 8,000 households and comprised of a good representation of minorities, primarily African Americans and Hispanic Americans. The survey contains information on demographics, health and disability status, housing, family dynamics, career history, retirement plans, financial status, and insurance.

An important finding of the HRS study is the changing demographics with regards to minorities. The future population of older adults will be comprised of significantly more minorities. If we use the year 2030 for those persons aged 65 and above, we can note that the Caucasian population will increase at a rate of 90%, the African American population by 250%, and the Hispanic American population by 400%. In essence, we will see the percentage of minorities rise from 15% today to 25% by the year 2030 and then to 33% by the year 2050 (U.S. Senate, 1991).

Employer Responses to Retirement

As we have mentioned, the term "retirement" is defined many ways today. When a person defines himself as "retired," we can no longer assume he has ceased work altogether. But, only about 3% of the entire workforce are working past the age of 65 and only about 11% of those 55–64 are still working (Porterfield, 1992). It was recognized that when the Social Security Program was initiated in 1935, the age of 65 was the "normal" age of retirement. The life expectancy in 1935, however, was only 45. Today our life expectancy exceeds 75 and those at age 65 are more healthy and educated as compared to 60 years ago. In 1935, the term retirement was synonymous with rest or respite after many years of hard work. But demographic changes have altered our view of retirement. Since 1935, there has been a decrease in the employment of older adults and an earlier availability of pension income. A recent trend, however, has been reflected by nearly 25% of all people who begin to receive Social Security benefits continuing to work for about one to three years. For the purpose of this chapter, we can safely assume that the term "retirement" is not synonymous with rest or respite or complete cessation of economic productivity.

Labor Force

We are experiencing an aging labor force which is middle-aged with fewer younger workers entering the workforce. By the year 2000, we may see youth workers (ages 16–24) account for only 16% of the workforce in specific industries. As a result, we will see the median age of the workforce increase from age 36 in the 1980s to age 39 or 40 at the end of the decade (Hardy, 1996). Other dramatic changes in the workforce are occurring as we shift away from product manufacturing toward a system based provision of services. A decline in medium-wage jobs in manufacturing caused by automation has also been experienced.

What are the potential impacts of these labor force changes? Some industries are feeling the pinch of not being able to hire enough younger workers to fill specific positions. Industries particularly affected are retailers, eating and drinking establishments, and other industries who have historically relied on entry, non-skilled labor. Many of these companies now have older workers who may not be as concerned about entry level pay or shorter hours of work. Some of the most notable company examples of this practice are McDonalds, Wal-Mart, and grocery food chains. Conversely, many manufacturing organizations have a high percentage of older workers, but are needing to "downsize" because of increased automation, merging of corporations, and fiscal prudence. The possible repercussions for older workers has been reliance by employers on early retirement packages, perhaps before the employee is financially or psychologically prepared to retire. However, if the financial package is attractive enough for older workers, many of these employees may opt to retire from the company. The employer may be faced, in turn, with losing many technically skilled employees who may be difficult to replace. In a study that was completed by the American Society for Personnel Administrators, Coberly (1991) found that: (1) 42% of the companies could not recruit qualified employees with good verbal and communicative skills and (2) 43% indicated that the applicants did not have good writing skills.

Early Retirement

Retirement may have been viewed 20 years ago as a single event or an activity that we were entitled to enjoy after years of faithful service to a company. But we did not anticipate that our public policies would change to encourage older adults to work longer than the usual age of 65, that people who are economically capable would actually retire much earlier than age 65, that many corporations would encourage early retirement incentive packages, that comparable replacement jobs at the age of 50 and over would be difficult to find, and that more women and minorities would retire to singlehood. Contrary to popular belief, the majority of older workers voluntarily retire early. When surveyed about why they chose to leave the workforce, Coberly (1991) found that retirees gave three principle reasons: (1) availability of full private pensions before age 65, (2) early retirement incentive programs, and (3) increased leisure. But, many retirees would like to continue working in some capacity. Coberly (1991) identified the following reasons as to why older adults would like to continue working past the age of 62 or 65: (1) 34% suggested financial reasons to pay for essentials, (2) 13%

needed to pay for medical expenses, (3) 17% would like to continue working to have extra spending money, and (4) 18% wanted something useful to do. Economists strongly suggest that the older worker's decision to work or retire is based primarily on the calculation of financial gains and losses associated with working. When older workers are asked if they would continue to work if their work schedule were flexible or they could work part-time, the over-wheeling majority indicated they would like to work part-time (68%), but only 6% to 8% wanted to work full-time (Jackson, 1996).

The continued decline in the average retirement age has forced employers to reassess current hiring and retention policies. By the age of 62, almost half of all men are considered out of the labor force. The early retirement scenario has taken some businesses by surprise because of the large cost of providing pensions and retiree health benefits for longer periods of time. One such study found that lowering the retirement age from 65 to 60 increased the benefit costs of a typical private pension by 69% (Jackson, 1996).

Facilitating the Needs of the Older Workers

Given the chance, more older adults would like to work if their work environment were flexible. Businesses and industry are evaluating how to best meet the needs of their older workers, while still meeting their own companies' economic challenges. Some of the creative work strategies employed by businesses include the following:

- Phased retirement—allowing the worker to retire gradually by decreasing the full-time employment over a set number of months or years.
- Partial retirement—part-time employment with no defined time limitation.
- Second career programs—offer partial payment of the older worker's salary for a determined amount of time for the employee to pursue an academic degree in a specified field. For example, IBM offers partial payment of the salary for two years while the individual who retires can pursue a degree in a technical or scientific field.
- Retirement rehearsal—to give a leave of absence for employees to "try out" retirement for usually 3 to 6 months and then they can make a determination to retire altogether or continue working.
- Part-time or job share—split one's position between two persons who want to work part-time.
- Retiree job bank—when the employer is short staffed, they can call in retirees instead of using temporary workers.
- Retirees as consultants—retain retirees as technical or managerial consultants.
- Volunteer opportunities—provide volunteer opportunities for those retirees who do not want a paid job.

Some of the well-known and innovative retirement programs are run by John Deere, Polaroid, IBM, Varion Associates, Motorola, and AT&T. These employers realize that older adults represent a very large group of people who possess wisdom, knowledge and skill level, and civic commitment. Today's older adults are healthy and have many more years of productive work to provide both to the workplace and the social community. When the "baby boom" generation enters their own "retirement age" in the years 2010–2030, we will see an even greater number of older adults desiring employment or volunteerism in their later years. Nearly 14 million older Americans aged 60 and over participate in volunteer work, much of which is done through religious organizations, health care facilities, senior citizen centers, and other service and civic organizations. It is estimated that such volunteer efforts represent over 1.1 million full-time employees and contribute about $17 billion annually to the American economy.

Research on retirement has increasingly illustrated the importance of examining retirement as an on-going process which involves a series of job changes rather than a single departure from a long-term career job. By examining job patterns, we notice that many older adults are working, but they may be involved in more non-traditional opportunities such as part-time work, self-employment, or volunteer work. We are also seeing an increase in older students returning to the universities to begin training for an entirely new career or attending university-sponsored Elderhostels, a non-credit educational-based experience.

If an older worker is involved in a sequence of part-time positions later in life, they may be trying to make a subtle transition from full-time paid employment to eventual ceasing of full-time employment. This type of transition has been called "bridge jobs." Most likely, part-time employment will be used to supplement a retiree's income and to facilitate more social interactions. Part-time work is viewed as more positive than full-time employment by older workers since it provides more leisure time to enjoy in their retirement. Many older workers use one or more bridge jobs between career employ-ment and complete retirement. Self-employment has also been a popular transitional stage in retirement. One reason that self-employment is more common among older workers is that those already self-employed in their career jobs tend to retire later than do wage and salary workers. Some of these part-time and self-employment opportuni-ties are bridge jobs between career work and retirement. Preliminary results from the 1992 HRS indicated the following: (1) There is a wide variety of retirement behaviors to be studied; (2) Bridge jobs continue to provide an important intermediate step in the retirement processes of a significant minority of older Americans; (3) There is a flow of workers into self-employment late in life, perhaps as a means of acquiring flexible hours and retiring gradually; (4) Women are more likely than men to utilize bridge jobs; (5) There are significant differences in current labor force status by ethnicity, with African Americans or Hispanics less likely than Anglos to be employed in the traditional retirement years; and (6) Much of the difference in retirement patterns by gender and some of the differences by race/ethnicity disappear when we concentrate only on those with a full-time, long-duration career job.

Economics of Retirement

Nearly two-thirds of American workers say they have saved something for retirement, but only one-third indicate that they have tried to determine what they will need according to a survey conducted by the Employment Benefit Research Institute and Greenwald and Associates (White House Conference Hearing, 1995). Of those persons surveyed, the majority of workers think that their lifestyle will improve with retirement, but when retirees were interviewed, they felt their lifestyle actually declined. Of those persons who admitted to not saving at all for retirement, 50% said that they expected a comfortable retirement. Yet, a careful review of financial planning assets for retirement does not support this viewpoint.

Income for retirement is usually divided into four areas: (1) Social Security, (2) Pensions, (3) Asset income, and (4) Employment earnings. At the retirement age of 65, pensions account for approximately 19% of retirement income (about $5,230 at the median for those receiving a private pension) and asset income accounts for about 19% (about $1,720 at the median) of the retirement income (White House Conference Hearing, 1995).

As illustrated in Table 13-1, Social Security and earnings make up the majority of retirement income. But many people do not realize that only 45% of retirees receive income from pensions. About 55% work for employers who provide a pension, but only 43% are vested in the plan so they can draw benefits (White House Conference Hearing, 1995). Moreover, about three out of every ten women participate in a basic pension plan because their working career has historically been more sporadic. The workers who are most likely to be covered by pension plans are from large firms (representing 1,000 or more employees) in the public sector and those in manufacturing jobs.

The predominate type of pension that employers provide has changed over the years. Since 1970, the proportion of defined contribution plans in the private sector has grown from 67% to 82%. In the defined contribution plans, the risk lies with the workers. If funds are adequately invested and managed successfully, then upon retirement, a worker can conceivably have a large sum of money to help finance their retirement. About 33% of those retirees, age 65 and over, have a pension income, with a median value of $6,240 (White House Conference Hearing, 1995). For those retiring with a defined contribution plan, the average value is about $98,500 with $4,800 being the average yearly retirement benefit.

Because of the uncertain financial future for baby boomers, there will be a need for future retirees to improve their retirement income security. There will undoubtedly be an increase in tax-deferred savings as education improves with this next age cohort. While these workers may not be able to influence the types of pensions their employers offer, they will be able to set up personal savings plans in response to the type and level of pension benefits they expect. Moreover, there are considerable differences between Caucasians and other minorities with regard to earnings or income. Minorities consistently have less earnings or income and are less likely to own a home. If they do own a home, their net equity will likely be less.

Table 13-1. Retirement income sources for older households

	Age 62-64	Age 65-69	Age 75-79	Age 85+
Social Security	13.5%	29.8%	46.2%	50.5%
Earnings	56.4	28.9	8.5	3.8
Pensions	14.8	18.8	19.1	12.6
Asset Income	11.1	18.7	22.3	28.1
Other	3.8	3.0	3.0	4.2

Other income includes Veterans' benefits and public assistance; Pensions include private and public sector pensions. Among households 65-69 years old, Social Security makes up 29.8% of total income. (Source: U.S. Department of Labor, 1994).

Approximately 26% of the total income for the elderly comes from assets, more than double the percentage two decades ago. Since minorities traditionally have less assets, they will continue to experience retirement with less resources and will have less private resources for future health care costs. Also, we must consider the lack of available and adequate health insurance coverage for minorities because of economic variances. Hispanics have extremely low levels of health insurance coverage, even more than other minority groups, with the lack being more pronounced for Mexican Americans. There are few alternatives for the working poor who hold jobs that do not provide health insurance and who do not qualify for Medicaid. Health and wellness in retirement is directly related to higher income and proper medical care (Hardy, 1996; Myers, 1996; Shea, 1996).

Changing Trends in Family Dynamics

Families are experiencing a change in many different areas with respect to marital status and lowered economic levels. These changes are pronounced for minorities. In 1960, 53% of all women in the United States, aged 65 and above, were widowed. Today, only 37.2% of women are widowed. This change is due to the declining mortality among men which has outweighed the higher probability that women would survive after their spouse's death. Other trends are in the areas of divorce. In 1960, only 1.5% of older women were divorced as compared to 13.2% in 1990. The negative effect on the incomes of women who are either widowed or divorced are very much alike because women marry less quickly than do men and spend longer years without the economic advantages of marriage. Even for those women who do remarry, they may find themselves economically disadvantaged because men in second marriages may hold premarital assets separately from their spouse, may have already split assets with the first spouse, and may leave a share of other assets to children in a previous marriage. Only a quarter of African American households are in a marriage that is the first for both spouses. Currently, the combined percentage of households experiencing a divorce or widowhood is greater than the number of traditional lifetime married households; a significant change from two decades ago. We do realize now that the stability of a marriage through the survivorship of both partners characterizes only one of two Caucasian women and is not the norm for African American women. Women and African Americans spend more years outside marriage, with African Americans experiencing higher rates of early marriage separations and less percentages of remarriage. Since gerontologists are now aware of this information, they may begin to instruct minorities and women on how best to prepare for their future retirement years (Holden, 1996).

Disability and Retirement

Chronic conditions may be occurring at younger ages for non-Anglos. The HRS indicates that the likelihood of poor health for both African American men and women is greater than their Caucasian counterparts. The ability of African Americans to work until older age is diminished, which probably forces them to have greater dependence for public assistance in post-retirement years (Wray, 1995). African Americans in poor health are much more likely to leave the labor force at an earlier time than Caucasians in poor health. Since many African Americans are in more physically demanding jobs, they may be unable to continue working with chronic problems and have more difficulty finding other work once their health has been compromised.

In the HRS, the following information was gathered with regards to self-reporting of physical functioning. Slightly over one-half of African American women reported some difficulty in physical functioning as compared with one-third of men. Those difficulties in physical functioning reported were alcohol abuse, body mass, arthritis, and respiratory illnesses. Also, the women reported having a greater prevalence and severity in six of nine chronic diseases and more pain. For men, the physical functioning difficulties were reported as alcohol abuse, smoking, body mass, diabetes, heart disease, cerebrovascular disease, arthritis, and pain. It should be noted that for both groups these conditions are preventable and manageable. However, many minorities do not have the financial means to retire early because of lack of pension plans or other financial assets, but they may have no choice if they are unable to physically work because of their chronic illnesses. Even at higher levels of wealth, African Americans are more likely to report being in fair or poor health and less likely to report being in excellent health. Those in poor health have dramatically lower wealth than those in better health (Shea, Miles, & Hayward, 1996).

Because of the many societal changes that were referred to at the beginning of the chapter, we realize that "retirement" is not a single event, but a fluid process that will be unique to every person who is experiencing it. We realize that "business as usual" in facilitating the needs of the future generation of retirees will not work in the 21st century. For some, retirement is a new stage of life altogether with its own unique organizations such as the American Association of Retired Persons (AARP), with its own economic and legal infrastructure. To others, retirement may indicate only a slight change from their normal routine of their past working career as they replace these full-time positions.

PRE-RETIREMENT EDUCATION

The objectives of pre-retirement education or planning are to help participants retain independence, cope with the physiological changes of aging, and enhance or maintain one's quality of life in later years. Yet, it is predicted that less than one quarter of employees will receive any type of pre-retirement training from their employers. Most employees are forced to seek retirement assistance from such specialists as attorneys, insurance agents, accountants, and stockbrokers. Even when sponsored by employers, pre-retirement planning takes on many different formats. Some of the larger corporations may offer comprehensive planning courses over a period of several days for employees as young as 40, while others may provide a "crash course" for a few hours to those about ready to retire. Key areas addressed in comprehensive sessions include finances, legal issues, private insurance and Medicare, Social Security, benefits, and social concerns. Of those employers who do offer some training, they usually say they do so to ease a retiree into early retirement, for good-will, or to make certain the employee is aware of the retirement benefit options. Many employers utilize in-house staff to cover the areas of benefits and some finances, but may invite outside specialists in the areas of Social Security, law, health, or social concerns. In this section, we discuss the content/format of corporate programs and six key issues for pre-retirement education.

Content/formats of Corporate Pre-retirement Programs

Like other educational ventures, corporate pre-retirement programs can be measured by content and format. Ossofsky (1980) graded programs on a content continuum of narrow to broad. Programs covering topical areas of three or less were defined as "narrow"; four to seven, "intermediate" and eight or more, "broad". Table 13-2 identifies the actual topics covered.

Program format was graded similarly. "Narrow" programs tended to heavily emphasize printed materials and counseling. "Intermediate" programs, while also relying on printed materials, were more likely to be conducted in a group rather than in private settings. "Broad" programs not only used printed materials and both individual and group sessions, but also included continued contact with retirees through follow-up activities and social clubs. Table 13-3 summarizes the formats of the companies surveyed.

In discussing program content and format, it is important to differentiate between pre-retirement programs that focus on counseling and those that focus on planning. Counseling programs are designed to develop favorable attitudes toward retirement and thus promote good adjustment in retirement. Planning programs serve as an information-disseminating and planning stimulant instrument. Regardless of this differentiation, both types of programs are generally conceived of as being charged with a counseling function. However, the overwhelming majority of pre-retirement programs consist of a brief lecture series that serves only the dissemination objective.

Table 13-2. Topics covered by retirement-preparation program as reported by personnel directors.

	= reported by more than 50% (of respondents)		
	Narrow	Intermediate	Broad
Social Security and Medicare	77%	87%	98%
Financial benefits and options	73	85	97
Physical and mental health	14	81	100
Leisure	9	76	100
Legal aspects	23	68	98
Employment	0	28	92
Housing	0	40	90
Community resources	5	49	88
Options for employment after retirement	18	19	83
Interpersonal relations	9	25	68
Life planning	14	21	61
	*	*	*
	(22)	(53)	(59)

*Adds up to more than 100 percent because individuals gave more than one answer.
Source: Developed by J. Ossofsky, "Retirement Preparation: Growing Corporate Involvement," *Aging and Work*, Winter 1980, p. 8. Used by permission of The National Council on the Aging, Washington, D.C.

Table 13-3. Formats of retirement-preparation programs as reported by personnel directors

	= reported by more than 50% (of respondents)		
	Narrow	Intermediate	Broad
Printed materials	78%	95%	100%
Individual counseling	57	64	91
Lectures and seminars	17	79	97
Outside experts	9	75	94
Audio-visual materials	9	67	91
Discussion groups	4	61	94
Continuing contact after retirement	35	47	91
Follow-up individual programs	9	35	66
Social clubs for retirees	4	19	63
Surveys to measure effectiveness of programs	4	28	63
Simulation exercises	0	10	28
	*	*	*
	(23)	(81)	(32)

*Adds up to more than 100 percent because individuals gave more than one answer.
Source: Developed by J. Ossofsky, "Retirement Preparation: Growing Corporate Involvement," *Aging and Work*, Winter 1980, p. 8. Used by permission of The National Council on the Aging, Washington, D.C.

Proponents of pre-retirement programs tend to lobby for counseling-oriented programs. It is their thesis that in a work-oriented society the individual who suddenly shifts from work to non-work life undergoes a transitional crisis and counseling is needed to deal with this crisis.

The evidence from the 1992 HRS and other researchers suggests that pre-retirement planning is still in a developmental stage and just now beginning to receive the attention it deserves. A statement made in the early 1960s by the U.S. Civil Service Commission is still appropriate today: "Many employers, both public and private, have a watchful, wait-and-see attitude, accompanied by a strictly limited program or none at all, because they think that the right and wrong answers have not been found in this relatively new area of personnel management" (1961, p. 6).

Six Issues of Pre-retirement Education

Because of all the social, psychological, and economic ramifications of retirement, it is essential to plan for this life stage. Enrollment in pre-retirement education programs is often the pre-retiree's first serious step in acknowledging these ramifications. As Wampler noted in his prepared statement before the Subcommittee Hearing on Retirement Income and Employment, "Prospective retirees who prepare for their needs and demands usually meet retirement with realistic expectations and are more capable of making their retirement years challenging, satisfying and rewarding" (1978, p. 2).

Yet there continues to be resistance to participating in pre-retirement education programs. This resistance is consistent whether the programs are conducted in community, educational, or corporate settings. Even though the "aging myths and barriers" have lessened, some older workers may not be ready to accept their own "aging process" and, subsequently, will opt not to participate in a scheduled pre-retirement education program. Breaking down people's resistance to pre-retirement planning will require destroying the myths and stereotypes about aging and retirement. The key is to emphasize the concept that retirement can be an opportunity to take up new challenges. In order to stress the "challenge" concept, pre-retirement education programs must address six issues: (1) How should pre-retirement programs be conducted to stimulate planning awareness and development? (2) What should be the relative roles of the community, education, government, and the corporate sector in delivering pre-retirement programs? (3) What needs should be met by an adequate retirement education program? (4) What is the role of the pre-retirement program coordinator? (5) How can we motivate people to participate? (6) Are there any good prepackaged retirement education programs?

How Should Pre-retirement Education Programs Be Conducted?

To make pre-retirement educational sessions valuable, the materials presented, both verbal and written, have to be delivered in a challenging way. The responsibility of the pre-retirement facilitator is to structure an environment where the received information can be manipulated in novel situations that meet the personal needs of the participants.

The environmental factors that need to be considered are: (1) program format, (2) location, (3) program length, (4) participant age, and (5) program size.

Program Format. Program formats are generally classified as group seminars or forum discussion groups. A comprehensive pre-retirement program will make use of both of these format types. The group seminar is used to provide an introduction to broad-based informational concepts. Smaller forum discussion groups are then formed to allow pre-retirees to apply this information to their own planning needs. Feedback in small settings is less intimidating and more natural since they allow the program to become the property of the participants and workshop leader. The more intimate nature of the discussion groups encourages give and take among pre-retirees so that they can learn from one another's experiences. Spouses or significant others are encouraged to join both the seminars and the forum discussions in order to facilitate couple strategy. It is not uncommon for smaller companies to provide only one-to-one retirement benefit counseling without incurring the time and expense of more lengthy programs.

Location. The location choice is simply to offer the pre-retirement program on or off the company premises. There are advantages to using either location. Advantages for conducting the program on the company premises include (1) lower cost because of the avoidance of potentially expensive meal costs and rental fees for meeting rooms and audio-visual equipment, (2) convenience, and (3) the introduction of the pre-retiree's spouse (or friend) to the employee's work environment. Advantages for locating the program outside the company include (1) feeling of ease in delving into personal matters that may be inhibited by the work environment, (2) fewer work interruptions, and (3) feelings of receiving a special fringe benefit because the program is conducted away from the job.

Choosing a location involves more than just tallying advantages and disadvantages. The key is to provide a nonrestrictive environment that will freely allow pre-retirees to confront their personal retirement needs.

Length of the Program. Two distinct lengths for pre-retirement education programs tend to be popular: (1) 8-week programs and (2) one or two 8-hour sessions. The 8-week programs consist of weekly two-hour sessions generally presented in consecutive weeks. If the number of sessions offered during the 8-week period is sufficient, in-depth discussions of novel retirement situations are possible.

The consecutive 8-week program presents logistical drawbacks in that a facility must be made available for a long period of time. Absenteeism and the possibility that a spouse or friend may not be able to make such a long-range commitment are also factors that must be considered. But it is our opinion that the 8-hour session has a more severe drawback. It requires conveying too much material in a very short period of time. A tendency in the intensive-length program is to laden the participants with too many questionnaires and material, with insufficient time for them to learn to apply this information in personal or novel situations. It is for this reason that most experts recommend sessions be confined to 2 hours.

Age of Participant. At what age should people be offered pre-retirement education? The answer depends on the content of the program entirely. Financial advisors would like to see people exposed to this aspect of planning in their 30s or 40s. Leisure educators also believe people in that age range should begin making plans about their leisure lifestyle. However, since retirees can possibly live many years after retirement, the attitude is becoming more prevalent that it is never too late to make retirement plans even if the person has already retired from one job. But most people do not show interest in retirement planning until they are in their mid 50s. Moreover, many companies do not provide planning programs until one to two years before the individual is scheduled to retire. Because of the many different circumstances that may either hasten or slow down predicted retirement dates for employees in corporations, proper retirement education planning may never be carried through satisfactorily. Prevailing attitudes suggest that those under age 50 are not yet interested in retirement, and those over age 65 are already retired and the retirees may erroneously perceive it as being too late for much of the planning.

Program Size. Retirement education programs have been conducted for individuals, groups as small as 8, or as large as 500. For the most interactive format, the ideal group size is between 10–25 participants. Group seminar programs that present generic material can handle much larger numbers of participants. However, reliance on group discussions should limit the size of groups to no more that 20 participants.

What Should Be the Relative Roles of the Public and Private Sectors?

The modern labor force is characterized by diversification and specialization. Thus no one institution or segment of the workforce can effectively design and implement a pre-retirement program to satisfy the whole. The needs of the employees who are blue-collar and white-collar, low income, high income, and ethnically diversified must be taken into consideration. Therefore federal, state, and local government, labor and management industry, public and private educational institutions and community-based organizations such as recreation or senior centers all play an integral role.

Because retirement preparation programs are still in the developmental stage, there is at present no real coordination among government, industry, educational, and community-based agencies. Many of these agencies claim they have the ideal approach for retirement planning, but because the retirement process is so complex, it is evident that a coordination of the aforementioned agencies will strengthen most pre-retirement educational programs.

What Needs Should Be Met by Any Adequate System of Pre-retirement Preparation?

The purposes of pre-retirement education programs are to provide current and factual information, to encourage active planning, and to inspire positive thinking about the retirement process. The fundamental premise governing pre-retirement programs is that obstacles are much easier to overcome in retirement when the individual has some idea of what to expect beforehand. Some common barriers that may exist for retirees are the following: (1) the change of relationships as a result of geographic moves, death, loss of close friends, (2) changes in relationships that are needed for one's emotional stability, and (3) lack of planning for retirement to develop alternative lifestyle habits.

The basic areas of concerns that are usually covered in the planning workshops include (1) financial planning which includes pension benefits, Social Security, investments, insurance, and estate planning, (2) legal planning which includes wills, estate planning, gifts, and bequests, (3) health and welfare which includes physical health, mental health, social health, spiritual health, housing, and transportation, and (4) leisure which includes alternative careers, community service, volunteerism, formal and informal educational opportunities, leisure activities, and hobbies.

The coordinator of these sessions is not expected to be knowledgeable in all the program topics associated with these areas of concern. Instead, the coordinator should familiarize herself with the speaker resources available within the community. Physicians, registered nurses, financial planners, bankers, attorneys, Social Security representatives, insurance agents, educators, community health centers, clergy, and private gerontology consultants are only a few possible resources available for the program. These sources will vary from community to community, but usually the reception is positive for using these outside "experts."

What Is the Role of the Pre-retirement Program Coordinator?

Coordinators often despair at not being able to cover all pertinent topics. It should be remembered, however, that the pre-retirement program is the initial, not the complete, effort to acquaint the pre-retiree with retirement options and alternatives. The coordinator is charged with setting the program sequence so that it is tailored to meet the needs and backgrounds of a particular group. A flexible action-oriented and experience-based learning model should be designed. Pre-retirement Planning Center, Inc., describes the five phases of an action-oriented program: (1) audience analysis, (2) establishing objectives, (3) design of the learning situation, (4) field research, and (5) feedback on the preceding four phases.

Audience analysis involves carefully researching the knowledge, attitudes, values and needs of program participants. Using this background information, objectives are established according to the areas of concern listed earlier in this section. Sub-objectives for these areas of concern are used to create the instructional outline, and materials are collected, prepared, and tested (design). A pilot run of the program is used to make revisions and refinements. When the coordinator is satisfied with the program content, field research is conducted to determine the effectiveness of the instruction among program participants. The fifth and final phase is feedback on the other four phases. This feedback process allows further evaluation and refinement of the program material and instructional design.

How Can We Motivate People to Participate in Pre-retirement Programs?

John Anderson, one of the first to be concerned with encouraging adults to prepare for retirement, advocated the premise that one motivates the adult learner in the same way that one motivates the very young learner; namely by structuring educational experiences so that the participant experiences success and accomplishment.

The reasons adults fail to become involved in pre-retirement programs may include: (1) lack of interest until on the verge of retirement, (2) suspicion that involvement will somehow hasten their retirement, (3) negative stereotypes of the aging process, or (4) corporation's failure to recognize pre-retirement education programs as a necessary expense. As one would surmise, the success of the program will be based on the quality of the program format, the atmosphere and the teaching style of the educators, and the way in which the process of aging and retirement is portrayed.

Are There Model Pre-retirement Education Programs?

There are many programs that have been successful in the past and newer ones that have emerged in later years. Some of the most notable ones are from large organizations that specifically delve with older adult issues such as: American Association of Retired Persons (AARP), The National Council on Aging (NCOA), The American Society on Aging (ASA), and the Retirement Research Foundation. Literally thousands of planned programs have been initiated in the past 10 years which usually cover the basic five topics for retirement education, provide audio/videotapes, trainers' manuals, and participant workbooks. Many of these programs are a good foundation, but the cost can be extremely high. Usually the best approach is to have a guidebook to work with, but develop an individualized pre-retirement planning session based on the needs of the specific audience.

CHAPTER SUMMARY

Retirement is no longer viewed as a simple termination of people's working years, as a single life event, or as an end to productive life. Increasingly, it is seen as a dynamic transition and process for many years to come and it signifies that a person is eligible for a pension, if one is available. The segment of the American population that is retired from work will continue to expand well into the 21st century. Many of these Americans can expect to enjoy 20–30 years of living after formerly retiring. Our focus so far has been on pre-retirement education. A number of experimental retirement education planning programs have been developed. We can expect continued efforts to identify ways and means to encourage the appropriate use of the talents and skills of older Americans.

Americans who are now in their 30s and 40s may live longer than today's retirees, may not retire as early (or may be unable to retire at all), and may not be able to rely as heavily on Social Security and private pensions. The important point is that during the past half century, we have changed the ground rules for old-age security. In creating the social institution of retirement, we have created new responsibilities for the individual. The individual must plan for that significant portion of his or her life called retirement because we have greatly curtailed both the opportunity and the right to work for the older person.

Retirees are expected to remain independent and make it on their own in a complex society. Because dependency is scorned by both the individual and American society, retirement poses a major threat to the individual. Pre-retirement programs are needed not just to maintain financial security in later life, but also to preserve dignity and meaning in those years. Preparation therefore should be a joint effort by the employer and the employee. The benefits of joint planning between the corporation and the employee are reflected by the major goals of pre-retirement programs.

Robert Atchley notes that the "ritual of retirement" is not standardized like weddings, funerals and graduations. We experience varying degrees of celebration of one's retirement from grand ceremonies to a simple "thank you" as the retiree leaves their full-time employment. Too often the speeches given by the management staff during the retirement celebration are a reminder of the worker's past and very little about the rite of passage a person may experience during retirement years, which could easily be another 20–30 years. A retiree's health and well-being physically, financially, and socially contributes vitally to the success of the "third age of life" or the retirement process. The process, just as any other time of life, is varied and not the same for everyone. Retirement success will be dependent on the time and effort the retiree and the family spent in planning for the third age.

CHAPTER 14

ETHNICITY AND HEALTH PROMOTION

As our population both grows older and becomes more ethnically diverse it becomes important to recognize the increasingly significant relationship between cultural diversity and health status. One's ethnicity suggests a common history and effects an individual's beliefs about family rules, role status, and values. More specifically, one's ethnic background may play a major role in their choice of food, rituals, relationships and responses to major life transitions. For elderly individuals and their families, ethnic background may have an impact on decisions about nursing homes, frequency of contact with family members, and even decisions about health care (McGoldrick, 1988). Interestingly, the reasons for certain choices informed by one's ethnicity may occur outside of that individuals awareness (McGoldrick, 1988). For example, the relationship of an Asian American eldest son toward his father might at times defy explanation for those unaware of cultural rules.

It also appears to be true that as individuals age they increase their identification with their culture (Gelfand, 1982). This increased focus on cultural beliefs may even create distance between the elderly individual and their children who have not yet reached that developmental stage, and could potentially result in generational friction (Markides & Black, 1996). Thus, as our population ages and becomes more ethnically diverse it seems to be critical that health professionals recognize the importance of ethnicity and cultural beliefs when developing programs.

Culturally sensitive and knowledgeable professionals should first understand the belief systems of ethnically diverse populations. This knowledge will help them develop programs which can build upon the strengths of diverse groups and increase the likelihood of positive outcomes. Yet, despite advances in health care delivery and an increased awareness that the United States is a multicultural society, substantial differences in the health of racial groups in this country persist.

ETHNICITY AND THE CURRENT HEALTH CARE SYSTEM

This section will be an examination of the relationship between the expanding minority population in the United States and their treatment by the health care system. Between 1980 and 1990 the United States experienced a 107% increase in the Asian American population, a 53% increase in the Hispanic/Latino population, and a 13.2% increase in the number of African Americans. All of these increases clearly exceed the total population growth of 9.8% since 1980. While there has been an increase in the number of minority individuals living in this country the overall health status of African Americans and other minorities continues to be poor (Braithwaite & Lythcott, 1989). According to Heckler (1985) between 1950 and 1980 African American males and females had a 40–70% higher age adjusted all-cause mortality rate when compared with whites. The report of the United States Department of Health and Human Services (1985) goes on to point out that in 1982 white males had a life expectancy of 71.5 years compared to a life expectancy of 64.9 years for black males. There also appeared to be a significant difference between white females with a life expectancy of 79 years and black females with an expectancy of approximately 72 years. More recently (Thomas, 1990) found that the life expectancy for African Americans was 6.2 years less than for whites. The data seems to suggest that while the population of minority individuals continues to grow, the disparity in preventable death and/or extending life between minority and white populations continues to exist.

African Americans have higher mortality rates from heart disease, stroke, cancer, diabetes, and cirrhosis of the liver (Yee & Weaver, 1994). The majority of deaths from these causes (54%) occurs before age 65 for African American males.

The six leading causes of death combined, accounted for more than 80% of the mortality observed among African American and other minority groups. Of these causes: cancer, cardiovascular disease and stroke, chemical dependency, diabetes, homicides, accidents, and infant mortality all are causes of death which might be impacted by comprehensive health promotion programs. Thomas (1990) argues that the risk factors for each disease category are potentially modifiable but in some cases appear to be resistant to change. In addition to the biologics and factors related to mortality he lists "unemployment, crime, the high cost of living, inadequate education and racism" as sources of excess death among minority groups (Thomas, 1990).

It appears, however, that current health care and promotion efforts are ineffective in eliminating these differences. Thomas (1990) and more recently Wallerstein (1992) suggest that traditional health promotion activities focused on voluntary personal change behavior alone may not be effective. Programs that primarily focus on viewing illness as a result of the continuation of negative behaviors by unmotivated individuals will continue to fail. The belief is that this type of individual approach alone ignores many of the systemic issues that contribute to poor health in minority communities and only blames the victim for their current condition. Wallerstein (1992) calls for empowerment education programs that build upon community participation, cooperation, and control. Neighbors, Braithwaite and Thompson (1995) seem to agree, arguing that it is impossible to improve health and health promotion activities among the powerless. They suggest that one method for empowering communities is to give them control and full participation in the development of health promotion programs.

The use of outreach activities and health information campaigns may also serve to provide minority groups with knowledge about health care problems. Minority populations may be less knowledgeable or aware about some specific health care problems and this lack of knowledge may be at least one factor related to different health outcomes (Heckler, 1985). More specifically, African Americans and Hispanics have less information about cancer and heart disease. It also appears that minority group members tend to underestimate the prevalence of cancer, give less credence to the warning signs of cancer, get fewer screening tests and as a consequence are diagnosed at later stages than nonwhites. Hispanic women seem to have less information about breast cancer and only 25% of Hispanic women have heard of breast self-examination. In addition, many hypertensive Japanese women are less aware of their hypertension than nonminority women and among Mexican Americans, cultural attitudes regarding obesity and diet are often barriers to achieving weight control (Heckler, 1985). Examining all of this information suggests the need for the development of programs providing health information targeting these underserved groups.

The relationship between health care outcomes and the development of comprehensive health promotion programs was examined by Williams (1990) who argued that medical care alone accounted for only 10% of the variation in health status. For example, reductions in cigarette smoking and cholesterol were responsible for 54% of the decline in heart disease mortality while medical interventions were responsible for only 40%. Thus, it appears to be possible to have a greater impact on morbidity and mortality through additional expenditures on formal education than through additional expenditure on medical care alone.

According to Julia (1996) many ethnic groups were also chronically underserved by the health care community. For example, Escarce et al. (1993) found that white elders received more procedures and diagnostic tests and appeared to have greater access to more advanced technology than African Americans. They concluded that these differences could not be explained by "differences in the prevalence of specific clinical conditions" and that "Race may exacerbate the impact of other barriers to access (p. 948)."

There also appeared to be a number of other differences in the delivery of health care to minority populations. For example, a higher percentage of African Americans and Hispanics reported that they have no usual source of medical care. This lack of continuity of care seems to be particularly critical when most major killers of minority individuals are chronic not acute. It appears that African Americans and Hispanics use physician offices less often then hospitals and emergency rooms as their usual source of medical care. Thus, follow-up care suffers. In general, this type of inconsistent care is more expensive and less effective. In addition, this lack of continuity and years of less than optimal treatment have resulted in minority individuals having a mistrust of the medical system.

What one finds based on the available literature is a system that has failed to address the distinctive needs of minority groups. The reasons for this failure are many but include systemic racism, a lack of awareness about cultural differences on the part of health care professionals, few minority health professionals and a refusal of the system to be flexible enough to build upon the strengths of each community it serves.

ETHNICITY AND AGING

While there has been some research done on the relationship between health care and ethnicity there appears to be few studies examining the health status of minority elders and the health promotion and disease prevention programs directed toward them. Research, however, does suggest that ethnic and racial minorities are more likely to develop chronic health conditions and suffer disabilities as they age (Jackson, Lockery, & Juster, 1996). In a recent study (Gold, Pieper, Westlund, & Blazer, 1996) examining a large group of older adults as part of the Established Populations for Epidemiologic Studies of the Aging at Duke University, the authors found that minority individuals were at greater risk for hypertension. Others have pointed out that minority elders tend to underutilize services that could enhance their health status and quality of life (Mui & Burnett, 1994). In addition, they often have to travel further to get medical care at facilities often viewed as intimidating (Coke & Twaite, 1995).

Ethnic minority elders have a variety of cultural health beliefs that must be addressed by any health promotion program and a lack of recognition of cultural health beliefs only serves as a barrier for delivering effective programs. One cultural problem exposed by Coke and Twaite (1995), is that many health care systems are staffed by whites who lack the ability to communicate effectively with older African Americans. When these beliefs however, are taken into account they can serve as a powerful tool for helping minority elders adopt new health practices (Yee & Weaver, 1994).

AWARENESS OF DIFFERENT CULTURES

One significant step for health promotion specialists working with multicultural groups is to become aware of specific group characteristics and beliefs that can be useful when structuring programs or during interactions. In general according to Holmes and Holmes (1995) there are a number of differences in life experiences, behaviors, and beliefs between minority and white cultures. For example, they state that minority individuals see old age as more of a reward than a disaster. They suggest that minority elders have fewer anxieties about old age and are considered less prone to commit suicide. They describe minority families as being more tolerant of behavioral peculiarities in elderly persons and more willing to expect greater participation from elders in family matters. Overall, while minority individuals also feel less integrated into society they appear to participate to a larger extent in religious organizations.

The purpose of this section is not to stereotype different groups but to sensitize health providers to the range of behaviors and beliefs held by different groups. The hope is that with increased awareness health providers will be in a better position to improve the quality of their care and act in a culturally sensitive fashion.

American Indians

Native Americans come from 460 distinct tribal groups that have different disease patterns (Morley, 1992). The available literature examining health promotion activities for American Indian elderly appears to be quite sparse. Overall, the health status of American Indians is below that of the general population. The five leading causes of death for those over 65 are:

1. heart disease
2. cancers
3. cerebrovascular diseases
4. pneumonia
5. diabetes

The diversity of Native American tribes, however, may make it difficult to generalize from population specific data. For example, diabetes mellitus appears to be particularly prevalent in the Pima, Papago, Seminole, Upland Yuman, and Seneca (Ghodes, 1986). According to Williams and Boyce (1989) elderly Navajo patients are particularly at risk for protein-energy malnutrition.

In addition, alcohol abuse continues to be a leading cause of health problems among American Indians and Alaskan Natives (Yee & Weaver, 1994). The issue of alcohol abuse within the American Indian population should, however, be addressed prior to older age.

Any health promotion program targeting a Native American population must take into account a belief system that focuses on the relationship between person, nature, and the universe. Healing requires a restoration of balance between mind, body, and spirit. As people age their diseases may be seen as part of a developmental process, not necessarily something to be remedied. Issues that health promotion programs must focus on include an examination of the reasons for poor compliance with medical regimens and cultural beliefs that affect nutrition (Yee & Weaver, 1994). Since it also appears that Native Americans physiologically age earlier than other populations, preventive services need to be provided to them in their mid-fifties (Morley, 1992).

African Americans

African Americans are the largest minority group in the United States and have proportionally more older adults than any other minority group (Winbush, 1996). Overall, the health status of African Americans appears to be worse than whites and they suffer higher mortality rates from heart disease, stroke, cancer, diabetes, and cirrhosis of the liver. Unfortunately, according to Yee and Weaver (1994), the majority of these deaths (at least 54%) occurs before age 65 for African American males. According to Kerner et. al. (1993) the life expectancy of an African American male growing up in Harlem is lower then that of a male growing up in Bangladesh. For females the same comparison is accurate once they reach 5 years of age.

The primary institutions within the African American community are the family and the church followed by social and political organizations. For many individuals religion appears to be related to health beliefs and prayer is seen as a common method for treating health-related concerns, particularly among the middle class and older adults (Winbush , 1996).

African Americans appear to be less likely to have a primary care physician and are most likely to receive their care in hospital outpatient departments, emergency rooms, and health centers. These findings, however, may be due to income rather than ethnicity yet they nonetheless have consequences for the health of many in the African American community who do not have access to regular health care. When compared to whites proportionally twice as many African Americans are without health insurance. Of those who had no insurance, 35% did not see a physician during the past 12 months compared to 22% for those who did have insurance (Heckler, 1985). Thus it appears that if you do not have insurance you are left without health promotion information and easy access to the health care system. In addition, when you do get sick you head to the emergency room and ultimately increase the cost of care.

The health belief system in African American communities suggests that illness is often caused by the neglect of one's own body, following an inappropriate diet or ingesting impurities (Yee & Weaver, 1994). For many who also believe in traditional cultures there is a strong belief in spiritualism that might attribute illness to demons or evil spirits (Winbush, 1996). Elderly individuals may delay medical care due to cost, mistrust of the system, and/or a belief that there is not much that can be done. Feeling fine translates into being cured and with certain illnesses such as hypertension, these beliefs may result in increased levels of noncompliance.

Overall, there remains a large gap in morbidity and mortality when comparing African American to white populations. There appears to be a need for the development of culturally sensitive health promotion programs in order to narrow and ultimately close that gap.

Asian Americans

Asian and Pacific Islander elders appear to be generally healthier then all other groups including whites. They do, however, have higher rates of TB, hepatitis, anemia, and hypertension. There appears to be a bimodal distribution when examining issues of health with the success of some masking the severe problems of others (Tanjasiri, Wallace, & Shibata, 1995).

Since Asian Americans are an extremely heterogeneous population coming from a broad geographic region with multiple identities there are certain subgroups whose health appears to be poor. Asian Americans fled their countries due to war and resettled in the United States with about 40% living in California. According to Chung (1996) there has been a trend toward a second migration from state to state as individuals look for better jobs, family reunification, familiar climate, and well-established

Southeast Asian communities. This has resulted in an increase in the size of Asian communities in such diverse places as California, Washington, New York, and Minnesota (Chung, 1996).

The family is regarded as an important system in Asian American culture. A child learns to respect lines of authority and fathers are the autocratic head of the family. Firstborn sons are viewed as the inheritor and caretaker of the family particularly when both parents become older. Elderly parents, Aunts and Uncles hold honored positions and are the main support system through which advice and counsel can be found. Children are expected to care for aging parents in their own home and "to raise a son is to protect themselves from old age" (Chung, 1996, p. 84).

One of the main barriers to health care for Asian Americans is language with over 100 Asian languages being spoken in the United States at this time. Since there is a good chance that different languages will be spoken it is important for the health professional to recognize culturally specific non-verbal behaviors. For example, a head nod might not signify agreement or understanding but could simply be a sign of deference to one in authority (Yee & Weaver, 1994). In these situations the health care professional must be cautious, making sure the patient understands any directions before they leave the office or program. At the same time the health care professional must always treat the Asian Elder with respect and decorum. This often means calling them by their last names.

Health is achieved for elderly Asian Americans if they can achieve balance. An imbalance occurs when the body experiences an excess of one behavior or a deficiency in another, such as too much work, too little rest, boredom, tension, too much eating, or not enough eating. Herbal and other traditional medicines and eating certain foods are seen as methods for staying healthy and balanced.

"Gaman" or self-control can cause Japanese patients to react to pain and suffering with stoicism. The combination of stoicism and a reluctance to see health care professionals may result in Asian Americans developing serious illnesses.

When a health care professional does work with an Asian American patient they need to recognize that, culturally, using children to interpret may not be acceptable. In addition using a male to interpret for an Asian woman may be inappropriate due to modesty.

Acculturation appears to be having a negative impact on health in Asian American communities. According to Markides and Black (1996) increased acculturation may also be linked to intergenerational conflict and unfulfilled expectations. Each generation that has lived in this country may be at greater risk for cardiovascular disease, diabetes, and certain cancers. For example, Japanese men who were acculturated had 3–5 times the coronary heart disease rate compared to those whose upbringing was more traditional (Chen,1993). Acculturation also appears to be related to increased smoking in females, ischemic heart disease, high blood pressure, and higher blood cholesterol levels. It appears that with each succeeding generation Asian Americans modify certain behaviors putting themselves at greater risk for certain illnesses. Due to these changes there is a need for health promotion programs which focus on smoking cessation and diet modification particularly targeting younger acculturated groups. It is interesting to note, however, that a review of the Healthy People 2000 report only lists eight objectives which target Asian American populations (Chen & Hawks, 1995). Thus, acculturation may result in an increased need for health promotion activities targeted at Asian Americans, while strategic objectives have not yet identified these programs as necessary.

While Asians and Pacific Islanders constitute the fastest growing racial group aged 65 and older in the United States today, they have been neglected as a research population. This lack of study may be due to the great diversity of this group or simply benign neglect. Whatever the reason, since by the year 2050 Asian and Pacific Islanders over 65 will account for almost 8% of all elderly, this omission must be rectified (Tanjasiri, Wallace, & Shinata, 1995).

Hispanic Americans

By the year 2000 it has been estimated that Hispanics will be the largest minority group in the United States (Burgos-Ocasio, 1996). The leading causes of morbidity and mortality in Hispanic groups are:

1. heart disease
2. diabetes
3. cancer
4. hypertension

The principal health risk behaviors for Hispanic elders include:

1. obesity
2. poor eating habits
3. lack of exercise
4. smoking
5. alcohol

It is interesting to note that all of these negative behaviors are modifiable with intervention using effective health promotion programs including physician office counseling. Hispanic adults, however, do not seek out physicians or participate on a regular basis with the health care system. For those between 45 and 64 the number of physician visits per year was 4.8 while for non-Hispanic blacks it was 5.6 and 6.5 for non-Hispanic whites (COSSMHO, 1995).

Hispanic families appear to be strong with two-parent families remaining the most common structure (COSSMHO, 1995). A majority of children live with their biologic mother and father and although more than one in four live in poverty (26.5%) strong family ties seem to persist.

Health care decisions are usually the responsibility of the "wisest" family member, usually an elder who is knowledgeable about folk remedies. Traditional home remedies are often used before any medical care is sought or preventive medicine provided. Using folk medicine and the integration of spirituality into health promotion programs may be one method for getting Hispanic elders involved in preventive care.

As with Asian Americans, acculturation may have an impact on future health in Hispanic populations. For example, less acculturated Hispanics were three times more likely to report abstaining from alcohol (27%) compared with those who were more acculturated. Hispanics who still spoke Spanish in the home were considered to be less acculturated.

Overall, Hispanic Americans have little in common with the cultural traditions of Northern Europe. Programs based on a European model will not be effective with Hispanic individuals. Culturally sensitive programs should be offered in Spanish and focus on family as opposed to individual interventions.

DEVELOPING CULTURALLY SENSITIVE HEALTH PROMOTION PROGRAMS

In 1986, 1.1 billion visits were made to physicians in the United States with one-fifth of those visits made by people 65 years and older. These visits plus comprehensive health promotion programs create a significant opportunity for health professionals to provide health information and advice to their elderly patients. Developing culturally sensitive health promotion programs maximizes the chance that these interventions will be successful.

There are a number of key concepts which should be considered when developing culturally sensitive programs. The first involves meeting the language needs of each identified minority group. Working in the language of participants fosters a feeling of trust and increases the possibilities of learning. For example, Yee and Weaver (1994) suggest that communicating health promotion information to Spanish speaking populations would probably be more effective if done via Spanish language media.

The second key concept involves using specific minority community resources for developing and designing educational approaches. In minority communities this includes establishing organizations like the Chinese Community Cardiac Council in San Francisco. They target Chinese speaking individuals and work within the structure of the American Heart Association but still retain their own cultural identity.

A second example, involves older African American males and their participation in health promotion campaigns targeting common risky behaviors such as obesity, poor eating habits, and alcohol misuse. It appears that these programs have been most effective when information is communicated through individuals and community institutions important to elderly African Americans. In the African American community important organizations include churches and religious organizations. Programs targeting African Americans should be held in churches maximizing the possibility of community participation.

Using community leadership also appears to be an effective strategy for reaching minority populations. According to Chen et al. (1993), one culturally competent program first went to the community leadership to find strategies which would meet their approval. The strategy developed to reach a particular group of people following a discussion with community leadership included simply placing the promotional message on wall calendars. It appeared that this intervention was effective.

The first step when developing programs should thus focus on encouraging community participation and identifying local leadership. When possible it also appears to be useful to train and use community peer educators (Ratliff, 1996).

Involving communities also involves offering the health promotion program in that community. According to Ratliff (1996) people did not attend a specific dietary seminar due to the fact that classes were being held in the "white" part of town and they believed they would be taught traditionally white food preferences. Working within the targeted community is a sign of respect for their neighborhoods and again increases the possibility of increased participation.

The issue of course content also appears to be particularly important. Initially course developers should have community representatives respond to content outlines. For example, nutritional health promotion programs should tailor their message to the food preferences of participants. A barrier of dietary change seems to be the lack of experience health providers have in suggesting culturally appropriate dietary modifications which would increase the likelihood of successful outcomes (Chen & Hawks, 1995). Again working with community members, health promotion providers could develop a cookbook based upon the cultural food preferences of community members increasing the likelihood that they will adhere to the nutrition health plan.

The course content should also be commensurate with the educational level of the target population. Any developed material should first be examined by community members and piloted for appropriateness of educational level. Once again inclusion at all levels of program development is an empowerment strategy designed to optimize community participation.

Any culturally sensitive health promotion program will use the leadership of the targeted community and build a program with their support. Serving as consultants rather than supervisors will help health promotion experts use the strengths that exist within any given community. The role of consultant suggests that the health provider will solicit input from the local community often leaving final decisions about content design to those living in that community. This model is quite different from one that simply provides each community a similar health promotion package.

CHAPTER SUMMARY

This chapter examines the importance of understanding issues of cultural diversity when developing health promotion programs. Programs should recognize the need for using a number of strategies that will enhance the participation of people from diverse backgrounds.

For many ethnically diverse populations the health care system is cold and unfriendly, often insensitive to their cultural needs. Rather than joining with targeted groups, providers often view these individuals as noncompliant and unappreciative (Kerner, Dusenbury & Mandleblatt, 1993). Health consultants are often unaware of techniques for joining with diverse groups and may give up in anger when community members choose not to participate.

Thus, it is important to provide adequate culturally sensitive health promotion information to minority underserved groups in non-emergency settings. There is a need to encourage people to participate in preventive care activities and demonstrate to them the wisdom of health maintenance. If preventive care is difficult to access as it has been for many minority populations, then treatment may be delayed. On a societal level this delay will only mean more costly and time-intensive cases with fewer success-ful outcomes. For individuals it could mean early death and/or a decrease in the quality of their lives.

APPENDIX A

Recommendation: Assuring Comprehensive Health Care Including Long-Term Care:

IRDS 1 Promotion/Prevention

1.1 Assuming personal responsibility for the state of one's health

Be it resolved by the 1995 WHCoA to support policies that:

Ensure that all individuals, especially older adults and caregivers, have full access to wellness and health educational programs, services and facilities so that they may provide sufficient self care and know when to seek appropriate professional care;

Provide information to all persons, especially older adults, about disease prevention, detection, chronic disease management, accident prevention, the consequences of smoking, substance abuse, poor nutrition, emergency response technology, mental health and wellness programs;

Utilize and promote traditional and non-traditional means as well as new technologies and innovative approaches to distribute information to older adults, their families and caregivers, including the frail elderly and individuals who are homebound or institution-alized, with follow-up support;

Require geriatric/gerontological education and training for physicians, other health care providers, informal, and formal caregivers, with the emphasis on health care promotion, disease promotion and palliative care;

Ensure that approaches and materials are culturally and linguistically appropriate, and accessible to both urban and rural populations;

Ensure the development of a universal health care plan for all Americans including emphasis on health promotion and preventive services;

Direct National Institute of Health to conduct research on health promotion, intervention, including how attitudes and values act as barriers to good health habits;

Implement/expand the Indian Health Service Elder Health Program to provide geriatric/gerontological training and elder wellness programs, and require that all programs of the Indian Health Service include tribal and urban health programs and have access to prevention, promotion and wellness programs.

Source: From the 1995 White House Conference on Aging.

1.2. Prevention/wellness throughout one's lifespan

Therefore, be it resolved by the 1995 WHCoA to support policies that:

Extend health promotion/prevention programs to all, especially older adults and vulnerable populations, to improve overall well-being, prevent health problems, reduce health care costs, and help people cope with chronic conditions;

Shift the emphasis of our health system from illness care toward health management for people of all ages, particularly older adults, high risk individuals, and underserved populations;

Increase access to and participation in health prevention, promotion, and alternative care programs that improve quality of life, reduce premature death, disability, and overall cost;

Make available and affordable preventive health measures, early detection methods, and screenings;

Encourage a total wellness approach by emphasizing fitness programs, regular dental care, nutrition assessment and counseling, stress management, medication manage-ment, and mental wellness services;

Disseminate cultural, linguistic, and age appropriate information and educational mater-ials on medical self care and prevention programs;

Increase research on morbidity among underserved groups, such as various ethnic groups and older women;

IRDS 2 Access to Quality Care

2.2 Ensuring quality care, services, and treatment

Therefore, be it resolved by the 1995 WHCoA to support policies that:

Improve communication between providers of health care for older individuals in all phases of care, from prevention to acute and long-term care services, including the development of longitudinal health care records.

2.3 Ensuring the availability of appropriate care, services and treatment

Therefore, be it resolved by the 1995 WHCoA to support policies that:

Improve the availability of and access to appropriate physical and mental health care services to persons of all ages including those with mental and physical disabilities.

2.4 Reforming the health care system

Therefore, be it resolved by the 1995 WHCoA to support system-wide health care reform efforts that adhere to the following principles:

Americans of all ages should have health security, including access to affordable, quality, physical and mental health care and long-term care, choice of providers and health plans;

IRDS 3 Continuum of Care Integrating Community and Social Services

3.1 Ensuring the quality of a broad spectrum of services

Be it resolved by the WHCoA to support policies that:

Ensure an integrated and affordable system providing a seamless continuum of quality services that begins with prevention education for healthier living and includes: care management, acute and subacute care, rehabilitation, community-based services, nutrition services, assisted living, adult day care, home care, personal/assistance services, respite care, substance abuse counseling, senior centers, mental health services/counseling and institutional care; and which is easily accessible and promotes the greatest functional independence for older Americans;

Develop and implement comprehensive, coordinated and culturally relevant community wellness models on the local level that rely on and promote cooperative agreements between public and private agencies;

IRDS 4 Medicare/Medicaid/Older Americans Act

4.1 Ensuring the future of the Medicare program

Therefore, be it resolved by the 1995 WHCoA to support policies that:

Continue to protect older Americans and disabled Americans, especially those on low and fixed incomes, with respect to health care affordability and access, giving special consideration to the burdens imposed by co-payments, deductibles and premiums.

4.2 Preserving the nature of Medicaid

Be it resolved by the 1995 WHCoA to support policies that:

Preserve and strengthen the existing aging network to ensure a seamless continuum of quality services which includes: nutrition, home and community-based services (including but not limited to care management, senior centers, in-home services, assisted living, mental health), advocacy and elder rights protections, health promotion, transportation, volunteerism and employment;

Strengthen and maintain federal protections for physical and mental health and long-term care needs of vulnerable individuals.

4.3 Providing health care coverage that addresses basic needs, prevention, and chronic disease concerns;

Therefore, be it resolved by the 1995 WHCoA to support policies that:

Cover preventive medicine, prescriptions, vision and hearing aids, mental health services, and dental care;

Recognize prevention as an important cost cutting measure by providing immunizations, annual Pap smears, mammograms, nutrition screening, and other proven preventive methods through Medicare and Medicaid;

4.4 Providing services in full range of locations that encompasses: institutional care; home care/foster home care; community-based services

Therefore, be it resolved by the 1995 WHCoA to support policies that:

Ensure that community-based services such as nutrition/meals programs take medical, social, and cultural needs into consideration, including, but not limited to, diabetic, low-fat, low-salt diets, and kosher meals.

4.7 Preserving the integrity of the Older Americans Act

Therefore, be it resolved by the 1995 WHCoA to support policies that:

Preserve and strengthen the existing aging network to ensure a seamless continuum of quality services which includes; nutrition, home and community-based services (including but not limited to care management, senior centers, in-home services, assisted living, mental health), advocacy and elder rights protections, health promotion, transportation, volunteerism and employment.

4.8 Preserving advocacy functions under the Older Americans Act

Therefore, be it resolved by the 1995 WHCoA to support policies that:

Increase the Act's emphasis on self-directed care, encouraging and supporting independence and autonomy.

IRDS 5 Research and Education

5.1 Increase federal funding for research in the areas of the mechanisms of aging, diseases of older people, long-term care, systems and services research, and special population.

Therefore, be it resolved by the 1995 WHCoA to support policies that:

Achieve by the year 2000 an increased federal funding level for aging research equal to or at least 1% of federal health care expenditures for Older Americans, consistent with recommendations of the Institute of Medicine (1991), the Federal Task Force on Aging Research (1995) and others. The research program will include:

> Basic and applied biomedical, clinical, behavioral/social, health services and ethics research, including health promotion, disease prevention, and rehabilitation research;

> Population-based studies (rural and urban) of nutrition, physical activity and mobility, incontinence, dementia, and overall geriatric health promotion to understand and project future demands for health care and social services and to identify future aging research topics;

> Research to improve the quality, access and cost-effectiveness of long-term care, institutional, home-based, and community-based settings; Women, ethnic and racial minorities, other societal groups of older persons as appropriate in all aspects of aging research;

> Increased research on mental health, mental health services, and mental disorders of the elderly;

> An emphasis on outcomes based research on common geriatric conditions, health care delivery mechanisms, chronic illnesses, and impact of care on quality of life.

5.3 Strengthening the federal role in building and sustaining a well-trained work force grounded in geriatric and gerontological education.

Therefore, be it resolved by the 1995 WHCoA to support policies that:

Increase geriatric and gerontological training in medical and nursing schools, other health professional schools and programs, continuing education and in-service programs;

Integrate geriatrics and gerontology into the curricula of health care specialty programs;

Promoting Economic Security

IRDS 9 Poverty and Hunger

9.3 Expanding programs to assess and address malnutrition:

Therefore, be it resolved by the 1995 WHCoA to support policies that:

Facilitate public and private partnerships at the community level to develop nutrition screening and intervention programs;

Maximizing Housing and Support Service Options

IRDS 14 Linking support services to housing

14.2 Promoting innovative strategies to encourage new models of supportive housing, particularly housing which facilitates long-term care services:

Therefore, be it resolved by the 1995 WHCoA to support policies that:

Promote the independence of older persons in their homes through the provision of services such as case management/care coordination, transportation, in-home care, home repair, assisted technology, homemaker assistance, adult protective services, mental health, respite, home delivered meals and adult day care including those funded by the Older Americans Act;

IRDS 15 Consumer choice/decision making/promoting independence

15.3 Maximizing transportation choices:

Therefore, be it resolved by the 1995 WHCoA to support policies that:

Promote and prioritize the importance of older person's access to transportation as an essential component of a quality life;

Maximizing Options for a Quality Life

IRDS16 Resources for Older Persons (Community and Social Services/Activities)

16.1 Expanding, coordinating and targeting necessary services:

Therefore, be it resolved by the 1995 WHCoA to support policies that:

Provide services which address the nutritional, social, emotional, physical and cognitive needs of older persons at risk of becoming isolated and alienated from society, including the needs of rural elders;

Expand nutrition programs to include education, with special attention to culturally appropriate nutrition education;

Source: Official 1995 White House Conference on Aging, Background Materials. May 2-5, 1995, Washington, DC.

APPENDIX B

Six HHAs: Similarities and Differences

	Interhealth Life Extension	University of Wisconsin Stevens Point	U.S. Centers for Disease Control	Well Aware about Health	University of Florida	University of Wisconsin, Madison
Copyright date	1979	1980	Not copyrighted	1979	1978	Not copyrighted
Instrument cost	$12.50	$7.50	free	$25.00	free	$6.00
Suggested audience	literate adult	12th grade-level reader	literate adult	literate adult	literate teenagers	adult
Questionnaire length	67 qq.	266 qq.	34 qq.	108 qq.	102 qq.	58 qq.
Health attitudes measured	no	yes	no	yes	yes	no
Health knowledge measured	no	no	no	yes	no	no
Occupational risks identified	no	no	no	yes	no	no
Life crisis questions included	no	no	no	yes	no	no
Life expectancy projected	no	yes	no	no	no	no

Source: Adapted from W. L. Beery, E. H. Wagner, V. J. Schoenback & R. M. Graham, "A Shopper's Guide to Appraisal Instruments, Promoting Health, July-August 8, 1981, pp. 8-9. The reader may wish to consult the Beery et al. article as six additional health-hazard appraisals are compared. Beery et al. also provide additional criteria for comparing health hazard instruments, e.g., graphic devices used, feedback time frame, etc.

APPENDIX C

Physical Activity Readiness Questionnaire (PAR-Q)*

_____

Name of Applicant

_____

Date

PAR-Q AND YOU

PAR-Q is designed to help you help yourself. Many health benefits are associated with regular exercise, and the completion of PAR-Q is a sensible first step to take if you are planning to increase the amount of physical activity in your life.

For most people physical activity should not pose any problem or hazard. PAR-Q has been designed to identify the small number of adults for whom physical activity might be inappropriate or those who should have medical advice concerning the type of activity most suitable for them.

Commonsense is your best guide in answering these few questions. Please read them carefully and check (/) the [] YES or [] NO opposite the question if it applies to you.

YES NO

[] [] 1. Has your doctor ever said you have heart trouble?

[] [] 2. Do you frequently have pains in your heart and chest?

[] [] 3. Do you often feel faint or have spells of severe dizziness?

[] [] 4. Has a doctor ever said your blood pressure was too high?

[] [] 5. Has your doctor ever told you that you have a bone or joint problem such as arthritis that has been aggravated by exercise, or might be made worse with exercise?

[] [] 6. Is there a good physical reason not mentioned here why you should not follow an activity program even if you wanted to?

[] [] 7. Are you over age 65 and not accustomed to vigorous exercise?

If you answered YES to one or more questions

If you have not recently done so, consult with your personal physician by telephone or in person BEFORE increasing your physical activity and/or taking a fitness appraisal. Tell your physician what questions you answered YES on PAR-Q or present your PAR-Q copy.

PROGRAMS

After medical evaluation, seek advice from your physician as to your suitability for:

*   unrestricted physical activity starting off easily and progressing gradually;

*   restricted or supervised activity to meet your specific needs, at least on an initial basis. Check in your community for special programs or services.

NO to all questions

If you answered PAR-Q accurately, you have reasonable assurance of your present suitability for:

*   a GRADUATED EXERCISE PROGRAM--a gradual increase in proper exercise promotes good fitness development while minimizing or eliminating discomfort.

*   a FITNESS APPRAISAL--the Canadian Standardized Test of Fitness (CSTF).

POSTPONE
If you have a temporary minor illness, such as a common cold.

Developed by the British Columbia Ministry of Health. Conceptualized and critiqued by the Multidisciplinary Advisory Board on Exercise (MABE). Transition, reproduction and use in its entirety is encouraged. Modifications by written permission only. Not to be used for commercial advertising in order to solicit business from the public. Reference: PAR-Q Validation Report, British Columbia Ministry of Health, 1978. Produced by the British Columbia Ministry of Health and the Department of National Health and Welfare.

APPENDIX D

USEFUL MATERIALS ABOUT NUTRITION FOR OLDER ADULTS

- Age Pages: Be Sensible about Salt; Dietary Supplements: More is Not Always Better; Food; Staying Healthy after 65; Osteoporosis: The Bone Thinner. One-page information sheets. National Institute on Aging, Bethesda, MD. (301) 496–1752. Free.
- Are You at Risk for Bone Disease. Brochure. Dairy and Nutrition Council, Dayton, OH. (513) 223–6289. $0.20.
- Diet and Nutrition: Facts to Consider. Brochure. Local Arthritis Foundation. Free.
- Eating to Stay Well and Get Well. Booklet and videotape. Local chapter American Red Cross. Small charge--booklet. Loan--videotape.
- Good Nutrition in Later Years. Brochure. Channing L. Bete Co., Inc., South Deerfield, MA. (413) 665–7611. Free.
- Help Yourself to Better Health. Slide-tape program. Local chapter American Association of Retired Persons. Loan.
- Like Mother, Like Daughter: A Mature Woman's Guide to Bone Health. Dairy and Nutrition Council, Dayton, OH. (513) 223–6289. $0.20.
- Nutrition Publications for Older Americans. Food and Drug Administration, Rockville, MD. (301) 443–3190. Free.
- Supermarket Survival. Brochure. Dairy and Nutrition Council, Dayton, OH. (513) 223–6289. $0.20.
- Sodium: Facts for Older Citizens. Brochure. Food and Drug Administration, Rockville, MD. (301) 443–3170. Free.
- The All-American Guide to Calcium-Rich Foods. Brochure. Dairy and Nutrition Council, Dayton, OH. (513) 223–6289. $0.20.
- To Your Health: In Your Second Fifty Years. Brochure. Dairy and Nutrition Council, Dayton, OH. (513) 223–6289. $0.40.

FOR PROFESSIONALS

- Health Finder: Weight Control. Publication list. National Health Information Clearinghouse, Washington, DC. (800) 336–4797. Free.
- Nutrition Publications: A Selected Annotated Bibliography. National Health Information Clearinghouse, Washington, DC. (800) 336–4797. Free.
- Weight Reduction: A Counseling Protocol. Information package. Health Education Center, Pittsburgh, PA. (412) 392–3165. $5.00.

APPENDIX E

USEFUL MATERIALS ABOUT MEDICATION MANAGEMENT FOR OLDER ADULTS

- *Age Page: Safe Use of Medicines by Older Persons.* One-page information sheet. National Institute on Aging, Bethesda, MD.
- *Consumer Drug Digest.* A publication for patients of all ages with emphasis on drugs used by the elderly. Selected local bookstores.
- *Doctors, Patients Don't Communicate.* Brochure. Food and Drug Administration, Rockville, MD.
- *Drug Abuse Prevention for Older Americans.* Brochure. National Clearinghouse for Drug Abuse Information, Kensington, MD.
- *Food and Drug Interactions.* Brochure. Food and Drug Administration, Rockville, MD.
- *Health Finder: Understanding Your Medications.* Eight-page summary of publications dealing with frequently asked questions about drugs. National Health Information Clearinghouse, Washington, DC.
- *Here Are Some Things You Should Know About Prescription Drugs.* Brochure. Food and Drug Administration, Rockville, MD.
- *Knowing about Medicines: Family Health Series.* Booklet and videotape. Local chapter American Red Cross. Small charge for booklet. Loan for videotape.
- *Medication Awareness Test, Health Check Test and Self-Medication Awareness Test.* Printed materials and audiovisual program. American Pharmaceutical Association, Washington, DC.
- *Treating Yourself with Care.* Slide-tape program. Local chapter American Association for Retired Persons. Loan.
- *Understanding Your Prescription.* Pamphlet and film. National Pharmaceutical Council, Reston, VA.
- *Using Your Medicines Wisely: A Guide for the Elderly.* Brochure. National Clearinghouse for Drug Abuse Information, Kensington, MD.
- *You and Your Medicines: Guidelines for Older Americans.* Brochure. U.S. Government Printing Office, Washington, DC.
- *Using Your Medicines Wisely: A Guide for the Elderly.* National Institute on Drug Abuse, Elder-Ed., P.O. Box 416, Kensington, MD 10745.
- *Drugs and the Elderly.* Published papers. National Institute on Aging, Bethesda, MD.
- *Health Finder: Medications: Sources of Information.* Books, pamphlets, other information on drugs and drug issues. National Health Information Clearinghouse, Washington, DC.
- *Operation Brown Bag: How To Manual.* National Pharmaceutical Council, Reston, VA.
- *Resource Materials on Geriatrics and Drugs.* Bibliography. National Institute on Aging, Bethesda, MD.

APPENDIX F

Community Substance Dependency Programs

Type of Program	Program Purpose	Program Activities
Drug information & education	Assumes drug knowledge will deter drug use, impede escalation of drug misuse, and lead to well-informed rational choices.	Literature, discussion groups, films, and opportunities to examine and clarify values and attitudes, along with problem-solving and decision-making skills.
Alternatives program	Services are not designed to deal specifically with drug abuse problems. Instead, the focus is on using individual and group activities to meet many of the same needs that underlie drug abuse: (1) achieving altered states of consciousness, (2) risk simulations and real situations, and (3) personal growth.	Altered state activities include yoga, self-hypnosis, biofeedback, transcendental meditation. Rugged physical activities (e.g., mountaineering) are used for risk activities. Informal group discussion is used for personal growth.
Community activities	Preventive strategies that impede further drug involvement. Diversity provides development of a variety of skills and competencies. Intent is to produce feeling of belonging.	Diverse activities, games, sports, self-help projects, political involvement.
Brief counseling	Focuses on immediate crises rather than long-term behavioral problems. Service is typically "storefront" where counseling is provided on request.	Situational problems, educational, vocational, interpersonal conflicts, drug/alcohol abuse are dealt with in a relaxed "drop-in" basis.
Short-term	Shift is away from immediate, manifest problems to more long-range, generalized goals. Goal is to improve clients' self-image and ability to function, usually within one year of counseling.	One-to-one interviews with psychotherapy professionally trained counselors (psychiatric, psychology, social work). Passive (e.g., transactional analysis) or active (e.g., Gestalt) therapy may be used.
Family counseling therapy	One-to-one therapy expanded to include the family. Therapist seeks to improve	Families may be seen in individual or group sessions. Families may also be brought

Type of Program	Program Purpose	Program Activities
	functioning of family as a group. Assumption is that a client's behavior does not occur in a vacuum and can be subtly or overtly manipulated by other family members.	together in a crisis situation for an extended period of continuous confrontation.
Extended psychotherapy	Emphasis is on significant personal change, brought about through re-education of individual at both conscious and subconscious levels.	One-to-one intensive psychotherapy that is analytic in dealing with client's past life, present behavior, and neurotic patterns.
Group encounters (light)	Focus is on interpersonal behavior and current behavior patterns dealt with on a contemporary and situational level rather than a probing and analytical style.	Client does not contribute directly but is drawn out by the group. Atmosphere is largely supportive and emphasis is mainly upon client's positive attributes.
Group encounters (heavy)	Form of treatment is directed toward clients with rigid defense patterns. Objective is to get client to face own shortcomings and those of other group members.	Direct and sometimes violent verbal confrontations are used in a "No-Holds-Barred" group session. Participants cannot show support for other group members; one must learn to defend self.
Day-care activity programming	Programs directed toward clients who have demonstrated past abilities to involve themselves in one-to-one group relationships.	Informal services that include vocational and educational training, "Alternating" programs, and some forms of light therapy.
Ideological groups (non-residential)	Basic treatment goal is to bring client to realization that he/she is fundamentally good, can salvage own life, and help others do same.	Emphasis on a religious or ideological conversion in which participant gives him/herself to a cause. Strict behavioral standards are enforced and recreatonal activities are frowned on.
Structured, therapeutic day care	This modality intervenes more drastically on the client's life than the other approaches discussed thus far. Focus is on clients whose drug involvement has been relatively short and who have poorly developed social strengths.	Individual group psychotherapy, vocational and educational counseling, recreation activities, field trips, regular facility maintenance.

Type of Program	Program Purpose	Program Activities
In-patient detoxification/ counseling	Focus is on several groups of clients: (1) clients with well-developed social strengths, regular job/school involvement, and drug-free home environment; (2) clients referred to some other pre-determined drug treatment who need initial detoxification; (3) clients for whom no treatment referral decision can be made until withdrawal is at least partially attained.	Client is gradually withdrawn from drugs in a medical setting; dosage of client's own drug may be gradually lowered. However, must use methadone as drug withdrawal progresses.
Ideological groups (resident)	Clients must be able to make lifestyle changes for adjusting to settings. Intent is to enlighten client religiously or raise political conciousness. Clients with ability for strong group involvement but poorly developed social strengths do well here.	Focuses on some specific religious or political doctrine. Clients are residential, expected to participate in and contribute to program functioning.
Halfway or re-entry houses	Similar to ideological-based residential program. However, primary goal is introduction back into society rather than political/religious conversion. Clients with well-developed social strengths respond more positively to the "light" therapy introduced in this treatment form.	Independent, temporary living facilities that offer individual group counseling under voluntary basis, recreational activities, vocational and educational training, and drug treatment referral.
Residential therapeutic	Drug user seen as person whose emotions/ behavior not developed past childhood and must be treated in a punitive and authoritarian manner. The aim is to destroy the "street image" so that the client will be forced into personality change. This modality is recommended for clients with lengthy	Services generally same as "light" therapeutic community but community (heavy) delivery manner is much more rigid and structured. Heavy confrontation and attack psychotherapy is used.

Type of Program	Program Purpose	Program Activities
	history of serious opiate, sedative, or multi-drug use.	
Methadone to abstinence	Assumption is that client is capable of eventually abstaining from heroin and methadone. Client is expected to detoxify from methadone within a pre-specified time period. Program is recommended for clients with lengthy history of serious drug involvement but who have well developed social strengths.	Daily controlled doses of methadone are provided. Provides similar services as the aforementioned day-care programs.
Methadone treatment program	Goal is to allow client as much time as needed to establish life-style independent from heroin before facing methadone withdrawal. Program directed toward long-history opiate users who are presently involved in work/school and live in a drug-free environment.	Daily controlled methadone for an indefinite period of time. Other services offered in day-care programs also provided here.
Methadone-based residential theapeutic community	Directed toward heavy opiate users with multi-drug abuse problems. Two program types: (1) therapeutic community plus methadone; (2) residential community plus methadone usage.	Most comprehensive form of treatment for long-term opiate addiction. Drug-free environment, strong peer support, physical support of plus methadone.
Custodial care or hospitalization	Recommended for clients with serious medical/psychiatric complications that preclude less intense treatment and those with chronic disabilities that preclude treatment participation.	Custodial activities for general maintenance.

Source: Stephen Pittel et al., "Drug abuse treatment modalities: An overview," in *Addictive Behavior: Drug and Alcohol Abuse*. Englewood, Coloardo: Morton Publishing Company, 1985. Used by permission.

APPENDIX G

BASIC PROCEDURE - MUSCLE RELAXATION

Get in a comfortable position and relax. Now clinch your right fist, tighter and tighter, studying the tension as you do so. Keep it clinched and notice the tension in your fist, hand and forearm. Now relax. Feel the looseness in your right hand, and notice the contrast with the tension. Repeat this procedure with your right fist again, always noticing as you relax that this is the opposite of tension - relax and feel the difference. Repeat the entire procedure with your left fist, then both fists at once.

Now bend your elbows and tense your biceps. Tense them as hard as you can and observe the feeling of tautness. Relax, straighten out your arms. Let the relaxation develop and feel that difference. Repeat this, and all succeeding procedures at least once.

Turning attention to your head, wrinkle your forehead as tight as you can. Now relax and smooth it out. Let yourself imagine your entire forehead and scalp becoming smooth and at rest. Now frown and notice the strain spreading throughout your forehead. Let go. Allow your brow to become smooth again. Close your eyes now, squint them tighter. Look for the tension. Relax your eyes. Let them remain closed gently and comfortably. Now clinch your jaw, bite hard, notice the tension throughout your jaw. Relax your jaw. When the jaw is relaxed, your lips will be slightly parted. Let yourself really appreciate the contrast between tension and relaxation. Now press your tongue against the roof of your mouth. Feel the ache in the back of your mouth. Relax. Press your lips now, purse them into an "O." Relax your lips. Notice that your forehead, scalp, eyes, jaw, tongue and lips are all relaxed.

Press your head back as far as it can comfortably go and observe the tension in your neck. Roll it to the right and feel the changing locus of stress, roll it to the left. Straighten your head and bring it forward, press your chin against your chest. Feel the tension in your throat, the back of your neck. Relax, allowing your head to return a comfortable position. Let the relaxation deepen. Now shrug your shoulders. Keep the tension as you hunch your head down between your shoulders. Relax your shoulders. Drop them back and feel the relaxation spreading through your neck, throat and shoulders, pure relaxation, deeper and deeper.

Give your entire body a chance to relax. Feel the comfort and the heaviness. Now breathe in and fill your lungs completely. Hold your breath. Notice the tension. Now exhale, let your chest become loose, let the air hiss out. Continue relaxing, letting your breath come freely and gently. Repeat this several times, noticing the tension draining from your body as you exhale. Next, tighten your stomach and hold. Note the tension, then relax. Now place your hand on your stomach. Breath deeply into your stomach, pushing your hand up. Hold, and relax. Feel the contrast of relaxation as the air rushes out. Now arch your back, without straining. Keep the rest of your body as relaxed as possible. Focus on the tension in your lower back. Now relax, deeper and deeper.

Tighten your buttocks and thighs. Flex your thighs by pressing down your heels as hard as you can. Relax and feel the difference. Now curl your toes downward, making your calves tense. Study the tension. Relax. Now bend your toes toward your face, creating tension in your shins. Relax again.

Feel the heaviness throughout your lower body as the relaxation deepens. Relax your feet, ankles, calves, shins, knees, thighs, buttocks. Now let the relaxation spread to your stomach, lower back and chest. Let go more and more. Experience the relaxation deepening in your shoulders, arms and hands. Deeper and deeper. Notice the feeling of looseness and relaxation in your neck, jaws and all your facial muscles.

Shorthand Procedure

The following is a procedure for achieving deep muscle relaxation quickly. Whole muscle groups are simultaneously tensed and then relaxed. As before, repeat each procedure at least once, tensing each muscle group from five to seven seconds and then relaxing from 20-30 seconds. Remember to notice the contrast between the sensations of tension and relaxation.

1. Curl both fists, tightening biceps and forearms (Charles Atlas pose). Relax.

2. Wrinkle up forehead. At the same time, press your head as far back as possible, roll it clockwise in a complete circle, reverse. Now wrinkle up the muscles of your face like a walnut: frowning, eyes squinted, lips pursed, tongue pressing the roof of the mouth, and shoulders hunched. Relax.

3. Arch back as you take a deep breath into the chest. Hold. Relax. Take a deep breath, pressing out the stomach. Hold. Relax.

4. Pull feet and toes back toward the face, tightening shins. Hold. Relax. Take a deep breath, pressing out the stomach. Hold. Relax.

Special Considerations

1. If you make a tape of the basic procedure to facilitate your relaxation program, remember to space each procedure so that time is allowed to experience the tension and relaxation before going on to the next muscle or muscle group.

2. Most people have somewhat limited success when they begin deep muscle relaxation, but it is only a matter of practice. Whereas 20 minutes of work might initially bring only partial relaxation, it will eventually be possible to relax your whole body in a few moments.

3. Sometimes in the beginning, it may seem to you as though relaxation is complete. But although the muscles or muscle group may well be partially relaxed, a certain number of muscle fibers will still be contracted. It is the act of relaxing these additional fibers that will bring about the emotional effects you want. It is helpful to say to yourself during the relaxation phase, "Let go more and more."

4. Caution should be taken in tensing the neck and back. Excessive tightening can result in muscle or spinal damage. It is also commonly observed that over tightening the toes or feet results in muscle cramping.

Reprinted with permission.

Davis M., Eshelman E., McKay M., 1994 3rd Edition, *The Relaxation and Stress Reduction Workbook*.

BIBLIOGRAPHY

Abeles, R. P., Gift, H. C., Ory, M. G., (Eds). (1994). *Aging and the quality of life*. New York, NY : Springer Publishing Company.

Adams, F. (1988). Fluid intake: How much do elders drink? *Geriatric Nursing, 9,* 218, 6-24.

Adams, R. C., Daniel, A. N., McCubbin, J. A., & Pullman, L. (1982). *Games, sports and exercises for the physically handicapped*. Philadelphia: Lea & Febiger.

Adelman, R. D., Greene, M. G., & Charon, R. (1987). The physician-elderly patient-companion triad in the medical encounter: The development of a conceptual framework and research agenda. *The Gerontologist, 27,* 729-734.

Adelman, R. D., Greene, M. G., & Charon, R. (1991). Issues in physician-elderly patient interaction. *Aging and Society, 11,* 127-148.

Adelman, R. D., Greene, M. G., Charon, R., & Friedmann, E. (1992). The content of physicians and elderly patient interaction in the medical primary care encounter. *Communication Research, 19,* 370-380.

Adelmann, P. K. (1994). Multiple roles and psychological well-being in a national sample of older adults. *Journal of Gerontology, 49,* S277-S285.

Aerobic Research. (1990). *Reebok Instructor*. Dallas, TX.

Ajzen, I., & Fishbein, M. (1980). *Understanding attitudes and predicting social behavior*. Englewood Cliffs, NJ: Prentice-Hall, Inc.

Allen, J. A., & Allen, R. F. (1986). Achieving health promotion objectives through cultural change systems. *American Journal of Health Promotion, 1,* 42-49.

Allen, R. F. (1981). *Lifegain*. New York: Appleton-Century-Crofts.

Aloia, J. F. (1981). Exercise and skeletal health. *Journal of the American Geriatrics Society, 29,* 104-107.

Alter, M. J. (1996). *Science of flexibility and strategies*. Champaign, IL: Human Kinetics Press.

American Academy of Family Physicians. (1989*). AIDS: A guide for survival*. Harris County Medical Society and the Houston Academy of Medicine.

American Academy of Physical Education. (1989). *Physical activity and aging*. Paper No. 22. Champaign, IL: Human Kinetics Publishers, Inc.

American Association of Retired Persons. (No Date). *Healthy older adults*. The National Resource Center on Health Promotion and Aging, 1909 K Street, N.W., 5th Floor, Washington, DC.

American College of Sports Medicine. (1980). *Guidelines for graded exercise testing and exercise prescription*. Philadelphia, PA: Lea & Febiger.

American Heart Association. (1995). *Your heart: An owner's manual*. Englewood Cliffs, New Jersey: Prentice-Hall.

American Hospital Association. (1985). *Health promotion for older adults: Planning for action*. Chicago, IL: Center for Health Promotion.

American Medical Association. (1984). *Guide to health and well-being after fifty*. New York: Random House.

American Psychiatric Association (1994). *Diagnostic and statistical manual of mental disorders* (4th ed). Washington, DC: American Psychological Association.

Anderson, B. (1980). *Stretching*. Bolinas, CA: Shelter Publications, Inc.

Anthony, J. C., & Aboraya, A. (1992). The epidemiology of selected mental disorders in later life. In J. Birren, R. Sloane, & G. Cohen (Eds.), *Handbook of mental health and aging* (2nd ed.). San Diego: Academic Press.

Antoni, M. H. (1993). Stress Management: Strategies that work. In D. Goleman, & J. Gurin (Eds.), *Mind/Body Medicine*. Younkers, NY. *Consumer Reports Books*, 385-397.

Antonovsky, A. (1987). *Unraveling the mystery of health: How people manage stress and stay well*. San Francisco: Jossey-Bass.

Applegate, W. B. (1987). Use of assessment instruments in clinical settings. *Journal of American Geriatric Society, 35*, 45-50.

Ardell, D. (1986, Spring). *Spirituality and wellness*. The Ardell Wellness Report.

Arnold, S., Kane, R. L., & Kane, R. A. (1986). *Health promotion and the elderly: Evaluating the research*. In K. Dychtwald (Ed.), *Wellness and health promotion for the elderly*. Rockville, MD: Aspen Publication.

Aronson, S., & Mascia, M. F. (1981). *The stress management workbook*. New York: Appleton-Century-Crofts.

Ascione, F. J., & Shimp, L. A. (1988). Helping patients to reduce medication, misuse and error. *Generations, 12*, 52.

Augsburger, D. (1983). *Caring enough to confront*. Ventura, CA: Regal Books.

Averill, J. R., & Wisocki, P. A. (1981). Some observations on behavioural approaches to the treatment of grief among the elderly. In H. Sobel (Ed.), *Behavior therapy in terminal care: A humanistic approach*. Cambridge, MA: Ballinger.

Babchuk, N. (1978). Aging and primary relations. *International Journal of Aging and Human Development, 9*, 2, 137-151.

Baechle, T. R., & Groves, B. R. (1994). *Weight training instruction*. Champaign, IL: Human Kinetics.

Bailey, C. (1978). *Fit or fat*. Boston: Houghton-Mifflin Company.

Balke, B., & Ware, R.W. (1959). An experimental study of physical fitness of air force personnel. *U.S. Armed Forces Medical Journal, 10*, 675-688.

Baltes, P. B. (1991). The many faces of human aging: Toward a psychological culture of old age. *Psychological Medicine, 21*, 837-854.

Bandura, A. (1977). *Social learning theory*. Englewood Cliffs, NJ: Prentice-Hall.

Banta, W. F. (1987). *AIDS in the workplace*. Lexington, MA: Lexington Books.

Baric, L. (1969). Recognition of the "at risk" role: A means to influence health behavior. *International Journal of Health Education, 12*, 1, 29-35.

Barrett, S. (1980). *The health robbers*. Philadelphia, PA: George F. Stickley Company.

Barry, K., & Fleming, M. (1993). *The Alcohol Use Disorders Identification Test (AUDIT) and the SMAST-13: Predictive validity in a rural primary care sample*. Alcohol, 17:1188-1192.

Barry, P. P. (1994). Geriatric clinical training in medical schools. *The American Journal of Medicine, 97*, 4A-4S.

Bauer, C. (1991). *Acupressure for everybody*. Henry Hold and Company.

Beck, A. T., & Emery, G. (1985). *Anxiety disorders and phobias: A cognitive perspective*. New York: Basic Books.

Beck, A. T., Ward, C. H., Mendelson, M., et al. (1961). An inventory to measure depression. *Archives of General Psychiatry, 4*, 53-63.

Beck, M. (1989, March 20). Living with arthritis. *Newsweek,* 64-20.

Becker, P. M., & Cohen, J. H. (1984, Nov.-Dec.). The functional approach to the welfare of the elderly. *Journal of the American Geriatrics Society, 32*, 923-928.

Bedolla, M. A. (1995). The principles of medical ethics and their application to Mexican-American elderly patients. *Clinics In Geriatric Medicine, 11*(1), February, 131-136.

Beisecker, A. E. (1988). Aging and the desire for information and input in medical decisions: Patent consumerism in medical encounters. *The Gerontologist, 28*, 330-335.

Beisecker, A. E., & Beisecker, T. D. (1990). Patient information-seeking behaviors when communicating with doctors. *Medical Care, 28*, 19-28.

Beisecker, A. E., & Thompson, T. L. (1995). The elderly patient-physician interaction. In J. Nussbaum & J. Coupland (Eds.), *Handbook of communication and aging research*. Mahway, NJ: Lawrence Erlbaum Associates.

Bellingham, R., Cohen, B., Jones, T., & Spaniel, L. (1989). Connectedness: Some skills for spiritual health. *American Journal for Health Promotion, 4*(1), 18-20, 31.

Bennett, I. L. (1977). Technology as a shaping force. In J. H. Knowles (Ed.), *Doing better and feeling worse*. New York: W. W. Norton and Company.

Bennett, W., & Gurin, J. (1982). *The dieter's dilemma*. New York: Basic Books, Inc.

Benson, H. (1975). *The relaxation response*. New York, NY: William Morrow and Company.

Benson, H. (1993). The relaxation response. In D. Goleman, & J. Gurin, (Eds.). *Mind/body medicine*. Younkers, NY: Consumer Reports Books, 243.

Benson, H. (1996). *Timeless healing: The power and biology of belief*. NY: Schribner.

Berg, K. E. (1986). *Diabetic's guide to health and fitness*. Champaign, IL: Human Kinetics Press.

Berger, P., & Luckmann, T. (1966). *The social construction of reality*. New York: Doubleday.

Bergin, A. E., & Garfield, S. L., (Eds). (1994). *Handbook of psychotherapy and behavior change*, 4th Ed. New York, NY: John Wiley and Sons.

Berkman, L.F. (1985). The relationship of social networks and social support to morbidity and mortality. In: S. Cohen, & S. L. Syme (Eds.), *Social support and health*. Orlando, FL: Academic Press, 241-262.

Berkman, L. F., Seeman, T. E., Albert, M., et al. (1993). High, usual and impaired functioning in community-dwelling older men and women: Findings from the MacArthur Foundation Research Network on Successful Aging. *Journal of Clinical Epidemiology, 46*, 1129-1140.

Berkman, L. F., & Syme, S. L. (1979). Social networks, host resistance, and mortality: A nine year follow-up study of Alameda County residents. *American Journal of Epidemology, 109*, 186-204.

Bertakis, K. D., Roter, D., & Putnam, S. M. (1991). The relationship of physician medical interview style to patient satisfaction. *The Journal of Family Practice, 32*, 175-181.

Besdine, R. W. (1983, November). The educational utility of comprehensive functional assessment in the elderly. *Journal of the American Geriatrics Society, 31*, II, 651-656.

Bezon, J. (1988). Individualized drug assessment inventory: A tool for increasing awareness of how medication regimes work in the elderly person's body. Paper presented at GSA. CA: San Francisco.

Bild, B. R., & Havighurst, R. J. (1976). Senior citizens in great cities: The case of Chicago. *Gerontologist, 16*, 1, pt. 2.

Binstock, R. H.,& George, L. K., (Eds.). (1996). *Handbook of aging and the social sciences.* San Diego, CA: Academic Press.

Bjoen, E., & Nordemar, R. (1987). In J. S. Skinner (Ed.), *Exercise testing and exercise prescription for special cases.* Philadelphia: Lea & Febiger.

Blackwell, B. (1976). Treatment adherence. *British Journal of Psychiatry, 129*, 513-531.

Blanchard, C. G., Labrecque, M. S., Ruckdeschel, J. C., & Blanchard, E. B. (1988). Information and decision-making preferences of hospitalized adult cancer patients. *Social Science and Medicine, 27*, 1139-1145.

Blanchard, E. B. (1994). Behavioral Medicine and Health Psychology. In A. E. Bergin, & S. L. Garfield, (Eds.), 4th ed. New York : John Wiley and Sons, 701-733.

Bland, J. (1985). Services for the elderly with alcohol-related problems: A systems approach. In E. Gottheil, K. Druley, T. Skoloda, & H. Waxman (Eds.), *Alcoholism, drug addiction, and aging.* Springfield, IL: Charles C. Thomas.

Bleidt, B. A., Moss, J. T., & Pharm, D. (1989, August). Age related changes in drug distribution. *U.S. Pharmacist.*

Bloom, S. W., & Speedling, E. J. (1981). Strategies of power and dependence in doctor-patient exchanges. In M. Haug (Ed.), *Elderly patients and their doctors.* New York: Springer Publisher Company.

Bogardus, C., Ravussin, E., Robbins, D. C., Wolfe, R. R., Horton, E. D., & Sims, E.A H. (1984). Effects of physical training and diet therapy on carbohydrate metabolism in patients with glucose intolerance and non-insulin-dependent diabetes mellitus. *Diabetes, 33*, 311-318.

Bogaret-Tullis, M. (1985, June). A resource guide for drug management programs for older persons. Washington, DC: Administration of Aging, Department of Health and Human Services.

Bortz, W.M., II. (1982). Disuse and aging. *Journal of American Medical Association, 248*(80), 1203-1209.

Bortz, W. M. (1992). *We live too short and die too long.* NY: Bantam Books.

Bower, K. A. (1985). Compliance as a patient education issue. In K. M. Woldum, V. Ryan-Morrell, K. A. Towson, & R. Zander (Eds.), *Patient Education.* Rockville, MD: Aspen Publication.

Bower, S. A., & Bower, G. (1976). *Asserting yourself: A practical guide for positive change.* Reading, MA: Addison-Wesley Publishing Company.

Brady, E. S. (1978). Drugs and the elderly. In R. C. Kayne (Ed.), *Drugs and the elderly.* Los Angeles, CA: University of Southern California Press.

Braithwaite, R. L., Lythcott, N. (1989). Community empowerment as a strategy for health promotion for Black and other minority populations. *JAMA*, January 13, *261*(2):282-283.

Brandon, J. (1985). Health promotion and wellness in rehabilitation services. *Journal of Rehabilitation, 51*(4), 54-58.

Brandtstädter, J., & Greve, W. (1994). The aging self: Stabilizing and protective processes. *Developmental Review, 14,* 52-80.

Bratter, B., & Freeman, E. (1990, Winter). The maturing of peer counseling. *Generations, 14,* 1, 49-52.

Breslow, L. (1990, Summer). A health promotion primer for the 1990s. *Promoting Health,* 6-21.

Brimm, O. G. (1988, September). Losing and winning. *Psychology Today,* 48-52.

Brink, T. L. (1979). *Geriatric psychotherapy.* New York: Human Sciences Press.

Broadman, K., Erdmann, A. J., Lorge, I., et al. (1953). The Cornell medical index health questionnaire. The relation of patients' complaints to age, sex, race, and education. *Journal of Gerontology, 8,* 339-342.

Brockett, R. (1987). Life satisfaction and learner self-direction: Enhancing quality of life during the later years. *Educational Gerontology, 13,* 225.

Brody, J. (1982). *Jane Brody's nutrition book.* New York: Bantam Books.

Brown, B. B. (1985). *Between health and illness.* Toronto: Bantam Books.

Brown, V. (1995). The effects of poverty environments on elders subjective well being: A conceptual model. *The Gerontologist, 35*(4), 541-548.

Brozan, N. (1990, November 26). Less visible but heavier burdens as AIDS attacks people over 50. *The New York Times,* A1, A10.

Bruce, R. A., Kusumi, F., & Hasmer, D. (1975). Maximal oxygen intake and nomographic assessment of functional aerobic impairment in cardiovascular disease. *American Heart Journal, 85,* 546-562.

Bruch, H. (1973). *Eating disorders.* New York: Basic Books.

Buller, M. K., & Buller, D. B. (1987). Physicians' communication style and patient satisfaction. *Journal of Health and Social Behavior, 28,* 4, 375-388.

Burgos-Ocasio, H. (1996). Understanding the Hispanic community. In: M. Julia (ed.), *Multicultural awareness in the healthcare professions.* Boston, MA: Allyn and Bacon 111-130.

Burns, G. (1983). *How to live to be one hundred or more.* New York: Putnam's Sons.

Burton, L., Kasper, Shore, A., et. al. (1995). The structure of informal care: Are there differences by race? *The Gerontologist, 35*(6), 744-752.

Busse, E. W. (1975). Aging and psychiatric diseases of late life. In S. Arieti (Ed.), *American handbook of psychiatry,* (2nd ed., Vol. 4).

Butler, R. N. (1978). Myths and realities of clinical geriatrics. In S. S. Steury & M. Blank (Eds.), *Readings in psychotherapy with older people.* Rockville, MD: National Institute of Mental Health.

Butler, R. N. (1975). Psychotherapy in old age. In S. Arieti (Ed.), *American handbook of psychiatry* (2nd ed., Vol. 5).

Butler, R. N. (1978). The doctor and the aged patient. In W. Reichel (Ed.), *The geriatric patient.* New York: HP.

Butler, R. N., & Lewis, M. I. (1973). *Aging and mental health: Positive psychosocial approaches.* St. Louis: C.V. Mosby Company.

Calamari, J. E., Faber, S. D., Hitsman, B. L., & Poppe, C. J. (1994). Treatment of obsessive compulsive disorder in the elderly: A review and case example. *Journal of Behaviour Therapy and Experimental Psychiatry, 25,* 95-104.

Calasanti, T. M. (1996). Incorporating diversity: Meaning, levels of research, and implications for theory. *The Gerontologist, 36*(2), 147-156.

Califano, J. A., Jr. (1986). *America's health care revolution.* New York: Random House.

Calley, J. M., Dirken, M., Engalla, M., & Hennrich, M. L. (1980). The Orem self-care nursing model. In J.P. Riehl & C. Roy (Eds.), *Conceptual models for nursing practice.* New York: Appleton.

Campaigne, B. N., & Lampman, R. M. (1994). *Exercise in the clinical management of diabetes.* Champaign, IL: Human Kinetics.

Campbell, J. M., Mangeon, J., et al. (1976). The Canadian home fitness test as a predictor of aerobic capacity. *Canadian Medicine Journal, 44,* 680-682.

Campolo, T. (1986). *Who switched the price tags.* Dallas, TX: Word Publishing.

Cannon, W. B. (1932). *The wisdom of the body.* New York: W. W. Norton.

Capuzzi, D., Gross, D., & Friel, S. E. (1990, Winter). Group work with elders. *Generations, 14,* 1, 43-48.

Carlyon, W. H. (1984). Disease prevention/health promotion--bridging the gap to wellness. *Health Values: Achieving High Level Wellness, 8*(3), 27-30.

Carlyon, W. H. (1986). Myths, mindsets, and the medical model: Misunderstanding school health instruction. *Health Values: Achieving High Level Wellness. 5*(5), 207-216.

Carroll, D. (1992). *Health psychology: Stress, behaviour and disease.* Washington, DC: Falmer Press.

Carter, B., McGoldrick, M. (1988). *The changing family life cycle: A framework for family therapy,* 2nd. ed. New York; London: Gardner Press.

Cassell, E.J. (1985). *Talking with patients, 1 & 2.* Cambridge, MA: MIT Press.

Caplan, G. (1974). *Support systems and community mental health.* New York: Behavioral Publications.

Caplan, G., & Killilea, M. (Eds.). (1976). *Support systems and mutual help.* New York: Grune & Stratton.

Catania, J. A., Stall, R., Coates, T. J., Pelham, A. O., & Sacks, C. (1989). Issues in AIDS primary prevention. *Generations, 1,* 50-54.

Catania, J. A., Turner, H., Kegeles, S. M., Stall, R., Pollack, L., Spitzer, S. E., & Coates, T. J. (1985). HIV transmission risks of older heterosexuals and gays. In M. W. Riley, M. G. Ory, & D. Zablotsky (Eds.), *AIDS in an aging society.* New York: Springer Publishing Company.

Chan, A. W. K., Pristach, E. A., & Welte, J. W. (1996). Detection by the CAGE of alcoholism or heavy drinking in primary care outpaitents and the general population. *Journal of Substance Abuse, 6,* 123-135.

Chapman, L. (1986). Spiritual health: A component missing from health promotion. *American Journal of Health Promotion, 1,* 38-41.

Chapman, L. (1987). Developing a useful perspective on spiritual health: Well-Being, spiritual potential, and the search for meaning. *American Journal of Health Promotion, 1*(3), 31-39.

Chen, M. S. (1993). Cardiovascular health among Asian Americans/Pacific Islanders: An examination of health status and intervention approaches. *American Journal of Health Promotion, 7*(3), 199-207.

Chen, M. S., Jr., & Hawks, B. L. (1995). A debunking of the myth of healthy Asian Americans and Pacific Islanders. *American Journal of Health Promotion, 9*(4), March/April, 262-268.

Chen, M. S., Jr., Guthrie R., Moeschberger, M., et. al. (1993). Lessons learned and baseline data from initiating smoking cessation research with Southeast Asian adults. *Asian American and Pacific Islander Journal of Health, 1,* Autumn, 194-214.

Chen, M., Zaharlick, A., Kuun, P., et. al. (1992). Implementation of the indiginous model for health education programming among Asian minorities: beyond theory and into practice. *Journal of Health Education, 23*(7), 400-403.

Chernoff, R. (1990). Nutrition, health promotion, and aging. *Topics in Geriatric Rehabilitation, 6*(1), 19-26.

Chung, E. Asian Americans. In M. Julia, M. (Ed.). (1996). *Multicultural awareness in the healthcare professions.* Boston, MA: Allyn and Bacon.

Cinque, C. (1989, September). Back pain prescription out of bed and into the gym. *The Physician and Sportsmedicine, 17*(9), 185-188.

Cisar, C., & Kravitz, L. (1991, January). IDEA Today, 28-36.

Clark, W. B., & Midanik, L. (1982). Alcohol use and alcohol problems among U.S. adults: Results of the 1979 national survey. In Alcohol and Health Monograph, No. 1: Alcohol Consumption and Related Problems, pp. 3-52. Washington, DC: HHH Publication No. (ADM) 82-1190, USGPO.

Clayton, P. (1973). Anticipatory grief and widowhood. *British Journal of Psychiatry*, 122, 47-51.

Coe, R.M. (1987). Communication and medical care outcomes: Analysis of conversations between doctors and elderly patients. In R. Ward & S. Tobin (Eds.), *Health in aging.* New York: Springer Publishing Company.

Cohen, G.D. (1985). Toward an interface of mental and physical health phenomena in geriatrics: Clinical findings and questions. In C. Gaitz & T. Samorajski (Eds.), *Aging 2000: Our health care destiny: Biomedical issues* (Vol. 1). New York: Springer Publishing Company .

Cohen, G. D. (1992). The future of mental health and aging. In J. Birren, R. Sloane, & G. Cohen (Eds.), *Handbook of mental health and aging* (2nd ed.). San Diego: Academic Press.

Cohen, S. (1985). The aging social drinker. In S. Cohen (Ed.), *The substance abuse problems,* Vol. 2. New York: Haworth Press.

Cohen, S., & Syme, S. L. (1985). *Social support and health.* Orlando, FL: Academic Press, Inc.

Cohen-Mansfield, J. (1995). Assessment of disruptive behavior/agitation in the elderly: Function, methods, and difficulties. *Journal of Geriatric Psychiatry and Neurology, 8,* 52-60.

Cohler, B. J. (1982). Personal narrative and life course. In P.B. Balts & O.G. Brim (Eds.), *Lifespan development and behavior.* New York: Academic Press.

Coke, M. M. and Twaite, J. A. (1995). *The Black elderly, satisfaction and quality of later life.* New York: Haworth Press.

Cole, P. A., Pomerleau, C. S., and Harris, J. K. (1992). The effects of nonconcurrent and concurrent relaxation training on cardiovascular reactivity to a psychological stressor. *Journal of Behavioral Medicine, 15,* (4), 407-414.

Cole, W., Park, A., & Smilgis, M. (1995, June). The estrogen dilemma. *Time,* 46-53.

Coleman, P. G. (1974). Measuring reminiscence characteristics from conversation as adaptive features of old age. *International Journal of Aging and Human Development, 5,* 281-294.

Commission on Chronic Illness. (1957). *Chronic illness in the United States.* Cambridge, MA: Harvard University Press.

Conlin, M. M. (1980). Essentials of geriatric care. *Primary Care, 7,* 595-605.

Consumer Guide. (1988). Walking for health and fitness. Lincolnwood, IL: Publications International, Ltd.

Coons, S. J., Hendricks, J., & Shean, S. L. (1988, Summer). Self medication with non-prescription drugs. *Generations, 12,* 4.

Cooper, K. H. (1981). *The new aerobics.* New York: Bantam.

Cooper, K. H. (1982). *The aerobics program for total well-being.* New York: M. Evans & Company.

Corbin, D. E., & Corbin, J. M. (1983). *Reach for it: A handbook of exercise and dance activities for older adults.* Dubuque, IA: Eddie Bowers Publishing Company.

(COSSMHO),Policy and Research, National Coalition of Hispanic Health and Human Services Organizations, Meeting the Health Promotion Needs of Hispanic Comunities. *American Journal of Health Promotion,* Vol. 9(4), 1995, 300-311.

Cowley, G. (1990, December 10). In pursuit of a terrible killer. *Newsweek,* 66-68.

Cox, D. M., & Sachs, G. A. (1994, August). Advance directives and the patient self-determination act. *Clinics in Geriatric Medicine, 10*(3).

Cox, F. D. (1989). *The AIDS booklet.* Dubuque, IA: William C. Brown Publishers.

Critelli, J. W., & Ee, J. S. *Stress and Physical Illness: Development of an Integrative Model,* 139-159.

Crystal, S. (1989, Fall). New demands and economic consequences. *Generations,* 23-27.

Crystal, S. (1989). Persons with AIDS and older people: Common long-term care concerns. In M. W. Riley, M. G. Ory, & D. Zablotsky (Eds.), *AIDS in an aging society.* New York: Springer Publishing Company.

Crystal, S., & Jackson, M. (1988). The hidden epidemic: Public policy and the care of persons with AIDS-related complex. *AIDS Patient Care, 2*(4), 4-7.

Cunningham, W. R., & Brookbank, J. W. *Gerontology: The psychology, biology, and sociology of aging.* New York: Harper and Row Publishers.

Czikszentmihalyi, M. (1990). *Flow: The psychology of optimal experience.* New York: Harper and Row.

Davidson, D. M. (1991). *Preventive cardiology.* Baltimore, MD: Williams & Wilkens.

Davidson, P. O., & Davidson, S. M. (1980). *Behavioral medicine: Changing health lifestyles.* New York: Brunner/Mazel.

Davis, M., Eshelman, E. R., McKay, M. (1994). *The relaxation and stress reduction workbook.* 3rd ed. Oakland, CA: New Harbinger Publications.

Davis, M. A., Randall, E., Forthofer, R. N., Lee, E. S., & Margen, S. (1985, July). Living arrangements and dietary patterns of older adults in the United States. *Journal of Gerontology, 40*(4), 434-442.

Dean, K. (1986). Self-care behavior: Implications for aging. In K. Dean, T. Hickey, & A. Holstein (Eds.), *Self-care and health in old age.* London: Croom Helm.

Dennison, D. (1984, March-April). Activated health education: The development and refinement of an intervention model. *Health Values: Achieving High Level Wellness, 8*(2), 18-24.

deVries, H. A. (1982). *Fitness after 50.* New York: Charles Scribner's Sons.

Dible, L., Pardini, A., Bogaret-Tullis, M. (1985). A resource guide for injury control programs for older persons. Washington, DC: Administration on Aging.

DiDomencio, R. L., & Ziegler, W. Z. (1989). *Practical rehabilitation techniques for geriatric aides.* Rockville, MD: Aspen Publishers, Inc.

Dienstfrey, H. (1991). *Where the mind meets the body.* New York: HarperCollins Publishers.

Doherty, W. J., & Campbell, T. L. (1988). *Families and health.* Newbury Park, CA: Sage Publications.

Dominguez, R. H., & Gajda, R. (1982). *Total body training.* New York: Warner Books.

Dorland's Illustrated Medical Dictionary, 124th edition. (1965). Philadelphia: W.B. Saunders.

Douglass, M. E., & Douglass, D. N. (1980). *Manage your time, manage your work, manage yourself.* New York: AMACOM.

Dula, A. (1994, August). The life and death of Miss Mildred: An elderly Black woman. *Clinics In Geriatric Medicine, 10*(3), 419-430.

Dusek, D. (1989). *Weight management: The fitness way.* Boston, MA: Jones and Bartlett Publishers.

Dychtwald, K. (1981). Holistic approaches to healthy aging and programs for the elderly. In A. G. Hastings, J. Fadiman, & J. S. Gordon (Eds.), *Health for the whole person.* Westview Press.

Dychtwald, K. (1984). The aging of America and the implications for health promotion. *Promoting Health, 5*(4), 1-3.

Ebel, H., Sol, N., Bailey, D., & Schechter, S. (1983). *Fitness manual: The total guide.* Havertown, PA: Fitcom Corporation.

Ebersole, P., & Hess, P. (1990). *Toward healthy aging.* St. Louis: The C.V. Mosby Company.

Edelman, C., & Milio, N. (1986). Health defined. Promotion and specific protection. In C. Edelman & N. Milio (Eds.), *Health promotion throughout the lifespan.* St. Louis: C. V. Mosby Company.

Eisdorfer, C. (1977). Stress, disease and cognitive change in the aged. In C. Eisdorfer & R. B. Friedel (Eds.), *Cognitive and emotional disturbance in the elderly.* Chicago: Year Book Medical Publishers.

Ekblom, B., & Nordemar, R. (1987). Rheumatoid arthritis. In J. S. Skinner (Ed.), *Exercise testing and exercise prescription for special cases.* Philadelphia: Lea & Febiger.

Elder, T. (1995). *Water fun and fitness.* Champaigne, IL: Human Kinetics Press.

Elliot, R. S., & Breo, D. L. (1984). *Is it worth dying for?* New York: Bantam Books.

Emanuel, E. J., & Emanuel, L. L. (1992). Four models of the doctor-patient relationship. *Journal of the American Medical Association, 267,* 2221-2226.

Emmelkamp, P. M. G. (1994). *Behavior therapy with adults,* 4th ed. Bergin & Garfield (Eds.), 379-427. New York: Wiley & Sons.

Enck, P., Daublin, G., Lubke, H. J., et. al. (1994, October). Long-term efficacy of bio-feedback training for fecal incontinence. *Dis Colon Rectum,* 37(10), 997-1001.

Engler, J., & Goleman, D. (1992). *The consumer's guide to psychotherapy.* New York: Fireside.

Epstein, M. (1995). *Thoughts without a thinker: Psychotherapy from a Buddhist perspective.* New York: Basic Books.

Erikson, E. H. (1959). Identity and the life cycle. *Psychological Issues,* 1(1). New York: International University Press.

Escarce, J. J., Epstein, K. R., Colby, D. C., et. al. (1993, July). Racial differences in the elderly's use of medical procedures and diagnostic tests. *American Journal of Public Health, 83*(7), 948-954.

Estes, C. L., Fox, S., & Mahoney, C. W. (1986). Health care and social policy: Health promotion and the elderly. In K. Dychtwald (Ed.), *Wellness and health promotion for the elderly.* Rockville, MD: Aspen Systems Corporation.

Estes, C. L., Gerard, L. E., Zones, J. S., Swan, J. H. (1984). *Political economy, health, and aging.* Boston, MA: Little, Brown and Company.

Evans, W., & Rosenberg, I. H. (1991). *Biomarkers: The 10 determinants of aging you can control.* New York: Simon & Schuster.

Fabrega, H. (1975). The need for an ethnomedical science. *Science, 189,* 969-975.

Fahlberg, L. L., & Fahlberg, L. A. (1991). Spirituality and consciousness with an expanded science: Beyond the ego with empiricism, phenomenology, and contemplation. *American Journal of Health Promotion, 5*(4), 273-281.

Falvo, D. R. (1985). *Effective patient education.* Rockville, MD: Aspen Systems Corporation.

Farberow, N. L., & Moriwaki, S. Y. (1975). Self-destructive crises in the older person. *Gerontologist, 15,* 333-337.

Farrell, P., & Chalmers, K. (1985). Questioning: An intervention for health promotion. *Health Values: Achieving High Level Wellness, 9,* 7-9.

Feineman, N. (1991). Life in the fast lane. *Longevity, 7,* 74.

Ferguson, T. (1989, February/March). The guilt-free guide to a smoke-free life. *Modern Maturity,* 76-85.

Ferry, M. E., Lamy, P. P., & Becker, L. M. (1985). Physician's knowledge of prescribing for the elderly: A study of primary care physicians. *Journal of the American Geriatric Society, 33,* 616-621.

Festinger, L. (1957). *A theory of cognitive dissonance.* Stanford, CA: Stanford University Press.

Fillenbaum, G. G. (1985). Screening the elderly. *Journal of the American Geriatrics Society, 33*(10), 698-706.

Filner, B., & Williams, T. F. (1979). Health promotion for the elderly: Reducing functional dependency. In *Healthy People*. Washington, DC: U.S. Government Printing Office, 365-387.

Finelts, M. E. (1987). Factors associated with serious injury during falls by ambulatory nursing home accidents. *Journal of the American Geriatric Society, 35*(7), 644-648.

Fishback, J. B., & Lovett, S. B. (1992). Treatment of chronic major depression and assessment across treatment and follow-up in an elderly female. *Clinical Gerontologist, 12*(1), 31-40.

Fisher, E. B., Bishop, D., & Goldmuntz, J., et al. (1988). Complications for the practicing physician of the psychosocial dimensions of smoking. *Chest, 93*(2), 69s-78s.

Fitness Challenge in the Later Years. (n.d.). Washington, DC: President's Council on Physical Fitness and Sports.

Flatarone, M. A., Marks, E. C., Ryan, N. D., Meredith, C. N., Lipsitz, L. A., & Evans, W. J. (1990). High intensity strength training in nonagenarians. *Journal of the American Medical Association, 263*(22), 3029-3034.

Fleg, J., & Lakatta, E. (1984). How useful is digitalis in patients with congestive heart failure and sinus rhythm? *International Journal of Cardiology, 6,* 295-305.

Flegel, M. J. (1992). *Sport first aid.* Champaign, IL: Human Kinetics.

Florsheim, M. J., & Herr, J. J. (1990, Winter). Family counseling with elders. *Generations, 14*(1), 40-42.

Folstein, M. F., Folstein, S. E., & McHugh, P. R. (1975). "Mind-mental state," a practical method for grading the cognitive state of patients for the clinician. *Journal of Psychiatric Resources, 12,* 189-198.

Forsell, Y., Jorm, A. F., Von Strauss, E., et. al. (1995). Prevalence and Correlates of Depression in a Population of Nonagenarians. *British Journal of Psychiatry, 167,* 61-64.

Fossel, M. (1996). Reversing human aging. NY: William Morrow and Company, Inc.

Fox, R. (1986). Medicine, science, and technology. In L. Aiken & D. Mechanic (Eds.), *Applications of social science to clinical medicine and health policy.* New Brunswick: Rutgers University Press.

Fox, R.C. (1977). The medicalization and demedicalization of American society. In J. H. Knowles (Ed.), *Doing better and feeling worse.* New York: W. W. Norton.

Frankel, L. J., & Richard, B. B. (1977). *Be alive as long as you live.* Charleston, WV: Prevention Publications.

Frankel, R. T., & Owen, A. Y. (1978). *Nutrition in the community: The art of delivering services.* St. Louis, MO: Mosby.

Frankl, V. E. (1963). *Man's search for meaning.* New York: Simon and Schuster.

Franklin, B. A. (1986). Clinical components of a successful adult fitness program. *American Journal of Health Promotion, 1*(1), 6-13.

Freundenberg, N. (1978). Shaping the future of health education: From Behavior change to social change. *Health Education Monographs, 6*(4), 372-7.

Fries, J. F., & Crapo, L. M. (1981). *Vitality and aging.* San Francisco, CA: W. H. Freeman and Company.

Frisk, A. (1986). The pharmacist's role in health promotion and wellness for the elderly. In K. Dychtwald (Ed.), *Wellness and health promotion for the elderly.* Rockville, MD: Aspen Publications.

Fry, P.S. (1986). *Depression, stress, and adaptations in the elderly.* Rockville, MD: Aspen Publication.

Frye, B. A. Use of cultural themes in promoting health among Southeast Asian refugees. *The American Journal of Health Promotion, 9*(4), March/April.

Fuller, S. H., Pharm, D., & Underwood, E. S. (1989, August). Update on antidepressant medications. *U. S. Pharmacist.*

Fuller-Jonap, F., & Haley, W.E. (1995). Mental and physical health of male caregivers of a spouse with Alzheimer's disease. *Journal of Aging and Health, 7,* 99-118.

Galizia, V. J. (1989, June). How the patient's personality affects drug compliance. *U.S. Pharmacist.*

Gallagher, J. C., & Riggs, B. L. (1978). Nutrition and bone disease. *New England Journal of Medicine, 298,* 193-195.

Gallagher-Thompson, D., Hanley-Peterson, P., & Thompson, L.W. (1990). Maintenance of gains versus relapse following brief psychotherapy for depression. *Journal of Consulting and Clinical Psychology, 58,* 371-374.

Gallagher-Thompson, D., & Steffen, A. M. (1994). Comparative effects of cognitive-behavioral and brief psychodynamic psychotherapies for depressed family caregivers. *Journal of Consulting and Clinical Psychology, 62,* 543-549.

Gallo, J. J., Reichel, W., & Anderson, L. (1989). *Handbook of geriatric assessment.* Rockville, MD: Aspen Publications.

Gambert, S. R., & Guansing, A. R. (1980). Protein-calorie malnutrition in the elderly. *Journal of the American Geriatrics Society, 28,* 272-275.

Garfield, C. A. (1984). *Peak performance.* Boston: Houghton Mifflin Company.

Garmezy, N. (1991). Resilience in children's adaptation to negative life events and stressed environments. *Pediatric Annals, 20,* 459-466.

Garnet, E. (1982). *Movement is life: A holistic approach to exercise for older adults.* Princeton, NJ: Princeton Book Company.

Gasper, P. M. (1988). Fluid intake: What determines how much patients drink? *Geriatric Nursing, 9,* 221.

Gelfand, D. E. (1982). *Aging: The ethnic factor.* Boston, MA: Little Brown & Company.

Gelfand, D. E. (1994). *Aging and ethnicity.* New York: Springer Publishing Company.

Geller, A. M. D. (1996). Common addictions. *Clinical Symposia, 48*(1), 1-33.

Gelman, D. (1988, November 7). Body and soul. *Newsweek,* 86-92.

Genevay, B. (1990, Winter). A 'summit conference' model of brief therapy. *Generations, 14*(1), 58-60.

George, L. K. (1992). Community and home care for mentally ill older adults. In J. Birren, R. Sloane, & G. Cohen (Eds.), *Handbook of mental health and aging* (2nd ed.). San Diego: Academic Press.

George, L. K., Blazer, D. G., Winfield-Laird, I., Leaf, P. J., & Fishbach, R. L. (1988). Psychiatric disorders and mental health service use in later life. In J. Brody & G. Maddox (Eds.), *Epidemiology and aging.* New York: Springer Publishing Company.

Ger, G. C., Wexner, S. D., Jorge, J. M. N., et. al. (1993). Evaluation and treatment of chronic intractable rectal pain — A frustrating endeavor. *Dis Colon Rectum, 36,* 139-145.

German, P. (1988). Compliance and chronic disease. *Hypertension, 11, (Part 2, Suppl. II),* 56-60.

German, P. S. & Burton, L. S. (1989, February). Medication and the elderly. *Journal of Aging and Health,* 1(1), 4-34.

Getchell, B. (1983). *Physical fitness: A way of life.* New York: John Wiley & Sons.

Ghodes, D. M. (1986). Diabetes in American Indians: A growing problem. *Diabetes Care, 9,* 609-613.

Gibbs, N.R. (1988, February 22). Grays on the go. *Time,* 66-69.

Gingold, R. (1993, November). Prevention of health problems in later life. *The Medical Journal of Australia,* 158(15), 682-690.

Ginzberg, E. (1977). Health services, power centers, and decision making mechanisms. In J. H. Knowles (Ed.), *Doing better and feeling worse.* New York: W. W. Norton & Company.

Glantz, M. D. (1985). The detection, identification and differentiation of elderly drug misuse and abuse in a research survey. In E. Gottheil, K. Druley, T. Skolada, & H. Waxman (Eds.), *Alcoholism, drug and addiction and aging.* Springfield, IL: Charles C. Thomas.

Gold, D. T., Pieper, C. F., Westlund, R. E., et. al. (1996, May). Do racial differences in hypertension persist in successful agers? *Journal Of Aging and Health,* 8(2), 207-219.

Goldfried, M. R., & Davison, G. C. (1976). *Clinical behavior therapy.* New York: Holt, Rinehart & Winston.

Golding, L. A., Myers, C. R., & Sinning, W. E. (Eds.). (1973). *The Y's ways to physical fitness.* Chicago, IL: National Board of YMCA.

Goldwasser, A. N., Auerbach, S. M., & Harkins, S. W. (1987). Cognitive, affective, and behavioral effects of reminiscence group therapy on demented elderly. *International Journal of Aging and Human Development, 25,* 209-222.

Goleman, D., & Gurin, J. (Eds.). (1993). *Mind/body medicine: How to use your mind for better health.* New York: Consumer Reports Books.

Goodman, R. M., Steckler, A., Hoover, S., et. al. (1993, January/February). A critique of contemporary community health promotion approaches: Based on a qualitative review of six programs in Maine. *American Journal of Health Promotion,* 7(3), 208-220.

Goodstadt, M. S., Simpson, R. I., & Loranger, P. L. (1987, Winter). Health promotion: A conceptual integration. *American Journal of Health Promotion,* 1(3), 58-63.

Goodstein, R. K. (1981). Inextricable interaction: Social, psychologic and biologic stresses facing the elderly. *American Journal of Orthopsychiatry, 51,* 219-229.

Gordon, N. F. (1993). *Arthritis & your complete exercise guide.* Champaign, IL: Human Kinetics Press.

Gordon, N. F. (1993). *Breathing disorders: Your complete exercise guide.* Champaign, IL: Human Kinetics Press.

Gordon, N. F. (1993). *Diabetes: Your complete exercise guide.* Champaign, IL: Human Kinetics Press.

Gordon, N. F. (1993). *Stroke: Your complete exercise guide.* Champaign, IL: Human Kinetics Press.

Graedon, J., & Graedon, T. (1988). *50+: The Graedon's people's pharmacy for older adults*. New York: Bantam Books.

Graedon, J., & Graedon, T. (1995). *The people's guide to deadly drug interactions*. NY: St. Martin's Press.

Granger, C. V., Hamilton, A. A., Keith, R. A., Zielezny, K., & Sherwin, F. S. (1986). Advances in functional assessment for medical rehabilitation. *Topics in Geriatric Rehabilitation, 1*(3), 59-74.

Green, B. H., Copeland, J. R. M., Dewey, M. E., Sharma, V., & Davidson, I. A. (1994). Factors associated with recovery and recurrence of depression in older people: A prospective study. *International Journal of Geriatric Psychiatry, 9,* 789-795.

Green, L. W. (1978, Spring). Determining the impact and effectiveness of health education as it relates to federal policy. *Health Education Monographs, 6,* 28-66.

Green, L. W. (1984). Modifying and developing health behavior. *Annual Review of Public Health, 5,* 215-236.

Green, L. W. (1986). Evaluation model: A framework for the design of rigorous evaluation of health efforts in health promotion. *American Journal of Health Promotion, 1*(1), 77-79.

Greenberg, J. S. (1983). *Comprehensive stress management*. Dubuque, IA: Wm. C. Brown Company.

Greenberg, S. S., & Pargman, D. (1986). *Physical fitness: A wellness approach*. NJ: Prentice-Hall.

Greene, J. (July, 1985). Psychotropic drug use in older people: A review. *Journal of the Tennessee Medical Association, 78*(2), 431-435.

Greene, M. G., Adelman, R. D., Charon, R., & Friedmann, E. (1989). Concordance between physicians and their older and younger patients in the primary care medical encounter. *The Gerontologist, 29,* 808-813.

Greene, M. G., Adelman, R. D., Friedmann, E., & Charon, R. (1994). Older patient satisfaction with communication during an initial medical encounter. *Social Science and Medicine, 38,* 1279-1288.

Greene, M. G., Hoffman, S., Charon, R., & Adelman, R. (1987). Psychosocial concerns in the medical encounter: A comparison of the interactions of doctors with their old and young patients. *The Gerontologist, 27,* 64-168.

Greslamer, R. P., & Loeble, S. (1996). *The Columbia Presbyterian osteoarthritis handbook*. NY: Simon & Schuster.

Grimes, D. C., & Krasevee, J. A. (1983). *Hydrorobics*. Champaign, IL: Leisure Press.

Gryfe, B. M. (1984). Drug therapy of the aged: The problem of compliance and the roles of physicians and pharmacists. *Journal of the American Geriatrics Society, 34,* 1-4.

Guillemot, F., Bouche, B., Gower-Rousseau, C., et. al. (1995). Biofeedback for the treatment of fecal incontinence. *Dis Colon Rectum, 38,* 393-397.

Gutmann, D. (1969). The country of old men: Cross-cultural studies in the psychology of later life. Occasional papers in Gerontology, No. 5. Ann Arbor, MI: Institute of Gerontology, University of Michigan-Wayne State University.

Hafen, B. A., & Frandsen, K. J. (1985). Addictive behavior and dependence. *Addictive behavior*. Englewood, CO: Morton Publishing Company.

356

Hahn, R. A., Mulinare, J., Teutsch, S. (1992, January 8). Inconsistencies in coding of race and ethnicity between birth and death in U.S. infants. *JAMA, 267*(2), 259-263.

Hale, C. B. (1992). A demographic profile of African Americans. In R.L. Braithwaite, S. E. Taylor (Eds.), *Health issues in the black community*. San Francisco: Jossey-Bass Publishers, 6-19.

Haley, J. (1973). *Uncommon therapy: The psychiatric techniques of Milton H. Erickson, M.D.* New York: Norton.

Hall, J. A., Milburn, M. A., & Epstein, A. M. (1993). A causal model of health status and satisfaction with medical care. *Medical Care, 31*, 84-94.

Hall, J. A., Roter, D. L., & Katz, N. R. (1988). Meta-analysis of correlates of provider behavior in medical encounters. *Medical Care, 26*, 657-675.

Hamalainen, K. P. J., Raivio, P., Antila, S., et. al. (1996). Biofeedback therapy in rectal prolapse patients. *Dis Colon Rectum, 39*, 262-265.

Hanawalt, C. L. (1992). Physical Exercise and Chronic Disease. In M. L. Teague & V. L. McGhee (Eds.), *Health promotion: High-level wellness in later years*. Dubuque: Wm. C. Brown, Publishers.

Hansen, A. G., Jensen, H., Langesen, L. P., & Peterson, A. (1982). Withdrawal of antihypertensive drugs in the elderly. *Acta Medica Scandanavia, 676*, 178-185.

Hardin, G. (1968). The tragedy of the commons. *Science, 162*, 1243-1248.

Harris, B. A., Jette, A. M., Campion, E. W., & Cleary, P. D. (1986). Validity of self-report measures of functional disability. *Topics in Geriatric Rehabilitation, 1*(3), 31-42.

Harris, C. S. (1978). *The fact book on aging: A profile of America's older population*. Washington, DC: National Council on the Aging.

Harris, M. (1985). Prevalence of noninsulin dependent diabetes and impaired glucose tolerance. In Diabetes in America, Section 6, 1-31. U.S. Department of Health and Human Services Publication, NIH #85-1468.

Haskell, W. L. (1987). *Coronary heart disease. Exercise testing and exercise prescription for special cases*. Philadelphia: Lea & Febiger.

Haug, M., Belgrave, L. L., & Gratton, B. (1984). Mental health and the elderly: Factors in stability and change over time. *Journal of Health and Social Behavior, 25*, 100-115.

Haug, M. R., & Ory, M. G. (1987). Issues in elderly patient-provider interactions. *Research on Aging, 9*, 3-44.

Hawks, S., Hull, M., Thalman, R., et. al. (1995). Review of spiritual health: Definition, role, and intervention strategies in health promotion. *American Journal of Health Promotion, 9*(5), 371-378.

Healy, B. M. D. (1995). *A New prescription for women's health*. NY: Viking.

Hearing Before the Special Committee on Aging. (1987, July 20). Prescription drugs and the elderly: The high cost of growing old. Washington, DC: United States Senate.

Heckler, M. (1985, August). *Report of the Secretary's task force on Black and minority health*. U.S. Department of Health and Human Services. Executive Summary, Vol. 1.

Heidrich, S. M., & Ryff, C. D. (1993). Physical and mental health in later life: The self-esteem as mediator. *Psychology and Aging, 8*, 327-338.

Henderson, J. B., & Enelow, A. J. (1976). The coronary risk factor problem: A behavioral perspective. *Preventive Medicine, 5,* 128-148.

Henderson, J. B., Hall, S. M., & Lipton, H. L. (1979). Changing self-destructive behaviors. In G. E. Stone, F. Cohen, N. E. Adler and Associates, *Health psychology: A handbook.* San Francisco, CA.

Henderson, L. J. (1935). Physician and patient as a social system. *New England Journal of Medicine, 212,* 819-823.

Henig, M. R. (1988). *The myth of senility.* Glenview, IL: Scott, Foresman and Company.

Herr, J. J., & Weakland, J. H. (1979). *Counseling elders and their families.* New York: Springer Publishing Company.

Herzog, A.R., & House, J.S. (1991, Winter). Productive activities and aging well. *Generations, 15(1),* 49-54.

Hickey, T. (1986). Health behavior and self-care in late life: An introduction. In K. Dean, T. Hickey, & B. Holstein (Eds.), *Self-care and health in old age.* London: Croom Helm.

Hodgson, R., Abbasi, T., and Clarkson, J. (1996). Effective mental health promotion: A literature review. *Health Education Journal, 55,* 55-74.

Hoenig, H. (1993). Educating primary care physicians in geriatric rehabilitation. *Clinics in Geriatric Medicine, 9,* 883-893.

Hollon, S. D. and Beck, A. T. (1994). Cognitive and Cognitive Behavioral Therapies. In A. E. Bergin, & S. L. Garfield (Eds.), *Handbook of psychotherapy and behavior change*, 4th ed. New York: John Wiley and Sons.

Holmes, E. R. and Holmes, L. D. (1995). *Other cultures, elder years.* Thousand Oaks, London, England, (2nd ed.). Sage Publications.

Holmes, T. H., & Rahe, R. H. (1967). The social readjustment rating scale. *Journal of Psychosomatic Research, 11,* 213-218.

Houlihan, J. P. (1987). Families caring for frail and demented elderly: A review of selected findings. *Family Systems Medicine, 5,* 344-356.

House, J. S., Robbins, C., & Metzner, H. (1982). The association of social relationships and activities with mortality: Prospective evidence from the Tecumseh Community Health Study. *American Journal of Epidemology, 116,* 123-140.

House, J. S., Landis, K. R., & Umberson, D. (1988). Social relationships and health. *Science,* 540-545.

Houston, J. (1982). *The possible human.* Los Angeles: J. P. Tarcher, Inc.

Howley, E. T., & Franks, D. (1992). *Health fitness instructor's handbook.* Champaign, IL: Human Kinetics Press.

Hu, F., & Cartwright, W. S. (1986). Evaluation of the costs of caring for the senile demented elderly: A pilot study. *Gerontologist, 26,* 158-163.

Huey, L., & Knudson, L. R. (1986). *The waterpower workout.* New York: New American Library.

Hurley, O. (1988). Safe therapeutic exercises for the frail elderly. Center for Studies on Aging, 706 Madison Avenue, Albany, NY 10228.

Ike, R. W., Lampman, R. M., & Castor, C. W. (1989). Arthritis and aerobic exercise: A review. *The Physician and Sports-medicine, 17(2),* 128-137.

Imber-Black, E. (1991). Rituals and the healing process. In F. Walsh & M. McGoldrick, (Eds.). *Living beyond loss: Death in the family.* W. W. Norton & Company, New York, NY; and London, England, 207-223.

Jaccard, J. (1975). A theoretical analysis of selected factors important to education strategies. *Health Education Monographs, 78,* 152-167.

Jackson, J. S., Lockery, S. A., & Juster, F. T. (1996). Introduction: Health and retirement among ethnic and racial minority groups. *The Gerontologist, 36*(1), 282-284.

Jacobson, E. J. (1929). *Progressive relaxation: A physiological and clinical investigation of muscular states and their significance in psychology and medical practice.* Chicago, IL: University of Chicago Press.

Jacobson, E. J. (1938). Progressive relaxation (2nd ed.). Chicago: Chicago Press.

Jaffe, D. T., & Scott, C. D. (n.d.). *From burnout to peak performance.* New York: McGraw-Hill Paperbacks.

Jajich, C., Ostfeld, A., & Freeman, D. (1985). Smoking and coronary heart disease mortality in the elderly, *Journal of the American Medical Association, 252*(20), 2, 831-834.

Janis, I. L. (1975). "Reaction" to section titled "Public opinion, attitude research and health problems." In A. J. Enelow & J. B. Henderson (Eds.), Applying behavioral science to cardiovascular risk. New York: American Heart Association.

Jette, A. M. (1986, April). Functional disability and rehabilitation of the aged. *Topics in Geriatric Rehabilitation, 3,* 1-8.

Jones, N., Berman, L., Bartkiewicz, P., & Oldridge, N. (1987). Chronic destructive respiratory disorders. In James S. Skinner (Ed.), *Exercise testing and exercise prescription for special cases.* Philadelphia: Lea & Febiger.

Jones, T. (1984). Balance. *Esquire, 101*(5), 112-114.

Julia, M. C., Ed. (1996). *Multicultural awareness in the health care professions.* Allyn and Bacon. Boston, MA.

Jutras, S., & Lavoie, J. P. (1995). Living with an impaired elderly person: The informal caregiver's physical and mental health. *Journal of Aging and Health, 7,* 46-73.

Kabat-Zinn, J. (1982). An outpatient program in behavioral medicine for chronic pain patients based on the practice of mindfulness meditation: Theoretical considerations and preliminary results. *General Hospital Psychiatry, 4,* 33-47.

Kabat-Zinn, J. (1993). Mindfulness Meditation: Health Benefits Of An Ancient Buddhist Practice. In D. Goleman, & J. Gurin (eds.), *Mind/body medicine.* Younkers, NY: Consumer Reports Books, 259-276.

Kabat-Zinn, J., Lipworth, L., Burney, R. (1985). The clinical use of mindfulness meditation for the self-regulation of chronic pain. *Journal of Behavioral Medicine, 8,* 163-90.

Kabat-Zinn, J., Lipworth, L., Burney, R., Sellers, W. (1986). Four year follow-up of a meditation-based program for the self-regulation of chronic pain: Treatment outcomes and compliance. *Clinical Journal of Pain, 2,*159-73.

Kabat-Zinn, J., Massion, A. O., Kristeller, J., et al. (1992, July). Effectiveness of a meditation-based stress reduction program in the treatment of anxiety disorders. *American Journal of Psychiatry, 149*(7), 936-943.

Kahn, R. L. (1994). Social support: Content, causes and consequences. In Abeles, R. P., H. C. Gift, & M. G. Ory (Eds.), *Aging and the quality of life*. New York: Springer Publishing Company. 163-184.

Kamm, A. (1979). Senior olympics. *Journal of Physical Education and Recreation, 50*, 32-33.

Kaplan, S. H., Greenfield, S., & Ware, J. E. (1989). Impatient of the doctor-patient relationship on the outcomes of chronic illness. In M. Stewart & D. Roter (Eds.), *Communicating with medical patients*. Newbury Park, CA: Sage Publications.

Kart, C. S., & Metress, S. P. (1984). *Nutrition, the aged, and society*. Englewood Cliffs, NJ: Prentice-Hall, Inc.

Kasl, S. R., & Berkman, L. F. (1977). Some psychological influences on the health status of the elderly: The perspective of social epidemiology. In J. L. McGaugh & S. B. Keisler (Eds.), *Aging: Biology and behavior*. New York: Academic Press.

Katch, F. I., & McArdle, W. D. (1983). *Nutrition, weight control, and exercise*. Philadelphia, PA: Lea & Febiger.

Katz, S., Ford, A. B., & Moskowitz, R. W., et al. (1963). Studies of illness in the aged: The index of ADL. *Journal of the American Medical Association, 185*, 914-919.

Kazdin, A. E., & Wilson, G. T. (1978). *Evaluation of behavior therapy: Issues, evidence, and research strategies*. Cambridge, MA: Ballinger.

Keck, J. O., Staniunas, R. J., Coller, J. A., et. al. (1994). Biofeedback training is useful in fecal incontinence but disappointing in constipation. *Dis Colon Rectum, 37*, 1271-1276.

Kelman, H. C., (1969). In W. Bennes, K. Bennes, & R. Chin (Eds.), *Processes of opinion change: Readings in the applied behavioral sciences* (2nd ed.). New York: Holt, Rinehart & Winston.

Kent, K. L. (1990, Winter). Community mental-health centers. *Generations, 14*(1),19-21.

Kerner, J. F., Dusenbury, L., Mandelblatt, J. S. (1993). Poverty and cultural diversity: challenges for health promotion among the medically underserved. *Annual Review of Public Health, 14*, 355-372.

Kessler, R. C., Neighbors, H. W. (1986). A new perspective on the relationship among race, social class, and psychological distress. *Journal of Health and Social Behavior, 27*, 107-115.

Kiecolt-Glaser, J. K., & Glaser, R. (1993). Mind and immunity. In J. Goleman, Daniel, & Gurin (eds.). Mind/body medicine: How to use your mind for better health. *Consumer Reports Books*. New York, NY, 39-64.

King, R., & Herzins, W. F. (1968). *Golden age exercises*. New York: Crown Publishers.

Kirscht, J. P. (1974). The health belief model and illness behavior. *Health Education Management, 2*(4), 387-408.

Kirscht, J. P., & Rosenstock, I. ((1980). Patients' problems in following recommendations of health experts. In G. Stone, F. Cohen, & N. Adler (Eds.), *Health psychology*. San Francisco: Jossey-Bass Publishers.

Kiyak, A., Lians, J., & Kahana, E. (1976). *A methodological inquiry into the schedule of recent life events*. Paper presented at Symposium on Life Events. New York: American Psychological Association.

Klein, L. E., German, P. S., & Levine, D. M. (1981). Adverse drug reactions among the elderly: A reassessment. *Journal of the American Geriatric Society, 29,* 525-529.

Klein, L. E., Rola, R. P., McArthur, J., et al. (1985). Univariate and multivariate analysis of the mental state examination. *Journal of American Geriatric Society, 33,* 483-488.

Klein, W. H., Le Shan, E., Furman, S. S. (1966). *Promoting mental health of older people through group methods: A practical guide.* New York: Manhattan Society for Mental Health.

Klerman, G. L. (1986). Drugs and psychotherapy. In S. Garfield & A. Bergin (Eds.), *Handbook of psychotherapy and behavior change* (3rd ed.). New York: John Wiley & Sons.

Klerman, G. L., Weissman, M. M., Karkowitz, J. C., et al. (1994). Medication and psychotherapy. In A. Bergin & S. Garfield (Eds.), *Handbook of psychotherapy and behavior change* (4th ed.). New York: John Wiley & Sons.

Kneller, G. F. (1963). *Foundations of education.* New York: John Wiley & Sons.

Kobasa, S. (1979) Stressful life events, personality and health: An inquiry. *Journal of Personality and Social Psychology, 37*(1), 1-11.

Kobasa, S., Maddi, C., Salvatove, R., Kahn, S. (1979). Personality and constitution as mediators in the stress-illness relationship: Clarification. *Journal of Personality and Social Psychology, 37*(1), 1-11.

Kobasa, S., Maddi, C., Salvatove, R., Kahn, S. (1982). Hardiness and health: A prospective study. *Journal of Personality and Social Psychology, 42*(1), 168-177.

Kobasa, S., Maddi, C., Salvatove, R., Kahn, S. (1993). Hardiness and health: A prospective study clarification. *Journal of Personality and Social Psychology, 65*(1), 207.

Koenig, H. G., & Blazer, D. G. (1992). Mood disorders and suicide. In J. Birren, R. Sloane, & G. Cohen (Eds.). *Handbook of mental health and aging* (2nd ed.). San Diego: Academic Press.

Koff, T. H. (1986). Wellness and long-term care. In K. Dychtwald (Ed.), Wellness and health promotion for the elderly. Rockville, MD: Aspen Publication.

Kumanyika, S. K., & Charleston, J. B. (1992). Lose weight and win: A church based weight loss program for blood pressure control among Black women. *Patient Education and Counseling, 19,* 19-32.

Kuntzleman, C. T. (1980). *Rating the exercises.* New York: Penguin Books.

Labrecque, M. S., Blanchard, C. G., Ruckdeschel, J. C., & Blanchard, E. B. (1991). The impact of family presence on the physician-cancer patient interaction. *Social Science and Medicine, 33,* 1253-1261.

Laine C., & Davidoff, F. (1996). Patient-centered medicine: A professional evolution. *Journal of the American Medical Association, 275,* 152-156.

Lamy, P. P. (1980). *Prescribing for the elderly.* Littleton, MA: PSG Publishing Company, Inc.

Landin, R. J., Linnemeier, T. J., Rothbaum, D. A., et al. (1985). Exercise testing and training of the elderly patient. In N. K. Wenger (Ed.), *Exercise and the heart.* Philadelphia, PA: F. A. Davis.

Langer, E. J. (1989). Mindfulness. Reading, MA: Addison-Wesley.

Lawrence, P. (1981). Applying skills with special populations. In J.E. Myers (Ed.), *Counseling older persons*, Vol. 2. Basic helping skills for service providers. Falls Church, VA: American Personnel and Guidance Association.

Lazarus, R. S., & DeLongis, A. (1983). Psychological stress and coping in aging. *American Psychologist, 38,* 245-253.

Lazarus, R. S., and Folkman, S. (1984). *Stress, appraisal and coping.* New York: Springer-Verlag,.

Lee, D., Johnson, R. A., Bingham, J. B., et al. (1982). Heart failure in outpatients: A randomized trial of digoxin versus placebo. *New England Journal of Medicine, 306,* 699-705.

Lehrer, P. M., Carr, R., Sargunaraj, D., and Woolfolk, R. (1993). Differential effects of stress management techniques in behavioral medicine. In P. M. Lehrer, & R. L. Woolfolk (Eds.). *Principles and practices of stress management*, 2nd ed. The Guilford Press, New York, NY., London, England, 571-605.

Lehrer, P. M., Sargunaraj, D., Woolfolk, R.L. (1994). *Stress management techniques: Are they all equivalent, or do they have specific effects?* Plenum Publishing Corporation. Vol. 19, No. 4.

Lehrer, P. M., Woolfolk, R. L. (1993). Specific effects of stress management techniques. In P. M. Lehrer, & R. L. Woolfolk (Eds.), *Principles and practices of stress management*, 2nd ed. The Guilford Press New York, NY.; London, England, 481-520.

Lehrer, P. M., Woolfolk, R. L. (Eds.). (1993). *Principles and practices of stress management.* 2nd ed. The Guilford Press, New York, NY., London, England, 1.

Leon, A. (1987). Diabetes. In James S. Skinner (Ed.), *Exercise testing and exercise prescription for special cases.* Philadelphia: Lea & Febiger.

Leon, A. S., Connett, J., Jacobs, D. R., & Rauramaa, R. (1987). Leisure-time physical activity levels and risk of coronary heart disease and death. *Journal of the American Association of Medicine, 258*(17), 2388-2395.

Leonard, G. (1984, May). Balancing acts. *Esquire, 101*(5), 116.

LeSage, J., & Zwygart-Stauffacher, M. (1988, Summer). Detection of medication misuse in elders. *Generations,* XII, 4.

Leslie, D. K., & McClure, J. W. (1975). Exercises for the elderly. Des Moines, IA: Commission on Aging.

Leventhal, H., & Cleary, P. D. (1980). The smoking problem: A review of the research and theory in behavioral risk modification. *Psychological Bulletin, 88,* 370-405.

Leviton, D. (1974). Toward a humanistic dimension of HPER. *Journal of Physical Education and Recreation, 45,* 41-43.

Levy, J. A., & Albrecht, G. L. (1989). Methodological considerations in research on sexual behavior and AIDS among older people. In M. W. Riley, M. G. Ory, & D. Zablotsky, *AIDS in an aging society.* New York: Springer Publishing Company.

Lewis, C. B. (1989). *Improving mobility in older persons.* Rockville, MD: Aspen Publishers, Inc.

Lewis, M. (1985). Older women and health: An overview. *Women & Health, 10,* 1-16.

Lieberman, M. A. (1978). Social and psychological determinant of adaptation. *International Journal of Aging and Human Development, 9*(2), 115-126.

Lieu, T. A., Newacheck, P. W., and McManus, M. A. (1993, July). Race, ethnicity, and access to ambulatory care among U.S. adolescents. *American Journal of Public Health, 83*(7), 960-965.

Like, R., & Zyzanski, S. J. (1987). Patient satisfaction with the clinical encounter: Social psychological determinants. *Social Science and Medicine, 24,* 351-357.

Lindsay, R. (1989). Osteoporosis: An updated approach to prevention and management. *Geriatrics, 44*(7), 57-62.

Linn, M. W., Linn, B. S., & Stein, S. R. (1982). Satisfaction with ambulatory care and compliance in older patients. *Medical Care, 20,* 606-614.

Lissoni, P., Tisi, E., Barni, et. al. (1992). Biological and clinical results of a neuroimmunotherapy with Interleukin-2 and the pineal hormone melatonin as a first line treatment in advanced non-small cell lung cancer. *British Journal of Cancer, 149,* 936-943.

Lockette, K. F. (1994). Conditioning with Physical Disabilities. Champaign, IL: Human Kinetics Press.

Longe, M. E. (1986). Hospitals and health promotion for older adults. In K. Dychtwald (Ed.), *Wellness and health promotion for the elderly.* Rockville, MD: Aspen Systems Corporation.

Lorig, K., (1989). Holman Halsted. Long term outcomes of an arthritis self managment study: Affects of reinforcement efforts. Special Issue: Health self-care. *Social Science and Medicine, 29*(2), 221-224.

Luks, A., & Barbato, J. (1989). *You are what you drink.* New York: Villard Books.

Lundervold, D. A., & Poppen, R. (1995). Biobehavioral rehabilitation for older adults with essential tremor. *The Gerontologist, 35*(4), 556-559.

Lustbader, W. (1990, Winter). Mental health services in a community health center. *Generations, 14*(1), 22-23.

Lutwak, L. (1969). Symposium on osteoporosis: Nutritional aspects of osteoporsis. *Journal of the American Geriatric Society, 17,* 115-119.

MacNeil, R. D., & Teague, M. L. (1987). *Aging and leisure: Vitality in later life.* Englewood Cliffs, NJ: Prentice Hall.

Maddox, G. (1991). Aging with a difference. *Generations, 3,* 7-10.

Maddox, G. L., & Blazer, D. G. (1984). Alcohol and aging. *Center Report on Advances and Research, 8*(4), Duke University, Center for Study of Aging and Human Development. Durham, NC.

Mahoney, F. I., & Barthel, D. W. (1965). Functional evaluation: The Barthel index. *Maryland State Medical Journal, 14,* 61-65.

Maldok, G. L., & Blazer, D. G. (1984). Alcohol and aging. *Center Report on Advances and Research, 8*(4). Durham, NC: Center for Study of Aging: Human Development.

Maloney, S. K., Fallon, B., & Wittenberg, C. K. (1984). *Aging and health promotion: Market research for public education.* Office of Disease Prevention and Health Promotion. Washington, DC: U.S. Department of Health and Human Services.

Maloney, S.K., Fallon, B., & Wittenberg, C.K. (1984, Sept.-Oct.). Study of seniors identifies attitudes, barriers to promoting their health. *Promoting Health,* 6-8.

Manton, K. G., & Singer, B. (1989). Forecasting the impact of the AIDS epidemic on elderly populations. In M. W. Riley, M. G. Ory, & D. Zablotsky (Eds.), *AIDS in an aging society.* New York: Springer Publishing Company.

Marge, M. (1988, Spring). Health promotion for persons with disabilities: Moving beyond rehabilitation. *American Journal of Health Promotion, 12*(4), 29-35.

Markides, K. S., & Black, S. (1996). *Race, ethnicity and aging: The impact of inequality,* 153-170.

Maslow, A. (1959). Creativity in self-actualizing people. In H. Anderson (Ed.), *Creativity and its cultivator.* New York: Harper and Row Publishers, Inc.

Massion, A. O., Teas, J., Hebert, J. R., et. al. (1995). Meditation, melatonin and breast/prostate cancer: Hypothesis and preliminary data. *Medical Hypotheses, 44,* 39-46.

Maud, P. J., and Foster, C. (1995). *Physiological assessment of human fitness.*

May, P. A., Moran, J. R. (1995, March/April). Prevention of alcohol misuse: A review of health promotion efforts among American Indians. *American Journal of Health Promotion, 9*(4), 288-299.

McAtee, R. E. Facilitated stretching: PNF stretching made easy. Champaign, IL: Human Kinetics Press.

McClary, C. L., Zahrt, J. D., James, R. N., Montgomery, J. H., Walker, H., & Petry, J. R. (1985, Nov.-Dec.). Wellness: The mode in the new paradigm. *Health Values: Achieving High Level Wellness, 9*(6), 8-15.

McCune, D., & Sprague, R. (1990). Exercise for low back pain. In J. Basmajian & Steven Wolf (Eds.), *Therapeutic exercise.* Baltimore/Hong Kong/London/Sydney: Williams & Wilkins.

McDaniel, J. S. *Stressful life events and psychoneuroimmunology,* 3-36.

McDaniel, S., Campbell, T. L., & Seaburn, D. B. (1990). *Family-oriented primary care: A manual for medical providers.* New York: Springer-Verlag.

McDowell, B. J., Burgio, K. L., Dombrowski, M., et al. (1992). An interdisciplinary approach to the assessment and behavioral treatment of urinary incontinence in geriatric outpatients. *Journal of American Geriatrics Society, 40,* 370-374.

McFadden, S. H., & Gerl, R. R. (1990, Fall). Approaches to understanding spirituality in the second half of life. *Generations,* 35-38.

McGinnis, J. M. (1988). The Tithonus syndrome: Health and aging in America. In R. Chernoff & D. Lipschitz (Eds.), *Health promotion and disease prevention.* New York: Raven Press, Ltd.

McGinnis, J. M. (1988). Year 2000 health objectives for nation, surgeon general's workshop: Health promotion and aging. March 20-23, Washington, DC.

McGoldrick, M., Almeida, R., Hines, P. M., et al. (1988). *Mourning in different cultures,* 178-205.

McGoon, D. (1990). *The Parkinson's handbook.* New York/London: W. W. Norton & Company.

McGuigan, F. J. (1993). Progressive Relaxation: Origins, Principles and Clinical Applications. In P. M. Lehrer, & R. L. Woolfolk (Eds.). Principles and Practices of Stress Management, 2nd ed. The Guilford Press, New York, NY; London, England, 17-52.

McKinlay, J. B., Skinner, K., Riley, J. W., Jr., & Zablotsky, D. (1989). On the relevance of social science concepts and perspectives. In M. W. Riley, M. G. Ory, & D. Zablotsky (Eds.), *AIDS in an aging society.* New York: Springer Publishing Company, 127-146.

McKnight, J. (1982). Health in the medical era. *Perspectives, 13.*

McReynolds, W. T., Lutz, R. N., Paulsen, B. K., & Kohrs, M. B. (1976). Weight loss resulting from two behavior modification procedures with nutritionists as therapists. *Behavior Therapy, 7,* 283-291.

Mellins, C. A., Blum, M. J., Boyd-Davis, S. L., & Gatz, M. (1993, Winter/Spring). Family network perspectives on caregiving. *Generations, 17*(1), 21-24.

Messana, I., & Beizer, J. (1991, January/February). Diabetes in elderly. *Practical Diabetology, 10*(1), 1-4.

Michocki, R. J., Pharm, D., & Lamy, P. O. (1988). A "risk" approach to adverse drug reactions. *Journal of the American Geriatric Society, 36,* 79-81.

Miller, H., & Morley, D. (1987). Low functional capacity. In J. S. Skinner (Ed.), Exercise testing and exercise prescription for special cases. Philadelphia: Lea & Febiger.

Miller, J. J., Fletcher, K., and Kabat-Zinn, J. (1995). Three year follow-up and clinical implications of a mindfulness meditation-mased stress reduction intervention in the treatment of anxiety disorders. *General Hospital Psychiatry, 17,* 192-200.

Miller, N. H. (1995). Lifestyle management for patients with heart disease. Champaign, IL: Human Kinetics.

Miller, R. W. (1983, July-Aug.). Doctors, patients don't communicate. FDA Consumer.

Miller, T. W. (Ed.). (1996). *Theory and assessment of stressful life events.* Madison, WI: International Universities Press, Inc.

Minkler, M., & Fullarton, J. (1980). *Promotion, health maintenance and disease prevention for the elderly.* Background paper for the 1981 White House Conference on Aging prepared by for the Office of Health Information, Health Promotion, Physical Fitness and Sports Medicine. Washington, DC: Department of Health and Human Services.

Minkler, M., & Pasick, R. J. (1986). Health promotion and the elderly: A critical perspective on the past and future. In K. Dychtwald (Ed.), *Wellness and health promotion for the elderly.* Rockville, MD: Aspen Publication.

Mirkin, G., & Hoffman, M. (1978). *The sportsmedicine book.* Boston: Little, Brown and Company.

Mischel, W. (1974). Process in the delay of gratification. In L. Berkowitz (Ed.), *Advances in experimental psychology,* (Vol. 7). New York: Academic Press.

Mischel, W. (1979). On the future of personality and assessment. *American Psychologist, 34,* 740-754.

Mishara, B.L. (1985). What we know, don't know and need to know about older alcoholics and how to help them: Models of prevention and treatment. In E. Gottheil, K. Druley, T. Skolada, & H. Waxman (Eds.), *Alcoholism, drug addiction and aging.* Springfield, IL: Charles C. Thomas.

Mishler, E. G. (1984). *The discourse of medicine: Dialectics of medical interviews.* Norwood, NJ: Ablex Publishing Corporation.

Moberg, P. J., & Lazarus, L. W. (1990). Psychotherapy of depression in the elderly. *Psychiatric Annals, 20,* 92-96.

Moffatt, F., Mohr, C., & Ames, D. (1995). A group therapy programme for depressed and anxious elderly inpatients. *International Journal of Geriatric Psychiatry, 10,* 37-40.

Moffat, M.J., & Painter, C. (Eds.). (1974). *Revelations: Diaries of women*. New York: Random House.

Monahan, D.J., & Hooker, K. (1995). Health of spouse caregivers of dementia patients: The role of personality and social support. *Social Work, 40,* 305-314.

Montes, J. H., Eng, E., Braithwaite, R. (1995, March/April). A commentary on minority health as a paradigm shift in the United States. *American Journal of Health Promotion, 9*(4), 247-250.

Montoye, H .J., & Lamphiear, D. F. (1977). Grip strength in males and females, age 10 to 69. *Research Quarterly, 48,* 109-120.

Moran, M. J. (1990). Smoking cessation and the elderly: It's never too late to quit. *Topics in Geriatric Rehabilitation, 6*(1), 46-56.

Moreley, J. (1992). Ethnicity and Aging. *Journal of the American Geriatric Society,* 40(11), 1183-1184.

Morin, C. M., Kowatch, R. A., Barry, T., & Walton, E. (1993). Cognitive-behavior therapy for late-life insomnia. *Journal of Consulting and Clinical Psychology, 61,* 137-146.

Morse, C. E., & Smith, E. L. (1981). Physical activity programming for the aged. In E. C. Smith & R. C. Serfass (Eds.), *Exercise and aging: The scientific basis*. Hillside, NJ: Enslow Publications.

Morse, D. R. (1995). Stress: Clarification of a Confused Concept. *International Journal of Psychosomatics, 42*(1-4), 4-24.

Mosher-Ashley, P. (1993). Referral patterns of elderly clients to a community mental health center. *Journal of Gerontological Social Work, 20*(3/4), 5-23.

Moss, J. T., Pharm, D., & Bleidt, B. A. (1989, July). Effects of aging on the disposition of drugs. *U.S. Pharmacist*.

Mui, A. C.,& Burnette, D. (1994). Long-term care service use by frail elders: Is ethnicity a factor? *The Gerontologist, 34*(2), 190-198.

Murray, M. D., et al. (1986). Factors contributing to medication noncompliance in elderly public housing tenants. *Drug Intelligence and Clinical Pharmacy, 20,* 146-152.

Mustard, A. S. (1945). *Government in public health*. New York: Commonwealth Fund.

Nachemson, A. L. (1990). Exercise, fitness and back pain. In A. L. Nachemson (Ed.), *Exercise, fitness and health*, 533-540. Champaign, IL: Human Kinetics Books.

Nagle, F. J., Balke, B., Naughton, J. P. (1965). Graduational step tests for assessing work capacity. *Journal of Applied Physiology, 20,* 745-748.

Nash, J. M. (1990, November 26). A slow, savage killer. *Time,* 52-54, 59.

National Center for Health Services Research (1985). *Utilization of hospital in patient services by elderly Americans*. (DHHS Publication # PHS: 85-3351). Washington, DC: U.S. Government Printing Office.

National Institute on Drug Abuse. (1982). Treatment research report: Drug taking among the elderly. (DHHS Publication No. ADM 83-1229). Washington, DC.

National Institutes of Health Technology Assessment Panel on Integration of Behavioral and Relaxation Approaches Into the Treatment of Chronic Pain and Insomnia. *JAMA, 276*(4), 313-318, July 24/31, 1996.

Neighbors, H. W., Braithwaite, R. L., Thompson, E. (1995, March/April). Health promotion and African-Americans: From personal empowerment to community action. *The American Journal of Health Promotion, 9*(4), 281-287.

Nelson, A. (1974). Functional ambulation profile. *Physical Therapy,* 54, 1061.

Nelson, E. C., Roberts, E., Simmons, J., & Tisdale, W. A. (1986). *Medical and health guide for people over fifty.* Washington, DC: AARP.

Neugarten, B. (1982). Policy for the 1980s: Age or need entitlement? In B. Neugarten (Ed.), *Age or need.* Beverly Hills, CA: Sage Publications.

Newsom, J. T., & Schulz, R. (1996). Social support as a mediator in the relation between functional status and quality of life in older adults. *Psychology and Aging, 11*(1), 34-44.

Nichols, M. P., & Schwartz, R. C. (1991). *Family therapy: Concepts and methods* (2nd ed.). Boston: Allyn and Bacon.

Nicholson, N. L., & Blanchard, E. B. (1993). A controlled evaluation of behavioral treatment of chronic headache in the elderly. *Behavior Therapy, 24,* 395-408.

Nieman, D. C. (1990). *Fitness and sports medicine: An introduction.* Palo Alto, CA: Bull Publishing Company.

Notelovitz, M. & Tonnessen, D. (1993). *Menopause & midlife health.* NY: St. Martin's Press.

Notelovitz, M., & Ware, M. (1985). *Stand tall!* New York: Bantam Books.

Nowak, C.A. (1985). Life events and drinking behavior in later years. In E. Gottheil, K. Druley, T. Skoloda, & H. Waxman (Eds.), *Alcoholism, drug addiction and aging.* Springfield, IL: Charles C. Thomas.

O'Donnell, M. P. (1986, Fall). Definition of health promotion: Part I. *American Journal of Health Promotion, 1*(2), 6-9.

O'Donnell, M. P., & Ainsworth, T. A. (1984). *Health promotion in the workplace.* New York: John Wiley & Sons.

O'Donohue, W. T., Fisher, J. E., & Krasner, L. (1986). Behavior therapy and the elderly: A conceptual and ethical analysis. *International Journal of Aging and Human Development, 23,* 1-15.

Older American Resources and Services (OAES). (n.d.). Methodology: Multidimensional functional assessment questionnaire (2nd ed.). Durham, NC: Duke University Center for the Study of Aging and Human Development.

Omenn, G. S. (1990, Summer). Prevention and the elderly: Appropriate policies. *Promoting Health,* 80-93.

Ong, L. M. L., de Haes, J. C. J. M., Hoos, A. M., & Lammes, F. B. (1995). Doctor-patient communication: A review of the literature. *Social Science and Medicine, 40,* 903-918.

Opatz, J. P. (1985). *A primer of health promotion.* Washington, DC: Oryn Publications, Inc.

Orem, D. E. (1980). *Nursing concepts of practice.* New York: McGraw-Hill.

Ornis, D. (1990). *Reversing heart disease.* NY: Baltimore Books.

Ornish, D. (1991, May). Can life-style changes reverse coronary atherosclerosis? *Hospital Practice, 26,* 123-132.

Ornish, D. (1992). *Dr. Dean Ornish's program for reversing heart disease.* New York, NY. Ballantine Books.

Ornish, D., Brown, S., & Sherwitz, et al. (1990). Can lifestyle changes reverse coronary heart disease? *Lancet, 336,* 129-133.

Ostrom, J. R., Hammerlund, E. R., Christensen, D. B., et al. (1985). Medication usage in an elderly population. *Medical Care, 23,*157-164.

Ostrow, A. C. (1984). *Physical activity and the older adult.* Princeton, NJ: Princeton Book Company.

Paffenberger, R. S., Hyde, R. T., Wing, A. L., et al. (1986). Physical activity, all-cause mortality and longevity of college alumni. *New England Journal of Medicine, 314* (10), 605.

Pago, H. C., Schraeder, J. S., and Coghlin, T. (1996). *The stanford life plan for a healthy heart.* San Francisco: Chronicle Books.

Palmore, E. (1980). The social factors in aging. In E. W. Busse & D. G. Blazer (Eds.), *Handbook of geriatric psychiatry.* New York: Van Nostrand Reinhold Company.

Parsons, T. (1951). *The social system.* New York: Free Press.

Peck, M. (1978). *The road less traveled.* New York: A Touchstone Book.

Pelletier, K. R. (1981). *Longevity: Fulfilling our biological potential.* New York: Delacort Press/Seymour Lawrence.

Pelletier, K. R. (1993). Between mind and body: Stress, emotions and health. In D. Goleman, & J. Gurin (Eds.). Mind/body medicine. Younkers, NY: Consumer Reports Books, 19-38.

Pender, N. J. (1982). *Health promotion in nursing practice.* New York: Grant Waters of France, Inc., Appleton-Century-Crofts.

Perspectives in Health Promotion and Aging. (1990). National Resource Center Health Promotion and Aging, AARP, 1909 K Street, N.W., Washington, DC 20049, 5(1).

Peterman, T. R., Stoneburner, J. A., Jaffe, H., & Curran, J. (1988). Risk of HIV transmission from heterosexual adults with transfusion-associated infections. *Journal of the American Medical Association, 259,* 55-58.

Pirozzolo, F. J., & Maletta, G. J. (1981). *Behavioral assessment and psychopharmacology* (Vol. 2). New York: Praeger.

Piscopo, J. (1985). *Physical activity and aging.* New York: John Wiley & Sons.

Podolsky, D. (1991, May 20). Eat your beans. *U.S. News & World Report,* 77-72.

Policy and Research, National Coalition of Hispanic Health and Human Services Organizations (COSSMHO), Meeting the Health Promotion Needs of Hispanic Communities. *American Journal of Health Promotion, 9*(4), 1995, 300-311.

Pollock, M., & Schmidt, D. H. (1995). *Heart disease and rehabilitation.* Champaign, IL: Human Kinetics Press.

Pollock, M., Wilmore, J., & Fox, S. (1984). *Exercise in health and disease.* Philadelphia: W. B. Saunders Company.

Popoff, L. M. (1969). A single method for diagnosis of depression by the family physician. *Clinical Medicine, 76,* 24-29.

Posen, D. B. (1995, April). Stress management for patient and physician. In *The Canadian Journal of Continuing Medical Education,* Internet Mental Health Magazine Articles, July, 1996. [Online]. Available World Wide Web: http://www. mentalhealt... gl/p51-str.html#Head-4.

Powell, D. R. (1985, July-Aug.). Sizing up the packaged program. *Promoting Health, 4,* 5-11.

Pray, W. S. (1989). Help your patients avoid drug interactions. *U.S. Pharmacist.*

Price, J., Desmond, S., Losh, D., et al. (1988). Family practice physicians' perceptions and practices regarding health promotion for the elderly. *American Journal of Preventive Medicine, 4*(5), 274-281.

Primavera, J. P., Kaiser, R. S. (1992). Non-pharmacological treatment of headache: Is less more? *Headache, 32,* 393-395.

Procter, E. A., & Alwar, L. (1995). A therapeutic group in the community for the elderly with functional psychiatric illness. *International Journal of Geriatric Psychiatry, 10,* 33-36.

Pryor, D. (1990, Fall). Commentary: A prescription for high drug prices. *Health Affairs,* 101-109.

Public Health Service. (1980, April). Statement on hypertension in the elderly. Bethesda, MD: Department of Health and Human Services, Public Health Service, National Institutes of Health, Building 31, Room 4A18, Bethesda, Maryland 20892.

Public Health Service. (1986). The 1990 health objectives for the nation: A mid-course review. Washington, DC: U.S. Department of Health and Human Services.

Public Health Service. (1989). Promoting health/preventing disease: Year 2000 objectives for the nation. Washington, DC: U.S. Department of Health and Human Services.

Qualls, S. H. (1993, Winter/Spring). Family therapy with older adults. *Generations, 17*(1), 73-74.

Quill, T. E. (1983). Partnerships in patient care: A contractual approach. *Annals of Internal Medicine, 98,* 228-234.

Raab, D. M., & Smith, E. L. (1985). Exercise and aging effects on bone. *Topics in Geriatric Rehabilitation, 1*(1), 31-39.

Rabins, P. V. (1992). Prevention of mental disorder in the elderly: Current perspectives and future prospects. *Journal of the American Geriatrics Society, 40,* 727-733.

Radecki, S. E., & Cowell, W.G. (1990). Health promotion for the elderly. *Family Medicine, 22*(4), 299-302.

Radecki, S. E., Kane, R. L., Solomon, D. H., Mendenhall, R. C., & Beck, J. C. (1988a). Do physicians spend less time with older patients? *Journal of the American Geriatrics Society, 36,* 713-718.

Radecki, S. E., Kane, R. L., Solomon, D. H., Mendenhall, R. C., & Beck, J. C. (1988b). Are physicians sensitive to the special problems of older patients? *Journal of the American Geriatrics Society, 36,* 719-725.

Rakowski, W. (1986). Research issues in health promotion programs for the elderly. In K. Dychtwald (Ed.), *Wellness and health promotion for the elderly.* Rockville, MD: Aspen Publication.

Rankin, E.J., Gilner, F.H., Gfeller, J.D. (1993). Efficacy of progressive muscle relaxation for reducing state anxiety among elderly adults on memory tasks. *Perceptual and Motor Skills, 77,* 1395-1402.

Rapheal, B. (1977). Preventive intervention with the recent bereaved. *Archives of General Psychiatry, 34,*1450-1454.

Ratliff, S.S. (1996). The multicultural challenge to health care, in multicultural awareness in health care professions. In M. C. Julia (Ed.). Allyn and Bacon, Boston, MA, 183-200.

Renner, V. V., & Birren, J. E. (1980). Concepts and issues of mental health and aging. In J. E. Birren & R. B. Sloane (Eds.), *Handbook of mental health and aging*. Englewood Cliffs, NJ: Prentice-Hall, Inc.

Rice, D. P., & Estes, C. L. (1984). Health of the elderly: Policy issues and choices. *Health Affairs, 3*(4), 26-49.

Rice, P. L. (1992). *Stress and health*, 2nd ed. Pacific Grove, CA: Brooks Cole Publishing Company.

Rickard, H. C., Scogin, F., Keith, S. (1994). Briefly noted: A one-year follow-up of relaxation training for elders with subjective anxiety. *The Gerontologist, 34*(1), 121-122.

Ricocur, P. (1981). Hermencutics on the human sciences (trans.). Cambridge, MA: University Press.

Rieff, P. (1979). *Freud: The mind of the moralist*, 3rd ed. Chicago: University of Chicago Press.

Rieff, P. (1987). *The triumph of the therapeutic: Uses of faith after Freud*. Chicago: University of Chicago Press.

Riley, M. V. (1989). AIDS and older people: The overlooked segment of the population. In M. W. Riley, M. G. Ory, D. Zablotsky, *AIDS in an aging society*. New York: Springer Publishing Company.

Richardson, C. A., Gilleard, C. J., Lieberman, S., & Peeler, R. (1994). Working with older adults and their families--A review. *Journal of Family Therapy, 16*, 225-240.

Robbins, A. S. (1989). Hypothermia and heat stroke: Protecting the elderly patient. *Geriatrics, 44*(1), 73-80.

Rogers, R., Meyer, J., Judd, B., et al. (1985). Abstention from cigarette smoking improves cerebral perfusion among elderly chronic smokers. *Journal of the American Medical Association, 253*(20), 2, 970-1974.

Roos, N. P., & Shapiro, E. (1981). The Manitoba longitudinal study on aging: Preliminary findings on health care utilization by the elderly. *Medical Care, 19*, 644-657.

Roos, N. P., Shapiro, E., & Roos, L. L. (1984). Aging and the demand for health services: Which aged and whose demand? *Gerontologist, 24*, 31-36.

Rolland, J. S. (1984). Toward a psychosocial typology of chronic and life-threatening illness. *Family Systems Medicine, 2*, 245-263.

Rolland, J. S. (1988). A conceptual model of chronic and life-threatening illness and its impact on the family. In C. Chilman, E. Nunnally, & F. Cox (Eds.), *Chronic illness and disability*. Beverly Hills: Sage Publications.

Rolland, J.S. (1991). Helping families with anticipatory loss. In F. Walsh, & M. Mc Goldrick (Eds.), *Living beyond loss*. New York: W.W. Norton & Company.

Rorick, M. H., & Scrimshaw, N. S. (1979). Comparative tolerance of elderly from differing ethnic backgrounds to lactose-containing and lactose-free dairy drinks. *Journal of Gerontology, 34*, 191.

Rosenstock, I. M. (1975). Prevention of illness and maintenance of health. In J. Kosa, & I. K. Zola (Eds.), *Poverty and health: A sociological analysis*. Cambridge, MA: Harvard University Press, 193-223.

Rosow, I. (1974). Socialization to old age. New York: Free Press.

Roter, D. L. (1989). Which facets of communication have strong effects on outcome--A meta-analysis. In M. Stewart & D. Roter (Eds.), *Communicating with medical patients*. Newbury Park, CA: Sage Publications.

Roter, D. L., Hall, J. A., & Katz, N. R. (1988). Patient-physician communication: A descriptive summary of the literature. *Patient Education and Counseling, 12,* 99-119.

Rotter, J. B. (1966). Generalized expectancies for internal versus external control of reinforcement. *Psychological Monographs, 80*(1), 609.

Rowe, J. W., & Kahn, R. L. (1987, July). Human aging: Usual and successful. *Science, 237,* 143-149.

Ruben, D. H. (1990). *The aging and drug effects*. Jefferson, NC: McFarland and Company, Inc., Publishers.

Rubinstein, R. L., Jubben, J. E., & Mintzer, J. E. (1994). Social isolation and social support: An applied perspective. *The Journal of Applied Gerontology, 13,* 58-72.

Rutter, M. (1987). Psychosocial resilience and protective mechanisms. *American Journal of Orthopsychiatry, 57,* 316-331.

Ryan, A. (1975). Importance of physical activity for the elderly. *In Testimony on Physical Fitness for Older Persons*. Washington, DC: National Association for Human Development.

Ryan, R .S., & Travis, J. W. (1981). *Wellness workbook*. Berkeley, CA: Ten Speed Press.

Salzman, C. (1992). *Clinical geriatric psychopharmacology*, 2nd ed. Baltimore: Williams & Williams.

Salzman, C., & Nevis-Olesen, J. (1992). Psychopharmacologic treatment. In J. Birren, R. Sloane, & G. Cohen (Eds.), *Handbook of mental health and aging*, 2nd ed. San Diego: Academic Press.

Sapolsky, R. M. (1994). *Why zebras don't get ulcers: A guide to stress, stress-related diseases, and coping*. New York: W. H. Freemen and Company.

Schaie, K. W., Dutta, R., & Willis, S. L. (1991). Relationship between rigidity-flexibility and cognitive abilities in adulthood. *Psychology and Aging, 6,* 371-383.

Schlenker, E. D. (1984). *Nutrition and aging*. St. Lous: C. V. Mosby and Company.

Schneider, E. L., & Guralnik, J. M. (1990, May 2). The aging of America: Impact on health care costs. *Journal of American Medical Association,* 2335-2340.

Schneiderman, N., McCabe, P., & Baum, A. (1992*). Stress and disease processes*. Hillsdale, NJ: Erlbaum Associates.

Schoening, H. A., & Iverson, J. A. (1968). Numerical scoring of self-care status: Study of Kenney self-care evaluation. *Archives of Physical Medicine and Rehabililitaton, 49,* 221.

Scholl, N. (1980). Smoking habits in the Glostrub population of men and women, born in 1914. *Acta med. Scand., 208,* 245-256.

Schuman, L. M. (1981). Smoking as a risk factor in longevity. In D. Daner, N. W. Shock, & M. Marois (Eds.), *Aging: A challenge to science and society*. Oxford: Oxford University Press.

Schwartz, M. S., & Schwartz, N. M. (1993). Biofeedback: Using the body's signals. In D. Goleman, & J. Gurin (Eds.), *Mind/body medicine*. Younkers, NY: Consumer Reports Books, 301-313.

Sciacca, J., Seehafer, R., Reed, R., et al. (1993, May/June). The impact of participation in health promotion on medical costs: A reconsideration of the Blue Cross and Blue Shield of Indiana Study. *American Journal of Health Promotion, 7*(5), 374-383.

Scogin, F., Rickard, H. C., Keith, S., et al. (1992). Progressive and imaginal relaxation training for elderly persons with subjective anxiety. *Psychology and Aging, 7*(3), 419-424.

Scogin, F., & Rohling, M. (1989). Cognitive processes, self-reports of memory functioning and mental health states in older adults. *Journal of Aging and Health, 1*(4), 507-520.

Seeman, T. E., & Syme, S. L. (1987). Social networks and coronary artery disease. *Psychosomatic Medicine, 41*, 340-353.

Seipel, M. M. (1989). Health care strategies for Asian American patients. *Journal of Health and Social Policy, 1*(1), 105-114.

Selye, H. (1936). A syndrome produced by diverse nocuous agents. *Nature, 138*, 32.

Selye, H. (1956). *The stress of life.* New York: McGraw Hill Book Company.

Selye, H. (1974). *Stress without distress.* New York: J. B. Lippincott.

Semenchuk, M. (1994). Treatment of common mental health problems in the elderly. *Journal of Geriatric Drug Therapy, 9*, 3-27.

Serfass, R. C., Agre, J. C., & Smith, E. L. (1985). Exercise testing for the elderly. *Topics in Geriatric Rehabilitation, 1*(1), 58-67.

Shaffer, H., & Kauffman, J. (1985). The clinical assessment and diagnosis of addiction. In T. E. Bratter & G. G. Forrest (Eds.), *Alcoholism and substance abuse.* New York: The Free Press.

Sharkey, B. (1990). Physiology of fitness, 3rd ed. Champaign, IL: Human Kinetics Books.

Shepard, R. J. (1984). Management of exercise in the elderly. *Canadian Journal of Applied Sports Science, 9*(3), 109-120.

Shepard, R. J. (1984, May). Aerobics. *Esquire, 14*(5), 92-94.

Shepard, R. J. (1985). [The] Cardiovascular benefits of exercise in the elderly. *Topics in Geriatric Rehabilitation, 1*(1), 1-10.

Shepard, R. J. (1994). *Aerobic fitness and health.* Champaign, IL: Human Kinetics Press.

Sherman, I. W., & Sherman, V. G. (1983). *Biology: A human approach.* New York: Oxford University Press.

Sherman, S. S. (1993, February). Gender, health, and responsible research. *Clinics In Geriatric Medicine, 9*(1).

Shimp, L. A., & Ascione, F. J. (1988, Summer). Causes of medication misuse and error. *Generations,* XII, 4.

Shubla, H. C., Solomon, G. F., & Dosli, R. P. (1979). Psychoneurimmunolgy. *Journal of Holistic Health, 4*, 125-131.

Siegel, B. S. (1986). *Love, medicine and miracles.* New York: Harper and Row Publishers.

Simon, A. (1980). The neuroses, personality disorders, alcoholism, drug use and misuse, and crime in the aged. In J. Birren & R. B. Sloane (Eds.), *Handbook of mental health and aging.* Englewood Cliffs, NJ: Prentice Hall.

Skelly, J., & Flint, A. J. (1995). Urinary incontinence associated with dementia. *Journal of American Geriatrics Society, 43,* 286-294.

Smilkstein, G., Ashworth, C., & Montano, D. (1982). Validity and reliability of the family APGAR as a test of family function. *Journal of Family Practice, 15,* 303-311.

Smith, C. K., Polis, E., & Hadac, R. R. (1981). Characteristics of the initial medical interview associated with patient satisfaction and understanding. *Journal of Family Practice, 12*(2), 283-288.

Smith, E. L. (1984). Special considerations in developing an exercise program for the older adult. In J. D. Matarazzo, N. E. Miller, S. A. Weiss, et al.(Eds.), *Behavior health: A handbook of health enhancement and disease prevention.* New York: John Wiley.

Smith, E. L., DiFabio, R. P., & Gilligan, C. (1990). Exercise intervention and physiologic function in the elderly. *Topics in Geriatric Rehabilitation, 6*(1), 57-68.

Smith, E. L., & Gilligan, C. (1983) Physical activity prescription for the older adults. *The Physician and Sportsmedicine, 11,* 91-101.

Smith, E. L., Smith, K. A., & Gilligan, C. (1990). Exercise, fitness, osteoarthritis and osteoporosis. In C. Bouchard, R. J. Shephard, T. Stephens, J. A. Sutton, & B. D. McPherson (Eds.), *Exercise, fitness and health.* Champaign, IL: Human Kinetics Press.

Smith, G. D., Wentworth, D., Neaton, J. D., et al. (1996, April). Socioeconomic differentials in mortality risk among men screened for the multiple risk factor trial: II. Black men. *American Journal of Public Health, 86*(4), 497-504.

Smith, R. C., Hoppe, R. B. (1991). The patient's story: Integrating the patient-and physician-centered approaches to interviewing. *Annals of Internal Medicine, 115,* 470-477.

Smith, S. L., Sherrill, K. A., Colenda, C. C. (1995, January). Assessing and treating anxiety in elderly persons. *Psychiatric Services, 46*(1), 36-42.

Snider, E. L. (1980). The elderly and their doctors. *Social Science and Medicine, 14A,* 527-531.

Society for Public Health, Committee on Professional Preparation and Practice. (1977, Spring). Criteria and guidelines for baccalaureate programs in community health education. *Health Education Monographs, 5,* 90-98.

Sol, N. (1992). ACSM's Health/Fitness.

Solis, J. M., Marks, G., Garcia, M., Shelton, D. (1990). Acculturation, access to care, and use of preventive services by Hispanics: Findings from the HANES 1982-84. *American Journal of Public Health, 80*(suppl).

Solomon, H. A. (1984). *The exercise myth.* San Diego, CA: Harcourt Brace Jovanovich.

Somers, A. R., Klainmen, L., & Clark, W. (1982, Fall). Preventive health services for the elderly: The Rutgers medical school project. *Inquiry, 19,* 190-221.

Sorenson, G., & Pechacek, T. (1987). Attitudes toward smoking cessation among men and women. *Journal of Behavioral Medicine, 10*(2), 129-137.

Sova, R. (1995). *Water fitness after 40.* Champaign, IL: Human Kinetics Press.

Spackman, R. R. (1981). *Conditioning for senior citizens.* Carbondale, IL: Hillcrest House.

Spiegel, D. (1993). *Living beyond limits: New hope and help for facing life threatening illness.* New York: Times Books.

Spiegel, D. (1993). Psychological intervention in cancer. *Journal of the National Cancer Institute, 85,* 1198-1205.

Spiegel, D. (1993). Social support: How friends, family and groups can help. In D. Goleman & J. Gurin (Eds.). *Mind/body medicine.* Younkers, NY: Consumer Reports Books, 331-349.

Staudinger, U. M., Marsiske, M., & Baltes, P. B. (1993). Resilience and levels of reserve capacity in later adulthood: Perspectives from life-span theory. *Development and Psychopathology, 5,* 541-566.

Steckel, S. (1980). Contracting with patient-selected reinforcers. *American Journal of Nursing, 80*(9), 1596-1599.

Stewart, M. (1984). What is a successful doctor-patient interview? A study of interactions and outcomes. *Social Science and Medicine, 19,* 167-175.

Stewart, M. (1994). *Yoga over 50.* NY: Simon & Schuster.

Stewart, M., Brown, J. B., Weston, W. W., McWhinney, I. R., McWilliam, C. L., & Freeman, T. R. (1995*). Patient-centered medicine: Transforming the clinical method.* Thousand Oaks, CA: Sage Publications.

Stoyva, J. M., & Budzynski, T. H. (1993). Biofeedback methods in the treatment of anxiety and stress disorders. In P. M. Lehrer, & R. L. Woolfolk (Eds), *Principles and Practices of Stress Management,* 2nd ed. New York, NY; London, England: The Guilford Press.

Strain, J. J. (1993). Psychotherapy and medical conditions. In D. Goleman & J. Gurin (Eds.), *Mind/body medicine.* Yonkers, NY: Consumer Reports Books.

Street, R. L., Jr. (1991). Information-giving in medical consultations: The influence of patients' communicative styles and personal characteristics. *Social Science and Medicine, 32,* 541-548.

Strub, R. L., & Black, F. W. (1985). *The mental status examination in neurology,* 2nd ed. Philadelphia: F. A. Davis Company.

Stuart, R. B. (Ed.). (1977). *Behavioral self-management: Strategies, techniques and outcome.* New York: Bruner/Mazel.

Surgeon General. (1990). Executive summary: The health benefits of smoking cessation. U.S. Department of Health and Human Services, Public Health Service, Center for Chronic Disease and Health Promotion, Rockville, MD: 20857. DHHS Publication No. (CDC) 90-8416.

Sutherland, H. J., Llewellyn-Thomas, H. A., Lockwood, G. A., et al. (1989). Cancer patients: Their desire for information and participation in treatment decisions. *Journal of the Royal Society of Medicine, 82,* 260.

Swell, L. (1976). *Success: You can make it happen.* New York: Simon & Schuster.

Switkes, B. (1985). Armchair fitness. (Video cassette). Chevy Chase, MD: CC-M Productions.

Szasz, T. S., & Hollender, M. H. (1956). The basic models of the doctor-patient relationship. *Archives of Internal Medicine, 97,* 585-592.

Tanjasiri, S. P., Wallace, S. P., & Shibata, K. (1995). Picture imperfect: Hidden problems among Asian Pacific Islander elderly. *The Gerontologist, 35*(6), 753-760.

Tate, D. (1994). *Mindfulness meditation group training: Effects on medical and psychological symptoms and positive psychological characteristics.* Brigham Young University, Unpublished Doctoral Dissertation.

Teague, M. L., Cipriano, R., & McGhee, V. L. (1990). Health promotion as a rehabilitation service for persons with disabilities. *Journal of Rehabilitation*, 56(1), 52-56.

Teasdale, J. D., Segal, Z., and Williams, J. M. G. (1995). How does cognitive therapy prevent depressive relapse and why should attentional control (mindfulness) training help? *Behavioral Research and Therapy, 33*(1), 25-39.

Terry, P. E. (1987). The role of health risk appraisal in the workplace: Assessment versus behavioral change. *American Journal of Health Promotion, 2*(2), 18-21, 36.

Thomas, E. G., & Chambers, K. O. (1989). Phenomenology of life satisfaction among elderly men: Quantitative and qualitative views. *Psychology and Aging, 4,* 284-289.

Thomas, R. T. (1986). *Muscular fitness through resistance training.* Dubuque, IA: Eddie Bowers Publishing.

Thomas, S. B. (1990, Spring). Community health advocacy for racial and ethnic minorities in the United States: Issues and challenges for health education. *Health Education Quarterly, 17*(1), 13-19.

Thomas, S. B., & Quinn, S. C. (1993, May/June). An evaluation of HIV education messengers in a Black low income housing complex. *Journal of Health Education, 24* (3), 135-140.

Thomas, V. G. (1992, October). Explaining health disparitites between African-American and White populations: Where do we go from here? *Journal of the National Medical Association, 84*(10), 837-840.

Thompson, L. W., Gallagher, D., & Breckenridge, J. S. (1987) Comparative effectiveness of psychotherapies for depressed elders. *Journal of Consulting and Clinical Psychology, 55,* 385-390.

Thompson, M., & Heller, K. (1990). Facets of support related to well-being: Quantitative social isolation and perceived support in a sample of elderly women. *Psychology and Aging, 4,* 535-544.

Thomson, R. (1989, September). Curbing the high cost of health care. *Nation's Business*, 18-26.

Tideiksaar, A. (1989). Geriatric falls: Assessing the cause, preventing recurrence. *Geriatrics, 44*(7), 57-62.

Tinetti, M. E. (1986). Performance-oriented assessment of mobility problems in elderly patients. *American Geriatrics Society, 34,* 119-126.

Tullis, M. B. (1985, June). *A resource guide for drug management for older adults.* Washington, DC: U.S. Department of Health and Human Services.

Turner, M. S. (1992). Individual psychodynamic psychotherapy with older adults: Perspectives from a nurse psychotherapist. *Archives of Psychiatric Nursing, 6,* 266-274.

Tyne, P.J., & Mitchell, M. (1983). *Total stretching.* Chicago: Contemporary Books, Inc.

U.S. Department of Health and Human Services. A resource guide for drug management for older pesons. Washington, DC: DHHS Publication No. (OHDS) 87-20953.

U.S. Department of Health and Human Services. (1979). Healthy People: The surgeon general's report on health promotion and disease prevention. DHEW Publication No. (PHS) 79-55071. Washington, DC: U.S. Government Printing Office.

U.S. Department of Health and Human Services. *Report of the Secretary's Task Force on Black and Minority Health* [Executive Summary] No. U.S. Department of Health and Human Services, 1985a.

U.S. Senate Special Committee on Aging (1985*). America in transition: An aging society.* (1984-1985 edition, Serial #99-B). Washington, DC: U.S. Government Printing Office.

U.S. Senate Special Committee on Aging (1986). *Developments in aging: 1985* (Vol. 3). Washington, DC: U.S. Government Printing Office.

U.S. Senate Special Committee on Aging (1991). *Aging America--Trends and projections.* (USDHHS # (FCOA) 91-28001). Washington, DC: U.S. Government Printing Office.

Van Dijk, W. K. (1985). Complexity of the dependence problem. In *Addictive behavior.* Englewood, CO: Morton Publishing Company.

Van Gelder, N. (1987). *IDEA foundation aerobic dance exercise: Instructor manual.* San Diego, CA: International Dance Exercise Association.

Van Norman, K. A. (1994). *Exercise programming for older adults.* Champaign, IL: Human Kinetics.

Varela, F. J., Thompson, E., Rosch, E. (1991). *The embodied mind: Cognitive science and human experience.* Cambridge, MA: MIT Press.

Vinick, B. H., & Ekerdt, D. J. (1991). Retirement: What happens to husband-wife relationships? *Journal of Geriatric Psychiatry, 24,* 23-40.

Waitzkin, H. (1984). Doctor-patient communication: Clinical implications of social scientific research. *Journal of the American Medical Association, 252,* 2441- 2446.

Waitzkin, H. (1991). *The politics of medical encounters: How patients and doctors deal with social problems.* New Haven: Yale University Press.

Waller, J. B., Young, R., & Sowers, J. R., (1994). *Frail elderly.* Report to National Institutes of Health (NIA # 10428). Washington, D.C.: Government Printing Office.

Wallerstein, N. (1992, January/Feburary). Powerlessness, empowerment, and health: Implications for health promotion programs. *American Journal of Health Promotion, 6*(3), 197-205.

Wallis, C. (1983, June 6). Stress: Can we cope? *Time,* 48-55.

Wallis, C. (1991a, January 14). A puzzling plague. *Time,* 48-52.

Wallis, C. (1991b, January 14, 1991). The road to recovery. *Time,* 54-54.

Walsh, F. (1980). The family in later life. In E. Carter & M. Mc Goldrick (Eds.),*The family life cycle.* New York: Gardner Press.

Walsh, F., & McGoldrick, M. (Eds.). (1991). *Living beyond loss: Death in the family.* W. W. Norton & Company, New York, NY; London, England.

Walsh, W. B. (1990). Publisher's letter. *Health Affairs, 9*(3) 3.

Warren, R. (1993). The morbidity/mortality gap: What is the problem? *Annual of Epidemiology, 3,* 127-129.

Wassarus, J. D. (1984). *JARM: How to jog with your arms to live longer.* Port Washington, New York: Ashley Books, Inc.

Watson, D. L., & Tharp, R. G. (1972). *Self-directed behavior: Self-modification for personal adjustment.* Monterey, CA: Brooks-Cole.

Watson, R. R. (1988). Caffeine: Is it dangerous to health? *American Journal of Health Promotion, 2*(4), 13-22.

Waxman, H. M., Carner, E. A., & Klein, M. (1984). Underutilization of mental health professionals by community elderly. *The Gerontologist, 24,* 23-30.

Webb, T. (1986). *Rubberband workout.* New York: Workman Publishing.

Webber, D., Balsam, A., & Oehlke, B. (1995, March/April). The Massachusetts farmers' market coupon program for low income elders. *American Journal of Health Promotions, 9*(4).

Webster's *Seventh New Collegiate Dictionary.* (1963). Springfield, MA: G. & S. Merriam, 868.

Webster's *Seventh Non-Collegiate Dictionary.* (1969). Springfield, MA: G. & S. Meriam.

Weg, R. B. (1978). Drug interaction with the changing physiology of the aged: Practice and potential. In R. C. Kayne (Ed.), *Drugs and the elderly.* Los Angeles, CA: University of Southern California.

Weiler, P. G. (1986). Education and training in wellness for health care providers. In K. Dychtwald (Ed.), *Wellness and health promotion for the elderly.* Rockville, MD: Aspen Systems Corporation.

Weiler, P. G. (1989, Fall). AIDS and dementia. *Generations, 13,* 16-18.

Weiner, B. (Ed.). (1974). *Cognitive views of human motivation.* New York: Academic Press.

Wexner, S. D., Cheape, J. D., Jorge, J. M. N., et al. (1992). Prospective assessment of biofeedback for the treatment of paradoxical puborectalis contraction. *Dis Colon Rectum, 35,* 145-150.

White, M. (1995). *Water exercise.* Champaign, IL: Human Kinetics Press.

Whitney, E. N., & Hamilton, E. M. (1984). *Understanding nutrition.* St. Paul, MN: West Publishing Company.

Whitton, C. (1994, January). Depression in elderly people. *Professional Nurse, 9,* 248-252.

Widner, S., & Zeichner, A. (1993). Psychologic interventions for the elderly chronic pain patient. *Clinical Gerontologist, 13,* 4, 3-18.

Williams, D. R. (1990). Socioeconomic differentials in health: A review and redirection. *Social Psychology Quarterly, 53*(2) 81-99.

Williams, M .A. (1994). *Exercise testing and training in the elderly cardiac patient.* Champaign, IL: Human Kinetics.

Williams, R., & Boyce, W. T. (1989). Protein malnutrition in elderly Navajo patients. *Journal of American Geriatric Society, 37,* 397-406.

Williams, W. F. (Ed.). (1984). *Rehabilitation in the aging.* New York: Raven Press.

Williamson, J. W., German, P. S., Skinner, E. A., Weiss, R., & Royall, R. (1988). *National survey of primary practitioners.* Annals of Internal Medicine.

Williamson, P. Beitman, B. D., & Katon, W. (1981). Beliefs that foster physician avoidance of psychosocial aspects of health care. *Journal of Family Practice, 13,* 999-1003.

Wilson, G. T. (1980). Cognitive factors in lifestyle changes: A social learning perspective. In P.O. Davidson & S.M. Davidson (Eds.), *Behavioral medicine: Changing health lifestyles.* New York: Brunner/Mazel.

Wilson, G. T., & Evans, I. M. (1976). Adult behavior therapy and the therapist client relationship. In C. M. Franks & G. T. Wilson (Eds.), *Annual review of behavior therapy: Therapy and Practice*, Vol. IV. New York: Brunner/Mazel.

Winbush, G. B. (1996). *African-American Health Care: Beliefs, Practices, and Service Issues*, 8-22.

Windsor, R. A., Baranowski, T., Clark, N., & Cutter, G. (1984). *Evaluation of health promotion and education programs*. Palo Alto, CA: Mayfield Publishing Company.

Wiswell, R. A. (1980). Relaxation, exercise and aging. In J. E. Birren & R. B. Sloane (Eds.), *Handbook of mental health and aging*. NJ: Prentice-Hall, Inc.

Woldum, K. M., Ryan-Morrell, L., Towson, M. C., Bower, K. A., & Zander, K. (1985). *Patient education*. Rockville, MD: Aspen Systems Corporation.

Wolf, M. (1985). The meaning of education in late life: An exploration of life review. *Gerontological Geriatric Education, 5*(3), 51.

Wolfe, S. M., Fugate, L., Hulstrand, E. P., Kamimoto, L. E., and the Public Citizen Health Research Group. (1988). *Worst pills, best pills*.

Wolpe, J. (1973). *The practice of behavior therapy*, 2nd ed. New York: Pergamon.

Wong, P. T. P., & Watt, L. M. (1991). What types of reminiscence are associated with successful aging? *Psychology and Aging, 6,* 272-279.

Woods, R. T. (1993). Psychosocial management of depression. *International Review of Psychiatry, 5,* 427-436.

Woods, R. T., & Britton, P. G. (1985). *Clinical psychology with the elderly*. London: Croom Helm.

Woollacot, M. H., Shumway-Cook, A., & Nashner, L. M. (1982). Postural reflexes and aging. In J. A. Mortimer, F. J., Pirozolo, & A. J. Malletta (Eds.), *The aging motor system*. New York: Praeger Publishers.

Work, J. A. (1989, November). Strength training: A bridge to independence for the elderly. *The Physician and Sport Medicine, 17*(11).

World Health Organization. (1980). International classification of impairments, disabilities, and handicaps. Geneva.

Wray, L. A. The role of ethnicity in the disability and work experience of preretirement-age Americans. *The Gerontologist, 36*(3), 287-298.

Yanker, G. D. (1983). *The complete book of exercise walking*. Chicago: Contemporary Books, Inc.

Yeagle, P. L. (1991). *Understanding your cholesterol*. San Diego, CA: Academic Press, Inc.

Yee, B. W. K., & Weaver, G. (1994, Spring). Ethnic minorities and health promotion: developing a "culturally competent" agenda. *Preventive Health Care and Health Promotion for Older Adults,* 39-44.

Yesavage, J. A. (1984). Effects of relaxation and menmonics on memory, attention and anxiety in the elderly. *Experimental Aging Research, 10*(4), 211-214.

YMCA. (1994). *YMCA Healthy Back Book*. Champaign, IL: Human Kinetics Press.

YMCA of Canada. (1986). *A fitness leader's guide to osteoporosis*. 80 Gerrard Street, East, Toronto, Ontario M5B 1G6.

York, P. R. Z. (1985). *Nutrition's role in health promotion: Health promotion and the older adult*. Conference proceedings. Manhatten, KS: Regional Health Administration, Public Health Service.

Young, R. F. (1994, Spring). Older people as consumers of health promotion recommendations. *Preventive Healthcare And Health Promotion For Older Adults*.

Zarit, S. H., & Orr, N. K. (1984). *Working with families of dementia victims: A treatment manual*. Washington, DC: U.S. Department of Health and Human Services, publication No. 84-20816. U.S. Government Printing Office.

Zatsiorsky, V. M. (1995). *Science and practice of strength training*. Champaign, IL: Human Kinetics.

Zeiss, A. M., & Lewinsohn, P. M. (1986). Adapting behavioral treatment for depression to meet the needs of the elderly. *Clinical Psychologist, 39,* 98-100.

Zeman, S. (1990). Screening and health promotion in the older adult. *Topics in Geriatric Rehabilitation, 6*(1), 6-18.

Zimberg, S. (1985). Treatment of the elderly alcoholic. In E. Gottheil, K. A. Druley, T. E. Skolada, & H. M. Wismen. *Alcoholism, drug addiction and aging*. Springfield, IL: Charles C. Thomas, Publishers.

Zohman, L. R. (1974). *Beyond diet. Exercise your way to fitness and heart health*. Englewood Cliffs, NJ: CPC International, Inc.

Zola, I. K. (1972). Medicine as an institution of social control. *Sociological Review, 20,* 487-504.

Zung, W. W. K. (1980). Affective disorders. In E. Busse & D. Blazer (Eds.), *Handbook of geriatric psychiatry*. New York: Van Nostrand Reinhold Company.

End-of-Book Credits

Preface
Figure 1   From Michael P. O' Donnell, "Definition of Health Promotion in *American Journal of Health Promotion,* Vol. 1, No. 1, Michael P. O' Donnell Publishers, Rochester Hills, MI. Reprinted by permission.

Chapter 1
Figures 1.1, 1.2, 1.4, and 1.5   From E. L. Schneider and J. M. Guralnik, "The Aging of America: Impact on Health Care Costs" in *JAMA,* (263), May 2, 1990. Copyright 1990, American Medical Association.

Chapter 2
Figure 2.1   From K. Green, "Healthy Promotion: Its Terminology, Concepts, and Modes in Practice" in *Healthy Values: Achieving High-Level Wellness,* Vol. 9, No. 3, May–June, 1985. Copyright c PNG Publications, Star City, WV. Reprinted by permission.

Figure 2.2   From M. S. Goodstadt et al., "Health Promotion: A Conceptual Integration" in *American Journal of Health Promotion,* Winter 1987. Michael P. O' Donnell Publishers, Rochester Hills, MI. Reprinted by permission.

Figure 2.3   From M. S. Goodstadt et al., "Health Promotion: A Conceptual Integration" in *American Journal of Health Promotion,* 1(2), 1987. Michael P. O' Donnell Publishers, Rochester Hills, MI. Reprinted by permission.

Chapter 3
Figures 3.2 and 3.3   From P. E. Terry, "The Role of Health Risk Appraisal in the Workplace: Assessment Versus Behavioral Change" in *American Journal of Health Promotion,* 2(2), 1987.
Michael P. O' Donnell Publishers, Rochester Hills, MI. Reprinted by permission.

Chapter 5
Figure 5.1 Reprinted by permission from page 38 of *Nutrition: Concepts and Controversies* by E. N. Hamilton et al.; Copyright c 1988 by West Publishing Company. All rights reserved.

Chapter 7
Figure 7.1   Reprinted from *Addicted Behaviors,* W. K. Van Dijk, "Complexity of the Dependency Problem," page 31, Copyright 1985, with kind permission from Elsevier Science Ltd., The Boulevard, Langford Lane, Kidlington, OX5 1GB, UK.

Figure 7.2   From "Dangers of Smoking, Benefits of Quitting." Reprinted by the permission of the American Cancer Society, Inc.

Chapter 9
Figure 9.1   From *Why Zebras Don't Get Ulcers* by Sapolsky. Copyright   1994 by W. H. Freeman and Company. Used with permission.

Chapter 11
Figures 11.1 and 11.2   From M. Notelovitz and M. Ware, *Stand Tall!,* Copyright c 1985 Bantam Books. Reprinted by permission of Barbara Lowenstein Lt. Agency, New York.

Figure 11.3   From J. A. Catania et al., in M. W. Riley et al., *AIDS in an Aging Society.* Copyright c 1989 Springer Publishing Company, Inc., New York, NY 10012. Used by permission.